St Antony's Series

Series Editors
Halbert Jones
St Antony's College
University of Oxford
Oxford, UK

Matthew Walton
St Antony's College
University of Oxford
Oxford, UK

The St Antony's Series publishes studies of international affairs of contemporary interest to the scholarly community and a general yet informed readership. Contributors share a connection with St Antony's College, a world-renowned centre at the University of Oxford for research and teaching on global and regional issues. The series covers all parts of the world through both single-author monographs and edited volumes, and its titles come from a range of disciplines, including political science, history, and sociology. Over more than forty years, this partnership between St Antony's College and Palgrave Macmillan has produced about 300 publications.

More information about this series at
http://www.palgrave.com/gp/series/15036

Patricia O'Neill

Urban Chinese Daughters

Navigating New Roles, Status and Filial Obligation in a Transitioning Culture

palgrave
macmillan

Patricia O'Neill
Visiting Academic, Contemporary China Studies (SIAS)
University of Oxford
Oxford, UK

St Antony's Series
ISBN 978-981-10-8698-4   ISBN 978-981-10-8699-1   (eBook)
https://doi.org/10.1007/978-981-10-8699-1

Library of Congress Control Number: 2018937698

Cover illustration: Blackstation

Printed on acid-free paper

This Palgrave Macmillan imprint is published by the registered company Springer Nature Singapore Pte Ltd. part of Springer Nature.
The registered company address is: 152 Beach Road, #21-01/04 Gateway East, Singapore 189721, Singapore

To my mother, Lorraine Shipley O'Neill.

Acknowledgements

To the courageous women in this book, who so generously shared their time and allowed me to glimpse into their lives, my respect for you is immeasurable and I thank you with my whole heart. More than anything else, you are my heroines. I hope this work honours you and that others will learn from your experiences, as I have.

Profuse thanks to Halbert Jones, of RAI and St. Antony's College, Oxford University, for his incalculable support, advice and perseverance in moving this project forward, and to St. Antony's College for allowing me to become a part of its amazing series. Likewise, my deepest thanks to Rachel Murphy, Contemporary China Studies (SIAS), Oxford University, without whose support I would not have been able to complete the research for this book.

The years I spent in Asia doing fieldwork could be frustrating and exhausting at times, especially when I was struggling to find the right women to speak with. The herculean efforts of Cao Ting and Alice Chin, introducing me to their friends, acquaintances and colleagues, were indispensable to laying a proper foundation and I owe you both a huge debt of gratitude. In this same regard, I also wish to thank Mary Ong, Helen Lim, Teresa Chiu, Leo Liao and Laura Wang.

It takes time and effort to read and evaluate another's work. Norella Putney and Cheryl Svensson put aside their very busy schedules to do just that, and to offer helpful suggestions to make this work better. I am truly beholden to you. I also want to thank Sarah Harper, George Leeson, Kenneth Howse, Jaco Hoffman, Kate Hamblin, and Andreas Hoff at the Oxford Institute of Population Ageing; the Department of Sociology, Oxford University; and Mariam Bernard, Keele University for exceptional input and guidance on the path to developing this research. Further, appreciation is owed to John Moore, for interminable hours spent listening to my ideas and proof reading my many drafts.

Finally, if medals could be awarded to editors, surely Joanna O'Neill at Palgrave Macmillan would merit one. Thank you for educating me, putting up with my questions and changes and gently nudging me forward with this project in the kindest imaginable way. Many thanks are also due to Joshua Pitt at Palgrave for sage advice and sound counsel.

In the end, writing a book is a long, difficult and solitary journey. To be blessed with friendship, support and encouragement along the way is an immense gift, without which the journey could not be made. I will never be able to adequately thank all of you for joining me on this adventure, but I am so very grateful that you did.

Contents

List of Figures

List of Tables

1

Introduction

Thirteen years into the twentieth century, Lee Choo Neo wrote:

> As soon as she is thirteen or fourteen she has to undergo a course of train-
> ing in cooking and sewing. These two are essential achievements without
> which she has scant hope of securing a good match...The Chinese girl is
> seldom provided with adequate education.... Parents regard it as a waste of
> money to educate their daughters who are supposed to be incapable of
> maintaining the family in time of need. (Cheng 1977, quoting *The Life of
> a Chinese Girl in Singapore*, by Lee Choo Neo, published in 1913)

Although this was more than 100 years ago, the formula of dependency
Lee portrayed was quintessentially Chinese, and it lasted throughout a
Chinese female's life. As a child, she was dependent on her father, as an
adult she was dependent on her husband, and in old age she was dependent on her son (Blake 1994; Croll 1995; Deutsch 2006).

Dependency was reinforced through Confucianism and filial piety,
comprised of certain immutable elements: respect, gratitude and absolute
obedience, unconditional care and support for parents, producing a male
heir to continue the lineage, bringing honour to the family, and revering
all elders and ancestors. Children owed the performance of these

© The Author(s) 2018
P. O'Neill, *Urban Chinese Daughters*, St Antony's Series,
https://doi.org/10.1007/978-981-10-8699-1_1

obligations to their father, with primary responsibility residing in the eldest son and the others in turn (Chan and Lim 2004).

A daughter's filial duty was limited to nurturing an appropriate attitude and avoiding shame. Lacking formal education, these virtues were achieved through obedient dedication to and mastery of domestic skills, offered first to her family of origin, but more specifically to the family of her prospective husband (Holroyd and Mackenzie 1995). Once a girl 'married out', her husband's family obligations became her own and she assumed the duty of perfectly executing them on his behalf. With no possibility for a different outcome, a daughter was thus conscripted to a life of subjugation, either to her husband's family or if unmarried, to her own (Blake 1994; Croll 1995).

In this manner, for innumerable generations of Chinese families, filial piety has functioned as the standard for behaviour and 'old age insurance' for elderly Chinese. However, throughout the twentieth century and particularly since the Second World War, urbanisation, industrialisation, modernisation and Westernisation have reportedly mitigated the underpinnings of this once rigid system (Chan and Lee 1995; Mehta and Ko 2004; Wong 1986). If that is so, then one of the most salient features of the reconfigured Chinese ethos must be the changing roles and status of women (Holroyd 2001; Salaff 1976).

As it has been in other parts of the world, young urban Chinese women today have become increasingly well educated and employed, and many have achieved financial independence (Lee 2000). The synergistic relationship between these developments, together with delayed marriage and childbirth and lowered fertility have been widely observed. New economic value to the family has also earned daughters greater bargaining power, however, elevated status and growing self-sufficiency have not translated into a commensurate diminution of normative expectations regarding traditional gender roles. Even if they have been educated and work, most Chinese women still expect to be assigned the role of caregiver for children, husband, household and parents. Given the stress and curtailment of their freedom, engendered by juggling these multiple and often conflicting commitments, it is axiomatic that women today have a need to restructure the traditional caregiving model (Wong 2000). It is the goal of this book to explain this.

Aim of the Research

This book addresses the overarching question: Why are contemporary urban Chinese daughters still willing to undertake traditional parent caregiving activities considering their self-sufficient, modern lifestyles and attitudes and what are their coping strategies for accommodating the tension and conflict involved with discharging filial obligation?

Relevance of the Research

In 2010, Standard & Poor's reported that, 'no other force is likely to shape the future of economic health, public finances and policymaking as the irreversible rate at which the world's population is ageing' (Mrsnik 2010: 1). Due to declining fertility and increased longevity, Asia is ageing faster than any other region on earth. At the same time, the historical reliance on Confucian values and filial piety has contributed to a paucity of social welfare services throughout the region.[1] Although pensions, health care and other benefits have been on the rise, they have remained largely inadequate to support populations with life expectancies beginning to reach or exceed 80 years (Du 2013; Pei and Tang 2012; Zhang et al. 2012). As a result, the onus for parental care is likely to remain predominately on the family,[2] with the real burden of hands on care almost unquestionably and disproportionately imposed on women (Croll 2006).

This book is a glimpse into the lives of urban Chinese women living in three transitioning Asian societies: Hong Kong, Singapore and Kunming, Yunnan province, mainland China. These women explain how they have tried to operate within a deeply ingrained cultural ethos with thousands of years of history while living the ordinary lives of modern women. In transitioning societies, living up to the standards and expectations imposed by tradition, and 'enforced' by both others and self, can create tension and conflict, especially when juxtaposed with contemporary norms. Reflecting on this, many of the women interviewed for this book said they felt guilty much of the time.

The origins of this guilt have grown out of a rigid collective society in which individual needs and desires were sacrificed for the good of the whole.

Prior research has shown that this traditional Chinese norm, while undergoing change, has not disappeared (Wong and Chau 2006). Thus, despite the progress they have made, many Chinese women today are in a double bind. For those who elect to provide care, the consequences are potentially severe. On one hand, caregivers who remain in the workforce are reported to miss more days off work, have poorer health, more stress at home, more depression, and engage in more risk behaviour such as smoking and substance abuse. On the other, many women with extensive training and experience are forced out of the workplace due to caregiving obligations (Met Life 2010).[3] A single woman who forfeits her job and spends her savings (assuming there is one) to provide care for her parents may in her own old age end up broke, dependent and unhealthy with no one to care for her.[4] Conversely, women who choose or are forced by circumstances to avoid, limit or postpone filial obligation may be ridden with conflict when transitioning norms compete with what has been called the 'irredeemable obligation' some feel toward their families (Berman 1987: 25). The women interviewed for this book found caregiving to be more difficult when they were torn between their perceived duty to their family and a desire for greater freedom. This translated into a variety of mixed emotions, including bitterness and resentment, apathy, resignation, frustration and anger over the restrictive conditions imposed on them. In the worst extremes, even daughters who were devoted to their parents could be driven to commit acts of elder abuse,[5] over which they anguished afterward.

With these notable changes to their roles and status, and the new conditions under which they live, it is fair to ask if urban Chinese women are still willing or able to undertake filial obligation in the same manner and to the same extent as they have in the past. If not, who or what is going to fill the gap?[6] To address these issues, the following research questions are presented for consideration.

Central Research Questions

- *Why* would filial obligation remain a strong normative value among modern Chinese women and *why* would they be willing to provide care for ageing parents?

- Is there a relationship between how daughters feel toward their parents and in-laws and the amount and quality of care they are willing to provide to them? If so, does this represent a shift from traditional Chinese values of filial obligation?
- *How* do modern Chinese women negotiate the actual discharge of support and caregiving?
- If filial obligation remains a strong normative value among Chinese daughters, *why* would they delegate caregiving responsibilities to foreign domestic helpers and be willing to place elderly parents in nursing homes?

Scope of the Research

The Venues

This book is based on the narratives of Chinese women in Hong Kong, Singapore and Kunming, mainland China. Hong Kong and Singapore were selected because the traditional Chinese family caregiving paradigm was under investigation in the context of transitioning norms, particularly filial piety and Confucianism.[7] The literature suggests that these city-states have been on the leading edge of Asian cultural change (Croll 2006; Koh and Tan 2000; Lieber et al. 2004)[8] and the modernising influences underpinning it.[9] Kunming was selected for several reasons. It is the capital and largest city of Yunnan Province, with a major university and a population of over six million people. It hosts both industrial and agricultural economies and occupies a central location in Chinese trade. However, it has generally been considered a second-tier city, as opposed to first tier cities like Shanghai and Beijing.[10] Yunnan is also an interior, rather than a coastal province, bordering Vietnam, Myanmar, Laos and the Tibetan Autonomous Region. It has a widely diverse ethnic population living among the Han Chinese.[11] Finally, it is a city that has been undergoing rapid growth and change. Thus, it provided a middle ground for examining transitioning norms.

Together, Hong Kong, Singapore and Kunming offer a solid basis for comparing what has been happening among urban Chinese women and to see whether there are any implications for what appears to be a slowly emerging shift in filial obligation. For millennia, Confucian-based filial obligation has been a widely shared value throughout East and Southeast Asia.[12] However, in the culturally fluid environment in which it currently exists, the changing roles and status of urban women has been an underlying theme touching most families. This book illustrates how enduring social norms and cultural expectations may compete with the realities of the modern world, thereby necessitating a restructuring of priorities and a modification of filial obligation in the many societies that still adhere to it.

The Daughters

From 2011 to 2017, three generations of Chinese women were interviewed for this book: three women born before 1946; 39 women born between 1946 and 1964 (Baby Boomers) and 25 women born between 1965 and 1980 (Gen X). The selection of these women was based on their range of ages and the times in which they grew up and became adults. The time span from 1946 to 1980 represents a period of rapid change in all three locations where the research for this book was conducted. The time before the Second World War was characterised by traditional norms and used as a basis for comparison. The aggregate key demographic information of the three generations of women interviewed for this book (N = 67) are shown below in Table 1.1. The six foreign domestic helpers (FDHs) interviewed have deliberately been omitted from this table.

In the chapters that follow, to the extent their views are reasonably homogenous, the Baby Boomers and Gen X women, and the locations where they reside, (Hong Kong, Singapore, Kunming), will be considered collectively. Where meaningful generational or geographic differences are found, they will be highlighted. The older women (<1946) are included in the discussion as a comparison group, but are not referred to in the later chapters.

Table 1.1 Key demographic characteristics (N = 67)

	Baby boomers	Gen X	>65
	N = 39	N = 25	N = 3
Age at interview			
30–39	0	17	0
40–49	6	7	0
50–59	23	1	0
60–65	10	0	0
>65	0	0	3
Number of siblings			
0	0	4	0
1–2	11	15	1
3–4	18	4	0
5 or more	10	2	2
Education			
Primary only	1	0	0
Secondary only	11	2	2
Some college	1	2	0
Tertiary grad (nurse/teacher)	5	1	1
College degree only	10	9	0
Some post grad	4	5	0
Graduate degree	6	6	0
Marital status			
Never married	13	7	0
Married	24	13	3
Divorced/remarried	2	2	0
Divorced	0	3	0
Number of children			
0	14	11	0
1–2	21	12	2
3–4	4	2	1
5 or more	0	0	0
Employment			
Employed	24	25	1
Currently unemployed	15	0	2
Mother ever employed	21	17	Unknown
Living or lived with parents or in laws			
Single or divorced/living or lived with parents	11	9	0
Married/living or lived with parents	2	1	0
Married/living or lived with in-laws	8	5	0
Not living with parents or children	18	9	3
Married/living or lived with both parents & in-laws	0	1	0

Key Demographics

Marriage, Divorce and Singlehood

Among the Baby Boomers, the median age at first marriage was similar in all three locations: 24 in Singapore 25 in Kunming and 26 in Hong Kong. The median age for the Gen X women was 24 in Kunming, 26 in Hong Kong and 28 in Singapore. The median age at marriage of the over 65 age group was 27. In the main group, seven women divorced and four re-married. In the comparison group, two of the women separated from their husbands but never divorced. Among the 64 women in the main group, 20 never married. These were all in Singapore and Hong Kong. All the Kunming women in both generations were married, perhaps reflecting more traditional values.

Large Families to Small Families

Consistent with national demographic trends, among these women, family size became smaller after the Second World War. In the over 65 group two women came from nuclear families with 13 children. One woman's mother was the third of five wives, and she had 26 siblings or half-siblings.

Most of the Baby Boomers came from medium to large families. In all three venues, at least half the women had three or more siblings. In contrast, seven out of nine Gen X Singaporeans had only one sibling; in Hong Kong six out of nine had no more than two; and in Kunming, four Gen X daughters were only children.

The median age at first birth for Singapore and Hong Kong daughters was the same: 29 for Baby Boomers and 31 for Gen X. The mainland women bore children earlier: 26 for Boomers and 30 for Gen X. Despite their postponement of child bearing, among the 44 ever-married women, only five were childless, with one beyond childbearing age. The childless women were all from Singapore and Hong Kong. Every woman interviewed in Kunming had a child. Among those actually giving birth, the mean number of children born to Singapore Baby Boomers was 2.14; in

Hong Kong, it was 1.53; and in Kunming it was 1.0. Among the Gen X women, the mean number of children born to Singaporean daughters was 2.5, whereas in Hong Kong it was 2.0 and in Kunming it was 1.2. The latter may reflect China's One Child Policy, implemented circa 1979.

Generational Differences in Education, Employment and Occupational Status

Most of the women interviewed had at least a secondary education, and many had gone to college or technical schools. A greater percentage of Gen X women were college educated, as might be expected. The Kunming women achieved the highest educational levels. Every one of them had attended college even though some had grown up during the Cultural Revolution when education was suspended. Some of the Hong Kong women had been forced to quit school to work when they were teenagers but later completed their secondary education in night school. One 58-year-old woman graduated college in 2012.

Although 16 of the women were retired, and three had quit working to perform elder or childcare, all the women, including those in the over 65 age group had worked outside the home at one time or another. Most had professional careers, were employed by corporations or had office jobs. Many were administrators or managers. Several of the women were teachers or social workers. Five women were college professors; one was a pastor; one was a nurse; and one was a traditional Chinese medicine doctor.

Many of the mothers of these women had also worked, especially in the mainland. However, except for three who had been teachers, most had been employed as unskilled labourers in factories or fields, performed domestic chores or had taken in piecework at home.

Living with Parents and Parents-in-Law

Chinese daughters have traditionally remained at home with their parents until they married, and the same was true with the women in this book. Among the 20 never married daughters, 13 still lived with at least one parent at the time they were interviewed. Likewise, three divorced women lived with a parent. Traditional filial norms also prescribe that married Chinese women live with their in-laws. This was not a common practice among these women. Among the 39 married women, only ten lived or had lived with their in-laws; three had previously lived as adults with their own parents and one was living with her mother at the time of her interview.

The living arrangements of parents and in-laws who were living apart from their daughters varied. Many of the Kunming women lived a hundred or more kilometres from their parents or in-laws. They often related how they had moved away for school, work or marriage, and their parents had chosen not to relocate even though some or all of their children had left home. The parents lived alone or with a spouse, or they lived with a helper or other family member, usually a son. Among the Hong Kong daughters, more parents lived alone or with a helper and more in-laws lived alone or with another son. In Singapore, more parents lived with another son or daughter and more in-laws lived with their own daughter or alone. If for no other reason than geographic proximity, Hong Kong and Singapore daughters saw their parents and in-laws more often than most of the women in Kunming. That said, the Kunming women were no less close to their families. They visited when possible and spoke with them often. Some even indicated that their (own) parents had moved closer to them as they had grown older.

Development and Importance of the Typology

In much of the academic literature and the actual fieldwork for this book, the words 'care', 'caregiving', and 'caregiver' emerged as generic expressions covering a wide spectrum of behaviour. However, there is a difference between what is needed from and provided by a woman whose parents are still healthy and independent and one whose parents are frail, needy and dependent. Having a meal with one's family (support) and being a full time hands-on caretaker (care), which have often been regarded as interchangeable by both academics and the women who do it, are not the same.[13] By viewing them as such, overly broad, inaccurate and even misleading interpretations of the motivations underlying *why* care is pro-

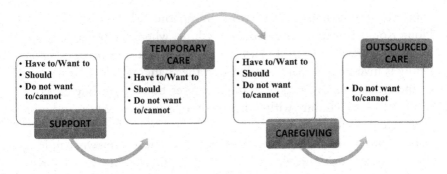

Fig. 1.1   The typology of support and care

vided, and the relationship between motivation and *how* care is discharged have resulted.

To allow for a more in depth exploration of the caregiving paradigm, a *typology of support and care* was developed for this book, comprised of two elements. To assess the amount of time and the commitment required, 'caregiving' was segregated into four distinct levels or **types** reflecting the parents' age and health status. These were designated: support, temporary care, full time caregiving, and outsourced care. Four key **analytic categories** of motivation were then superimposed on each level or type to ferret out how caregiving was driven by either relationships and/or obligation (Holroyd 2003a, b; Wong 2000; Wong and Chau 2006). These categories were designated: 'I have to' [duty]; 'I want to' [love, gratitude]; 'I should want to' [conflict]; and 'I do not want to/I cannot' [unwillingness/ inability]. The complete *typology* is shown in Fig. 1.1 below, representing a new and more accurate framework to measure the complex attitudes and behaviour of women living under transitioning conditions and norms. Throughout the rest of this book, this format will be used to move the discussion forward.

Summary of the Remaining Chapters

Chapter 2 frames the research through background and context. A review of the literature explores the ageing Asian demographic and explains how industrialisation, modernisation, urbanisation and Westernisation have contributed to changing filial norms throughout Asia and specifically in Hong Kong, Singapore and mainland China, where the research for this book was carried out. The contemporary restructuring of the Chinese family is investigated, with emphasis on the changing roles and status of Chinese daughters. Caregiving and caregiver burden are briefly scrutinised before concluding with a discussion of domestic helpers and long-term care facilities.

In Chap. 3, the core perspectives and theoretical framework guiding this study are introduced, and drawing on the literature, a heuristic framework is proposed within which the research questions are addressed. The chapter begins by discussing symbolic interactionism, the principal underlying theory of the research, and then turns to the key analytic concepts and how they have evolved, assessing the motivations for caregiving from both the Asian and Western perspectives. The different ways governments have manipulated the support and care discourse through social engineering and legislation [where significant differences are found] are also discussed, followed by the limitations on caregiving motivation. Thereafter, drawing from symbolic interactionism and the sociology of emotions, Arlie Hochschild's (1983) theory of emotion management is presented. The use of strategies of emotion management help to explain how daughters accommodate the stress and contradictions associated with caregiving for elderly parents, and how they resolve inner conflicts over whether they should provide care, or the duration and quality of care they should provide. Hochschild's 'gift exchange' is integrated into this discussion. Overall, the chapter illustrates why the concepts and theories utilised are the best ones to expand our knowledge of why Chinese daughters may or may not be willing to fulfil their traditional filial obligation to care for elderly parents, and if they do how they accommodate the competing demands and inherent contradictions of professional employment, family responsibilities and parent care.

Chapter 4 introduces the *typology of support and care* and provides the structural framework within which the empirical evidence is presented. It begins by reviewing the context and trends in which the research is embedded while addressing the potential for tension between traditional Chinese values and contemporary norms generated by changes to the world in which the Chinese daughters lived. As discussed above, the four stages of support and care emerging from the interviews have been organised into a typology and denominated 'support', 'temporary care', 'caregiving', and 'outsourced care'. In this chapter, each stage of support or care is examined through examples based on the daughters' actual accounts.

Having established the typology of support and care, the motivational and experiential aspects of contemporary filial obligation are reintroduced through the narratives of different daughters, illustrating the key analytic categories underlying support and care: structural norms [*I have to*]; relational norms [*I want to*]; how tension and conflict is managed in the discharge of filial obligation [*I should want to*]; and why negative relational motivation can impede or prevent support and care [*I do not want to/I cannot*].

The final function of Chap. 4 is to explain how the empirical chapters are structured. Chapters 5, 6, 7, and 8 each study one stage of support and care from within the typology. All of the key analytic categories are explored at each stage, with the exception of outsourced care, which investigates the relationship between Chinese daughters and their parents when domestic helpers are employed or parents are institutionalised in a hospital or nursing home. The traditional and contemporary norms underpinning these processes are featured throughout Chaps. 5, 6, 7, and 8, and in this manner the research questions are answered.

Chapter 5 considers the support of ageing parents through the women interviewed for this book. It examines the forces underpinning support; how support is discharged and the tension and conflict experienced in doing so; why support may not be undertaken, and the limitations and conditions that may be placed on it. In this chapter, the forces underpinning motivation for support and care [structural, relational] are emphasised and discussed. Role modelling, taught gender roles, the oral transmission of values, and the importance of domestic helpers to the support and care paradigm, are explored. Filial piety is distinguished from family obligation and filial belief is differentiated from filial behaviour. The women explain how they have straddled traditional and contemporary norms, and why they did not want to burden their own children with the same filial obligations that had been imposed on them. This chapter also examines the reasons why structural norms appear to be giving way to relationships, and how duty, love and gratitude are inter-related in the Asian context. The role of Christianity as support motivation is also featured. Finally, the ways in which support may be limited, how it is discharged, and why some may decline to undertake it, are all addressed through the women interviewed for this book.

Chapter 6 examines the temporary care of ageing parents, including dissimilarities in the kinds of stress experienced with in-home as opposed to hospital care. The motivations and forces underlying temporary care are discussed, and the types of tensions and conflicts that occur (and how they are distinct from support) are presented together with the conditions and limitations that may arise. Chapter 6 begins to address whether there are differences in motivation between parents and in-laws, and if so, why relationships may matter to support and care. The difference between employed and unemployed daughters is also explored, emphasising the differences between Hong Kong, Kunming and Singapore, particularly in the context of *Work-Life Balance*.

In Chap. 7 the length and intensity of care moves to the next stage in the typology. After addressing the motivations underlying it, the primary focus is on how the practice of filial obligation is sustained. This chapter explores some of the issues and obstacles intrinsic to the execution of caregiving and how these are navigated. It looks at whether the importance of relational norms and the intensity of emotion work increase as caregiving moves from temporary to long-term care. In Chap. 7, the question is posed whether motivation matters at this stage of the typology and if it can be considered a framing rule as defined by Hochschild (1983). It examines the relationship between framing rules and self-image; and how framing rules, feeling rules and self-image may all be implicated in the discharge of care. The discussion then focuses on the importance of emotion work and support to caregiving.

Chapter 8 raises the question of why caregiving is discontinued or not undertaken in the first place, and the rationale upon which decision-making relies. The motivation to discontinue caregiving is viewed from the perspective of those who have undertaken care and can no longer manage or are unwilling to manage it. This chapter also examines the difficulties of providing care without a domestic helper and then addresses the issues involved when a helper is employed. It probes the relationship between daughters and their parents once the helper becomes the primary caregiver, and looks at emotion work from the perspective of the helper. Further, it examines the extent to which contemporary norms may have influenced (if at all) the perception of outsourcing care as being unfilial behaviour in the context of traditional Chinese values.

Chapter 9 brings the discussions of the previous chapters together and attempts to answer the research questions. Throughout Chaps. 5, 6, 7, and 8, the accounts of the daughters in their interviews provide an evidentiary foundation for understanding the contemporary caregiving paradigm of Chinese daughters and their parents. Chapter 9 reflects on the typology of support and care by revisiting the meaning of these stories and in the context of the conceptual and theoretical framework, the literature and the findings, attempts to move the academic discussion forward. Implications of the research and its limitations are articulated before the concluding remarks.

Notes

1. Social welfare services across Asia, and particularly between the rural and urban areas and geographical regions of mainland China, are uneven.
2. 'Ageing in place' has been prioritized by the governments of Singapore, Hong Kong and mainland China. This refers to the intention to keep the majority of elderly citizens in their own homes. In mainland China the stated target is 90% in Beijing and Shanghai (McMillan and Danubrata 2012; Xu 2016).
3. The training of women who leave the workforce is a corporate expense that is not recaptured. The average additional health cost to employers for caregiver employees was 8% in the Met Life study.
4. Many of those interviewed for this book were supporting their parents, and even supporting their brothers. Others had no siblings, a pattern that will surely continue because fertility rates are currently less than the replacement level in Hong Kong, Singapore, mainland China and most of East Asia (Hong Kong: The facts June 2014; Statistics Singapore 2014; World Bank Fertility Rate 2014). As the parents of these women have become older and more disabled, some women have had to choose between continuing to work and providing care.

5. Specifically, verbal abuse, however, some physical abuse and abandonment also took place.
6. For example, will governments step in and assume more responsibility? Will more elderly parents be placed into nursing homes?
7. The literature suggests that these ideologies, while undergoing change, continue to be embedded in the cultural norms of Hong Kong, Singapore, mainland China and elsewhere in Asia (e.g., Taiwan, Japan, South Korea) to greater or lesser extents. Further, although Confucianism encountered formal opposition and disapproval following the establishment of the PRC in 1949, in the past few years it has enjoyed a resurgence in China, especially under the presidency of Xi Jinping.
8. Hong Kong and Singapore are widely believed to be the most progressive Asian societies, largely due to their historical ties with Great Britain and influence from the West. However, at the same time, both are essentially immigrant populations with very similar migration patterns originating for the most part in mainland China. Longstanding cultural ties and cross-border family relationships have subsequently been maintained, and of course in 1997 Hong Kong was returned to Chinese sovereignty.
9. Transitioning norms include education, global and professional employment and financial self-sufficiency for some women, resulting from the advance of industrialisation, urbanisation and globalisation throughout most of Asia over the past 30 years (Chan and Lee 1995; Mehta and Ko 2004).
10. This was originally a classification system of the Chinese government, but it has been widely interpreted by economists using a variety of factors, such as GDP.
11. China is geographically enormous and vastly diverse socio-economically and culturally. It would have been impossible to capture the attitudes and beliefs of all women-or even all urban women, and unwise to suggest that any one locale would be representative of the country as a whole. As discussed in the main text, Kunming had many salient features to recommend it.
12. Filial piety and Confucian values have predominated throughout the region for centuries, and because of this, the findings and methodology from this research could be considered in future studies beyond Hong Kong Singapore and mainland China, to Japan include South Korea, Vietnam, Myanmar and Thailand, who share similar norms. Cambodia and Laos also subscribe to Confucian norms, but they are ageing at slower rates. Other Southeast Asian countries (e.g., Philippines, Malaysia,

Indonesia, Brunei) have not historically embraced the Confucian culture, but enjoy other forms of familism (Help Age International 2014; United Nations Population Fund 2011; UN World Population Division 2008; World Bank 2016). There is no intention in this book to generalise its qualitative findings, but merely to present a snapshot in time/place meriting further exploration.

13. For example, a woman financially supporting her disabled parents and at the same time assisting with all of their activities of daily living is under significantly more stress and burden than one who spends a few hours once a week engaging in a pleasant activity.

References

Berman, H. J. (1987). Adult children and their parents: Irredeemable obligation and irreparable loss. *Journal of Gerontological Social Work, 10*(1-2), 21–34.

Blake, C. F. (1994). Foot-binding in neo-Confucian China and the appropriation of female labor. *Signs: Journal of Women in Culture and Society, 19*, 676–712.

Chan, H., & Lee, R. P. L. (1995). Hong Kong families: At the crossroads of modernism and traditionalism. *Journal of Comparative Family Studies, 26*(1), 83–99.

Chan, A. C. M., & Lim, M. Y. (2004). Changes of filial piety in Chinese societies. *International Scope Review, 6*(11), 1–16.

Cheng, S.-H. (1977). Singapore women: Legal status, educational attainment, and employment patterns. *Asian Survey, 17*(4), 358–374.

Croll, E. J. (1995). *Changing identities of Chinese women; rhetoric, experience and self-perception in twentieth-century China*. Hong Kong: Hong Kong University Press.

Croll, E. J. (2006). The intergenerational contract in the changing Asian family. *Oxford Development Studies, 34*(4), 473–491.

Deutsch, F. M. (2006). Filial piety, patrilineality, and China's one-child policy. *Journal of Family Issues, 27*(3), 366–389.

Du, P. (2013). Intergenerational solidarity and old-age support for the social inclusion of elders in mainland China: The changing roles of family and government. *Ageing and Society, 33*(01), 44–63.

HelpAge International. (2014). Ageing population in Myanmar. http://ageingasia.org/category/ageingpopulation-myanmar/

Hochschild, A. (1983, 2012). The managed heart: Commercialization of human feeling. Berkeley: University of California Press.

Holroyd, E. (2001). Hong Kong Chinese daughters' intergenerational caregiving obligations: A cultural model approach. *Social Science & Medicine, 53*(9), 1125–1134.

Holroyd, E. (2003a). Hong Kong Chinese family caregiving: Cultural categories of bodily order and the location of self. *Qualitative Health Research, 13*(2), 158–170.

Holroyd, E. (2003b). Chinese family obligations toward chronically ill elderly members: Comparing caregivers in Beijing and Hong Kong. *Qualitative Health Research, 13*(3), 302–318.

Holroyd, E. A., & Mackenzie, A. E. (1995). A review of the historical and social processes contributing to care and caregiving in Chinese families. *Journal of Advanced Nursing, 22*, 473–479.

Koh, E. M. L., & Tan, J. (2000). Favouritism and the changing value of children: A note on the Chinese middle class in Singapore. *Journal of Comparative Family Studies, 31*, 519–528.

Lee, W. K.-M. (2000). Women employment in colonial Hong Kong. *Journal of Contemporary Asia, 36*, 246–264.

Lieber, E., Nihura, K., & Mink, I. T. (2004). Filial piety, modernization, and the challenges of raising children for Chinese immigrants: Quantitative and qualitative evidence. *Ethos, 32*(3), 324–347.

McMillan, A. F., & Danubrata, E. (2012, October 1). Old age in China is a fledgling business opportunity. *The New York Times.* http://www.nytimes.com/2012/10/02/business/global/old-age-in-ch...

Mehta, K. K., & Ko, H. (2004). Filial piety revisited in the context of modernizing Asian societies. *Geriatrics and Gerontology International, 4*(Supp. 4), S77–S78.

MetLife Mature Market Institute, National Alliance for Caregiving and University of Pittsburgh Institute of Aging. (2010). *The MetLife study of working caregivers and employer health care costs; new insights and innovations for reducing health care costs for employers.* https://www.metlife.com/assets/cao/mmi/publications/studies/2010/mmi-working-caregivers-employers-health-care-costs.pdf

Mrsnik, M. (2010, October 10). *Standard & poor's: Global aging 2010: An irreversible truth.* Council on foreign Relations. http://www.cfr.org/aging/standard-poors-global-aging-2010-irrever...

Pei, X., & Tang, Y. (2012). Rural old age support in transitional China: Efforts between family and state. In S. Chen & J. L. Powell (Eds.), *Aging in China: Implications to social policy of a changing economic state* (International perspectives on aging 2, pp. 61–81). doi: https://doi.org/10.1007/978-1-4419-8351-0_5. Springer Science=Business Media LLC 2012.

Salaff, J. W. (1976). Working daughters in the Hong Kong Chinese family: Female filial piety or a transformation in the family power structure? *Journal of Social History, 9*(4), 439–466.

Wong, S.-I. (1986). Modernization and Chinese culture in Hong Kong. *The China Quarterly, 106*, 306–325.

Wong, O. M. H. (2000). Children and children-in-law as primary caregivers: Issues and perspectives. In W. T. Liu & H. Kendig (Eds.), *Who should care for the elderly* (pp. 297–321). Singapore: Singapore University Press.

Wong, O. M. H., & Chau, B. H. P. (2006). The evolving role of filial piety in eldercare in Hong Kong. *Asian Journal of Social Science, 34*(4), 600–617.

Xu, B. (2016). A silver lining to China's ageing population. *Australian Business Review; Business Spectator.* Retrieved from http://www.businessspectator.com.au/article/2016/1/27/china/silver-lining-chinas-ageing-population

Zhang, N. J., Guo, M., & Zheng, X. (2012). China: Awakening giant developing solutions to population aging. *The Gerontologist, 52*(5), 589–596.

Hong Kong

Hong Kong: The facts. (2014, June). http://www.gov.hk/en/about/abouthk/factsheets/docs/population.pdf

Singapore

Statistics Singapore. (2014). *Population Trends 2014. Life Expectancy.* http://www.singstat.gov.sg/publications/publications_and_papers/population_and_population_structure/population2014.pdf

Other

United Nations Population Fund. (2011). *UNFPA annual report 2011*. Retrieved from http://www.unfpa.org/publications/unfpa-annual-report-2011

United Nations World Population Division Department of Economic and Social Affairs, Population Division. (2008). *World population prospects. The 2008 revision*. Retrieved from www.un.org/esa/population/publications/wpp2...

World Bank. (2014). *Fertility rate, total (births per woman) data/table*. Retrieved from http://data.worldbank.org/indicator/SP.DYN.TFRT.IN?order...

World Bank. (2016). *Population ages 65 and above (% of total)*. Retrieved from http://data.worldbank.org/indicator/SP.POP.65UP.TO.ZS

2

Framing the Issues Through Historical Context

Introduction to the Chapter

This chapter integrates the historical narrative with traditional moral imperatives and kinship schemes in Hong Kong, Singapore and mainland China. It explores societal transitions and outcomes as they pertain to the Chinese family and particularly the changing roles and status of Chinese daughters. The challenges of caregiving and the alternatives to caregiving daughters, including the employment of domestic helpers and the institutionalisation of elderly parents, are also examined.

The Ageing Demographic

In 2016, 17.2% of the population of East and Northeast Asia were over the age of 60. By 2050 this is expected to become 36.8%. Likewise, Southeast Asia's over 60 population was 9.6% in 2016, but is projected to reach 21.1% by 2050 (United Nations, world Population Ageing 2016). East Asia is rapidly ageing.

In 2015, China alone was home to 130 million people over the age of 65 (World Bank 2016), representing 10.5% of the Chinese population

© The Author(s) 2018
P. O'Neill, *Urban Chinese Daughters*, St Antony's Series,
https://doi.org/10.1007/978-981-10-8699-1_2

(China Statistical Yearbook 2016). Projections for China suggest that by 2050, 36.5% of its population will be over 60 years of age and 8.9% will be over 80 (United Nations 2015). Life expectancy at birth in 2015 was 79.43 for females and 73.64 for males (China Statistical Yearbook 2016).

Likewise, in 2014, Hong Kong's over 65 population was 15%. By 2064 it is expected to reach 36%. Life expectancy at birth for Hong Kong women in 2014 was 86.9 and for men it was 81.2 (Hong Kong Census and Statistics 2015). Conditions were similar in Singapore. In 2016, the percentage of Singaporeans over 65 was 12.4% (Statistics Singapore 2016a), but this is expected to grow to 28.6% by 2050 (United Nations World Population Aging 1950–2050 2016). Singaporean males born in 2016 could expect to live to 80.6 and female life expectancy at birth for that year was 85.1 (Statistics Singapore 2016b).

As longevity has increased, fertility rates have fallen and remained below replacement. In 2014, the fertility rate was 1.123 in Hong Kong (Hong Kong Census and Statistics 2015) and 1.56 in mainland China (World Bank 2016). In 2016, Singapore's fertility rate was 1.24 (Statistics Singapore 2016a).

Low fertility has been ascribed to several factors. In the case of mainland China, it has primarily been the imposition of its One Child Policy, which has also resulted in a substantial gender imbalance currently estimated to be around 116 males for every 100 females (United Nations 2015). In Singapore, a 'stop at two' policy was similarly imposed from the mid-1960s to 1986. However, unlike China, gender asymmetry did not occur.

In addition to anti-natal policies, low fertility has been attributed to postponed marriage. In Hong Kong, the mean age of women at first marriage in 2015 was 29.3 (Women and Men in Hong Kong 2016).[1] Under the Women's Charter in Singapore,[2] the mean age of women at first marriage in 2015 was 28.6 (Statistics Singapore 2016c). In contrast, the mean age of first marriage for mainland women in 2010 was 22.8.[3] However, more educated women married later. For example, 41.2% of female university graduates and 62% of women with postgraduate degrees married between the age of 25 and 29 (Women and Men in China Facts and Figures 2012).

The postponement of marriage in mainland China has proven to be problematic for women, especially the highly educated. The term *shengnu*, or 'leftover women' has become a popular colloquial expression deliberately stigmatising urban professional women in their late twenties and older who are unmarried. Women who wait too long to marry have been characterised as 'too picky' or greedy. Older educated women might also find themselves competing for the attention of eligible men their own age with uneducated but physically attractive younger women (Fincher 2014), or women from Hong Kong (Women and Men of Hong Kong 2016). This is particularly ironic given the shortage of women in China.

Other explanations for declining fertility have included delayed child bearing, greater numbers of single women, and higher divorce rates. In 2015, the mean age at first birth of Singapore mothers was estimated to be 30.5 (CIA World Fact book 2016) and in Hong Kong it was 31.4 (Women and Men in Hong Kong 2016). Mainland China has been the exception. Consistent with marriage norms, in 2010 mainland women were having their first child at around age 23 (People's Daily, Sept. 2010).[4]

Further to declining fertility, divorce and singlehood have been on the rise, although to a much greater extent in Hong Kong and Singapore than in mainland China. In the 30–49-year-old age range, on average, 22.7% of women in Hong Kong and 17.3% of Singaporean women were unmarried in 2011 and 2010 respectively. In stark contrast, only 1.7% of mainland women were single in 2010. The crude divorce rates for Hong Kong, Singapore and mainland China in 2015 were 3.0, 6.6 and 2.8 respectively (Hong Kong Monthly Digest of Statistics, Marriage and Divorce Trends 1991–2013, January 2015).

As a practical matter, what this means for the future is that at a time when there will be more elderly people requiring care there will be fewer caregivers to provide it and fewer workers to support pensions and social welfare schemes. Increased longevity may also mean that individuals retiring in their 60s, or even later, may outlive their savings or find their pensions (if they have one) behind the curve of Asia's rising inflation. Combined with the current and projected dearth of services and institutional housing for elders, the outcome is likely to be that ageing Chinese will become increasingly dependent on their adult children whether they want to or not (Croll 2006).

Migration, Industrialisation, Modernisation, Urbanisation and Westernisation

> The Asian value system is actually the manifestation of the dynamic conflict of varying values [which are] not static but…change as economy, politics and society change. (Yin 2003)

China is a vast country with over 3000 years of history, characterised by more than two millennia of successive imperial dynasties, rising and falling throughout intermittent periods of stability and upheaval, expansion and contraction, and contacts with the West. For most of this time, Taoism, Confucianism and later Buddhism (separately and amalgamated) have underpinned and guided Chinese moral and philosophical thought, essentially defining appropriate conduct and the structure of all relationships within the society. Until 1912, this rigid and seemingly inalienable system was reinforced through an elite education scheme in which boys (primarily from upper class families) competed through national examinations for highly coveted government jobs or were otherwise prepared to ascend to their family's business. In such a way, Chinese erudition and culture rose to a level that was renowned for its elegance and sophistication. However, apart from this, and paradoxically, for most of its long existence, the greatest proportion of China's enormous landmass and population was, and until recently has remained, agrarian (Elman 2013; Keay 2009).

From an historical perspective, it is remarkable to think that China's traditional way of life and longstanding cultural ethos would be abruptly interrupted; however, that is exactly what happened. Early in the twentieth century a series of events diverted the country from its imperial past and ushered in more than a century of radical change. It began with the fall of the Qing Dynasty in 1912, and the nascent but short lived republic that replaced it. As this new form of government struggled to survive in the aftermath of World War I, Marxism from Russia infiltrated China and eventually gave rise to the Chinese Communist Party. Throughout the 1920s, until the Japanese invasion and occupation of the 1930s, political chaos and conflict arose from the competing ideologies of the

Communists and supporters of the republic. These tensions resumed at the end of the Japanese War in 1945, and civil war ensued, culminating in the establishment of the People's Republic of China (PRC) in 1949 (Fenby 2008; Keay 2009).

After 1949, concerted efforts were made by the PRC to replace the old ideologies with new dogmas and doctrines. Among other endeavours, land reform was undertaken, work units (*danwei*) were created, and Confucian norms were largely disavowed. Both directly and indirectly these reforms had implications for women, at least on paper. Following Mao's famous acclamation, 'women hold up half the sky,' women achieved new and supposedly equal rights with men in terms of marriage, education and work (Fenby 2008; Li 2004; Mingxia 2004; Wanhua 2004; Yongping 2004; Yu 2004). Although much of this has been subsequently tested, some parts have carried over to the present day.

Unfortunately, the founding of the PRC and the transformation of China from its imperial and essentially feudal past to a modern Communist model did not end its internal turmoil. As the new PRC government moved to solidify its power and unify the country, 'class struggle' was encouraged and more lives were lost (Fenby 2008). Some policies were implemented with devastating consequences. The Great Leap Forward of the 1950s, for example, was accompanied by massive deprivation, starvation and death (Dikötter 2013). The Cultural Revolution (1966–1976) that followed turned Chinese society upside down: families were torn apart both physically and emotionally; the society became divided; and the education system was either downgraded or suspended (Dikötter 2016).

With the death of Mao Zedong in 1976, the Cultural Revolution ended. Two years later new economic reforms further propelled China on its march toward modernisation and the rebuilding that continues. In conjunction with this, in 1986 nine years of universal compulsory education was legislated for all school aged children and adolescents beginning at age six, together with mandates for the construction of new schools and the development of a curriculum under the supervision of the government (China, Ministry of Education 2017). Although there have been difficulties with the practical implementation of this huge undertaking, particularly in rural areas, education has continued to evolve. China's literacy rate for individuals 15 and above in 2010 was 92.71 for women and 97.48 for men (Women and Men in China, Education 2012: 71).

Yet despite the progress China has made, after a century and a half of violence, political upheaval, economic instability, destroyed institutions and fluctuating norms, many Chinese citizens have abandoned aspects of their traditional culture and values, and some have even abandoned their homeland. In this way, the histories of Singapore and Hong Kong have been inextricably intertwined with events in mainland China. Due to migration, both city-states have emerged with predominately Chinese populations and cultural norms that are fundamentally Chinese. However, unlike the mainland, Singapore and Hong Kong have also experienced years of British governance and greater exposure to the West. Their geography and economic development have been more analogous to one another than to mainland China and their legal systems have grown out of the British Common Law. Both have become modern urban societies with, arguably, Western leaning views. Yet in terms of social policy, Singaporeans, like the mainland Chinese, have been subjected to more government control.

To be accurate, early migration of the Chinese into Singapore originated, not from the mainland but from Malaysia, and for the most part from Penang and the Malacca Straits after the East India Company infiltrated Singapore in 1819. Only after China ceded Hong Kong to Britain in 1841, did a second wave of Chinese flee south from the Fujian and Guangdong provinces of southern China into both Singapore and Hong Kong. Most of these early settlers were men, given that it was not until 1850 that women were permitted to leave the Chinese mainland. In any event, British trade assured that the influx of job seekers would last for the remainder of the nineteenth century (Evans 2008; Law 2007; Rudolph 1998; Song 2007).

Under British rule, Singapore and Hong Kong first became prominent seaports and later colonies of the British Empire. Further growth was fostered from 1912 onward by a swell of migrant workers emerging from the Xinhai Revolution during which China's Qing Dynasty was overthrown. The ensuing period of unrest in China helped to expand the population of both colonies exponentially until the depression and invasion of China by the Japanese in the 1930s and later during World War II (Fong and Lim 1982; Salaff 1976).

The end of the war and the fall of China to the Communists in 1949 generated yet another surge of mainland refugees (Chiu et al. 2005; Seng 2009). For the next 30 years, political instability on the mainland combined with economic opportunity in Singapore and Hong Kong incentivised large numbers of individuals to enter the colonies where factory jobs were plentiful. On the receiving end, the exploitation of cheap migrant labour contributed to the transformation of the city-states from entrepot trading ports to important centres of industry and manufacturing (Pong 1991; Salaff 1976; Seng 2009).

Beyond the labour market, the infusion of capital and educated entrepreneurs from Shanghai most likely gave Hong Kong an economic edge over Singapore in the early post war years (Young 1992). However, following mutual recessions in the 1960s and 1970s, Singapore began to catch up. From then on, both city-states ran nearly parallel development courses, with similar industries throughout the second half of the twentieth century. Hong Kong for the most part pursued a laissez-faire model whereas Singapore enforced a policy of rigid government control. Both enjoyed stellar success (Pereira 2005; Pong 1991).

Throughout this interval, prosperity accompanied by low wages and periodic labour shortages, generated a rise in labour force participation by family members of both sexes and all ages. Simultaneously, children began to benefit from education reform. In Hong Kong, heightened government interest in universal education was mobilised by fear of social instability from uneducated immigrants. By 1964, most children of primary school age were receiving some form of institutionalised instruction, and 14 years later, nine years of free, compulsory education for children aged six to 15 was legislated by the Hong Kong government. At the same time, in a push to solidify its control, the government replaced private institutions as the dominant education provider (Law 2007; Pong 1991). By 2016, Hong Kong's adult literacy rate was estimated to be 95.7% (Social indicators of Hong Kong 2017a).

Educational reform in Singapore was similarly propelled by a political agenda. In this case the catalyst was independence and statehood. Prior to World War II, education was dichotomous, with Chinese and Anglo schools (Rudolph 1998; Wong 2003; Yen 1981). From the end of the war, however, until well after Singapore gained independence in 1965, aspirations for decolonisation and ultimately successful statehood were indivisible from the creation of a Singaporean identity. This meant merging Singapore's Malay, Chinese and Indian ethnicities, using education as the medium (Wong 2003; Zhang et al. 2008). Conflict over what the system should look like was ubiquitous for decades. However, in 2003, compulsory education was introduced (Ministry of Education, Singapore 2017). By 2016, Singapore's literacy rate among citizens aged fifteen and older had achieved 97% (Statistics Singapore 2017a).

Today, in mainland China, Singapore and Hong Kong, education is generally viewed as a mechanism for achieving success and ascending the ladder of status and social pre-eminence. The right education combined with hard work is widely believed to correspond to better job opportunities and a more rapid progression on one's career path (Li and Bray 2006; Mok 2016; Wong 1981).

Parenthetically, it has been suggested that the availability of educational opportunity in Hong Kong and Singapore may have been due in part to public housing. Cheap rent enabling parents to save for higher education was an unintended benefit of what was essentially an accident of fate (Lee and Yip 2006). After 1949, floods of destitute worker refugees from mainland China, seeking housing near their employment, constructed villages of shabby wooden houses and lean-tos to shelter their families. Concerns eventually arose over sanitation and fire hazards. However, the outbreak of a succession of fires in Singapore during the 1950s, plus a colossal fire in 1961 and a fire leaving 53,000 homeless in 1953 Hong Kong prompted both governments to undertake subsidised public housing projects (Lee 2000; Peterson 2008; Salaff 1976; Seng 2009).

Since then, the effect of public housing has been substantial. In Singapore, preferential treatment on housing location, size and loans, has been used to encourage young couples to live with or near their ageing parents (Teo et al. 2003). In Hong Kong, part of its economic success has been attributed to the belief that public housing has enabled workers to accept poor working conditions and lower wages. This, it has been argued, has allowed competitive pricing while simultaneously acting as a safety net for families (Lee and Yip 2006).

Low-income housing has also been credited with promoting the initial inflow of housewives and children into the workforce, because they could perform 'outwork' in their own homes, which were located near factories (Lee and Yip 2006). In the context of these times, it has been argued that wage-earning women contributing to the household's well-being adopted new attitudes toward some traditional mores. Further, these women were said to have developed a desire for autonomy, gradually securing for themselves a degree of freedom and control over their own lives (Rajakru 1996; Salaff 1976; Wong 1981; Yip and Lee 2002). Nonetheless, as will be discussed below, public housing has also contributed to the breakdown of the traditional Chinese family.

Traditional Filial Piety (Xiao)

萧

The Chinese character for filial piety (*xiao*), i.e. 萧 consists of two components, one standing for 'child' and the other meaning 'old'. The character has the part symbolising the old *above* the part symbolising the child, meaning that the child both supports and succeeds the parent. This might also be taken to mean that the child is subservient to the parent, who is morphologically and by implication, socially 'higher'. (Singapore Management University Social Sciences & Humanities 2008: 5; *Emphasis in the original*)

Xiao, or filial piety, is a patriarchal, hierarchal and collective construct whose constituent parts combine to ensure the cohesion and perpetuation of the Chinese family and its name (Singapore Management University Social Sciences & Humanities 2008). Under *xiao*, family members subscribe to a strict moral and social ordering, featuring respect, obedience, loyalty and obligation. These commitments are explicitly owed to the head of household or elder male, with whom absolute authority resides. Children, notably male children, are expected to bear sons to carry on the line, to discipline themselves to uphold family honour and avoid shame, to work hard to ensure financial security, to care for their parents as they age and to revere their ancestors after death (Chan and

Lim 2004). Parents, in exchange, are expected to care and provide for their offspring as they move through childhood and adolescence, thereby creating, through a combination of love, duty and self-regulation, an unbreakable bond of interdependence (Croll 2006; Holroyd 2001; Lee and Kwok 2005; Ng et al. 2002).

Among siblings, the oldest son is generally expected to inherit the greatest portion of family wealth, bring honour to the family through his accomplishments and accept responsibility for his ageing parents (Hashimoto and Ikels 2005). Conversely, until recently, convention dictated that daughters be prohibited from working outside the home. Because their economic value to the family was negative, daughters were routinely 'married out' to become the property of their husband's parents. The husband's filial piety thus became ensured through his wife's labour (Croll 1995; Graham et al. 2002; Holroyd and Mackenzie 1995).

Filial piety predated Confucianism, but was later institutionalised by an amalgam of Confucianism, government policy and the family system, all of which became integrated into it. Simplified, the family contributed a path for moral behaviour and self-discipline, plus an economic foundation (Chow 1991). Confucianism provided order through a system of ethics and the five cardinal relationships: father-son, brothers, husband-wife, friends and emperor-officials (Chan and Lim 2004). Within this framework, filial conduct became prescribed both within and without the family, not only in terms of respect, obedience and support for parents, but for all elders. One functioned within the family (the 'inside sphere') and within the state (the 'outside sphere'). The community within which one lived became an extension of the family and an instrument for regulating behaviour. In this way, the misfeasance of one family member was imputed to all and failure to adhere to tradition could result in ostracisation from both the family and the community. The objective was the promotion of harmony without which it was believed neither family nor nation could function. To ensure the perpetuation of this helpful scheme, governments meted out rewards and punishments (Chow 1991).

Today, throughout most of Confucian Asia, the principal tenets of filiality are purported to persist (Wong and Chau 2006). However, societal change is widely perceived to have eroded it. The extent to which the deterioration of filial piety translates into behaviour has continued to lack clarity and consensus.

The Chinese Family in Transition

An old sage, Mencius, once taught that 'the root of the world is the nation and the root of the nation is the family'. (Chow 1991)

The Chinese family cannot be viewed in a vacuum. It is grounded in filial piety and is the product of both history and societal change. In the past, families were patrifocal and patrilineal. Filial piety imposed order on family members so that each understood their status and obligations from birth (Chan and Lim 2004). Families were large and incorporated extended kin networks for additional support. Intergenerational housing was the norm. Families were the principle source for the transmission of values. They also determined who would be educated and their resources controlled the quality of education. Often the employment of sons in the family business followed schooling and all children were placed into arranged marriages, whenever possible (Croll 1995; Graham et al. 2002; Hashimoto and Ikels 2005; Holroyd and MacKenzie 1995; Salaff 1995).

Today many of the traditional roles of the family have been usurped. The state has become the principle provider of education, which has become far more widespread and egalitarian than it was previously (Post 2004). International corporations have begun to dominate the workforce, commanding loyalty and obedience in their own right. Families have become smaller and women are working, thereby depleting essential resources for providing hands-on care to elderly parents. Marriages have almost universally become based on choice and singlehood and divorce have been rising. Further, multiple generations of family members no longer live together to the extent they once did, and families experience separations through employment obligations. The totality of this is that the intergenerational transmission of values that had previously taken place within the home has been marginalised or at least amended (Holroyd and Mackenzie 1995; Lam 2006).

Hong Kong, Singapore and mainland China have all experienced disruption to the traditional family structure. In 2016, Hong Kong's average domestic household size was 2.8 persons (Hong Kong Census and Statistics 2017). Mainland China and Singapore were close to this. In 2015, the average household size in the mainland was 3.1 (China Statistical Yearbook 2016), and in Singapore, it was 3.35 in 2016 (Statistics Singapore 2017b).

The adjustment to living arrangements has been attributed to different factors. Family members could choose to live apart. Older adults might favour privacy and autonomy over living with children, particularly if they are still relatively young and healthy. Adult children today have often become financially independent. They might prefer to provide parents with cash or its equivalent rather than living together. Intergenerational cohabitation might also depend more on the relationship between the parties than on filial obligation.

Employment has also contributed to the transformation of the Chinese family structure. Since 1979, rural to urban migration within mainland China has separated millions of working adults from their parents and children (Hu 2016). Similarly, China's prodigious industrial expansion in Guangdong province and its open-door policy with Hong Kong has allowed Hong Kong residents to spend the working week in southern China and return home on weekends (Chan et al. 2011). With globalisation, other adult children and their nuclear families have also begun to migrate overseas for work, often without taking their elderly parents (Mehta et al. 1995).

In Hong Kong and Singapore, the downsized family unit has been additionally linked to public housing. In 2015, 45.6% of Hong Kong's land-based non-institutional population lived in public permanent housing (Hong Kong Housing Authority 2016) and in 2016, 80% of all Singaporeans resided in Housing Development Board (HDB) subsidised flats (Statistics Singapore 2017c). Individual units in government-subsidised housing have tended to be small. Multi-generational families could be unable or unwilling to share space. Further, the choices of location where flats become available could be limited or away from established neighbourhoods where elderly parents or in-laws currently reside. Thus, public housing combined with jobs could separate families geographically. In Hong Kong for example, young adults might move to the New Territories for work, but due to the size of available housing, leave their parents behind in the city (Ng et al. 2002).

Whatever the reason, research has suggested that children living at greater geographic distance from their parents are less likely to provide regular instrumental and emotional support for them than those who co-reside (Lee and Kwok 2005; Ng et al. 2002).

Aside from geography, a generation gap has contributed to the restructuring of the family. This divide has emanated in part from the greater education and employment opportunities of the young in addition to modern technologies like the Internet. As S.-T. Cheng, Chan and Chan (2008) articulated, most of the older generation lived through the Second World War and/or the Chinese civil war when the pursuit of education and training were widely unavailable. Having survived the wars and in some cases famine, and having lived under harsh conditions, the individuals who migrated overseas predominantly did so without money, education or skills. For those left behind on the mainland, the disruption to their lives continued throughout the Great Leap Forward and the Cultural Revolution. Thus, whether they migrated from the mainland or remained, for many in that generation, the favourable circumstances later afforded their children were closed to them, especially if they were women. For example, in 2015, 22.7% of Hong Kong women and 6.8% of men over the age of 60 had no formal education (Women and Men in Hong Kong, Key Statistics 2016), and in the 2010 population census of mainland China, among those who had never been to school, 68.1% were females and 64.9% were males over the age of 60 (Women and Men in China 2012).

In contrast, in 2011, 61.66% of mainland females and 70.66% of males over the age of six had achieved at least a junior secondary education (Women and Men in China 2012). In 2015, 78.4% of Hong Kong females and 84.3% of males over the age of 15 had attained at least a secondary education (Women and Men in Hong Kong, Key Statistics 2016), and 95.5% of Singaporeans aged 25–34 had achieved the same (Statistics Singapore, Population Trends 2016a).

Lack of education could also explain the inability of many elders to master computer skills. In such cases, being denied access to the vast amounts of information available to Internet users, the relevance of elderly wisdom formed in a world that no longer exists might have been called into question. Notwithstanding the tendency toward nuclear families, generativity in the sense of nurturing and guiding the next generation, has been viewed as declining (Cheng et al. 2008). As Holroyd (2001: 1126) described it, in the urban context intergenerational relations today are largely governed by a culture of 'autonomy, modernity, youth, spontaneity and affection' rather than mores acquired largely through experience and oral transmission.

Elders, however, have appeared to be adapting. A series of focus groups conducted by S.-T. Cheng et al. (2008) with low income Hong Kong elders, revealed impressive resilience in adjusting to changing norms. Technology and lack of education were reported to be issues for these elders who said they were troubled by the disparity between the younger generations' knowledge and skills and their own, which they considered to be obsolete. The elders conveyed they had nothing to contribute, particularly because their efforts to dispense advice were often met with distain or disinterest. They said they were distressed over their lack of resources and often with the geographic distance from their children. However, they emphasised the importance of maintaining harmony within the family. Remaining silent was an option exercised to avoid conflict and they also attempted to refrain from making demands. They added that they had to respect the privacy and autonomy of their children and not interfere with their lives. The elders were willing to provide household help and babysitting to enable their children to work, contingent upon their own health. In that regard, they communicated the necessity of taking care of themselves and continuing to work so as not to become a burden, and importantly, they had lowered expectations for their children (Cheng et al. 2008; Ng et al. 2002).

Elderly focus group participants in Singapore verbalised similar sentiments. They did not want to be burdensome to their children and reflected on the reality that support from children was not within the scope of parental control. Filial piety was, in fact, considered to be a 'bonus'. Although some viewed their children as ungrateful and obsessed with money, the government was blamed for creating a 'take care of yourself' mentality (Mehta 1999).

Interviews with institutionalised elders in mainland China, also reflected parents' sensitivity and concern for overburdening their children. Parents suggested that living alone or in an institution were viable alternatives to intergenerational households. In addition to wanting to relieve their children (particularly their daughters) of caregiving and financial responsibility, other reasons cited were guilt for imposing on their children, the quality of life, the companionship of other elders and having adequate care (Chen 2011; Zhang 2017).

The above expressions tend to support the proposition that intergenerational relationships have been modified and even transposed within the Chinese family and that some may no longer embrace the culture of their ancestors. It does not, however, mean that the family has broken down, as has so frequently appeared in the literature. Restructuring has not necessarily equated with erosion. Going beyond the rhetoric, the condition of the modern family should be more accurately perceived as a correction or adjustment to norms in transition (Croll 2006; Koh and Tan 2000; Lieber et al. 2004; Yeh et al. 2013). As duty and obligation have waned, relational norms have been gaining in importance.

The Changing Roles and Status of Urban Daughters and Its Effect on the Chinese Family

The changing roles and status of urban daughters has affected the Chinese family in at least three important ways. First, daughters' access to education and participation in the workforce has made them less dependent on their parents and husbands and has given them increased autonomy and bargaining power (Salaff 1976). Second, greater financial independence has raised their value within the family as an alternate source of funding for parents (Graham et al. 2002). Third, employment has imposed new responsibilities on these women without releasing them from culture specific gender roles (Lee 2000).

Education has been driving this social reorganisation. As discussed above, the educational status of women in Singapore, Hong Kong and mainland China has changed significantly since the end of the Second World War.

There has also been a formidable presence of women in the labour market. In Singapore, 60.4% of females aged 15 and over were working in 2016 (Singapore Ministry of Manpower 2016). Hong Kong was similar, with 54.8% of women over the age of 15 employed in 2015 (Women and men in Hong Kong 2016). In mainland China, 45.9% of the labour force were women in 2012 (Women and Men in China 2012).

Working women are not new to Asia (Lee 2000; Rajakru 1996). However, educated working women are, and unlike earlier periods, women today have extensive exposure to other cultures and values. The urban environments in which they live, the mass media, the Internet and their employment by multi-national corporations have arguably created conditions in which their attitudes have been transformed and their perspectives enlarged (Salaff 1976). However, the real question is, has this translated into behavioural change?

Singlehood, postponed marriage and delayed childbirth have enabled women to remain in the workforce longer than they would have otherwise, and for better educated women it has given them opportunities to compete with men on the career path. Careers, in turn, have led to the historical predilection for sons as the providers of 'old age insurance' being extended to daughters. Until a woman is married, a substantial portion of her salary is contributed to her family, enabling younger siblings to be educated, family housing to be upgraded and money to be saved for important occasions, such as marriage. However, even after marriage, the financial support of parents may be expected or provided voluntarily by daughters (Graham et al. 2002; Holroyd and Mackenzie 1995; Mehta et al. 1995; Post 2004; Salaff 1995).

In exchange, daughters have gained some command over their lives. The choice of a marriage partner, or even whether to marry, for example, has mostly become an individual rather than a collective decision. Women have begun to exercise control over their disposable income after family obligations have been met. They have found their voice in minor family purchases and arrangements. It has even become possible for them to have a life outside the home and live outside the home before marriage, although few do. Women have generally become free to choose their place of employment and time of employment, contingent on family resources and their level of education (Salaff 1995). However, daughters' financial contributions and working status have not excused them from homemaking and caregiving.

Hong Kong, Singapore and mainland China have remained fundamentally patriarchal societies. With all the progress women have made, they are still not considered equal to men (Lee 2000; Post 2004; Wong 1981). Working women with husbands, children and parents to care for, whether they are factory workers or professionals, are required to balance the demands of family and job, each affecting the performance of the other. This can present a difficult dilemma that may not always be resolved favourably for the family. For example, in a study of 435 married Hong Kong Chinese nurses, Tang (2009) observed that women faced with conflict between work and family gave precedence to work more than the reverse.

A.K. Wong (1981: 450) asserted that education and work have resulted in greater 'role strain and psychological pressure' on Singapore women. According to her, professional women have been better able to cope because they have housekeepers and relatives to help them. In contrast, women engaged in manual labour might have to work plus take care of the house and children or ask for help from relatives or child care workers. Because they often take shift work in factories, these women might only see their husbands and children on weekends. To avoid this, the night shift has become a viable option, with the added benefit of paying overtime. However, this has left no time for rest so these women tire faster than others (Rajakru 1996). Tang (2009) observed that low-income working women have also been deprived of choice. They might prefer to stay home but could not make ends meet if they did.

Paradoxically, Rajakru (1996) argued that women working in factories receive better support from their husbands than working professionals do. The men to whom factory workers are married might have little choice but to participate in housework and childcare because they need their wives' salaries. By comparison, the husbands of professional women have given no indication they would share housekeeping or caregiving with their wives. Accordingly, although domestic help might have relieved some of these women from daily household chores, their availability has not appeared to have altered the traditional patriarchal structure in any meaningful way. Whether there is a causal relationship or not, among educated professional women, divorce rates have been on the rise (Lee 2000; Rajakru 1996).

Beyond the obstacles other working women have faced, mainland women migrating from the countryside to the city have endured problems unique to them. Due to the *Hukou* system,[5] they might not have adequate access to the healthcare, education, housing or other services that registered urban residents do (Hu 2016; Wen and Hanley 2015). Having grown up in the rural area, the quality and extent of their education and experience is likely to have been less than their urban counterparts (Li 2004; Zhou 1997). Further, most would be separated from their extended families of origin and deprived of their primary support networks back home while confronting a new and challenging environment.

Considering all of the ways in which the lives of Chinese women have changed, it must certainly have led to further modifications of filial piety, family structure and values. In a literature review, Yan, Tang and Yeung (2002) provided a glimpse into this. Citing their own unpublished study of Hong Kong college students, they noted that many did not believe filial devotion to parents would bring them good luck. Nor did they believe they should be bound to care for their mothers-in-law or that placing elders in assisted living was a breach of filial piety. However small these changes were, they represent a change from the past.

Caregiving and Caregiver Burden

As people age, they can become more dependent, possibly losing mobility, continence, cognitive function and the ability to carry out the simple activities of daily life. Chronic or acute illness, periodic hospitalisations and frequent doctor appointments often accompany the advancing frailty of old age. In response to this, family life can increasingly revolve around the needs of the elderly (Yan et al. 2002), requiring an indeterminate commitment of time and financial resources. A child who elects to care for a disabled parent may also be faced with the choice of whether to remain in employment, together with the consequences of that decision.

Once caregiving begins, it almost always increases in duration and intensity, leading to caregiver stress or burden. This emotional condition is regularly conjoined with fatigue, psychological problems, financial crisis, loss of independence, isolation and profoundly negative health (Ng et al. 2002; Wong 2005). In a recent study, Ho, Chan, Woo, Chong and Sham (2009) compared the health and quality of life of informal caregivers, principally family members, with non-caregivers in Hong Kong. Primary caregivers had poorer health than non-caregivers, evidenced by more doctor visits and weight loss. Women reported more osteoporosis, arthritis, digestive ulcers, headaches, dizziness, memory loss, heart palpitations, insomnia and emotionality. Men reported more bronchitis and arthritis. Both were more likely to be depressed; however, women reported worse quality of life than men. Adjusting for sex, age, education and work status, the decline in physical and especially mental health were strongly associated with the number of hours of caregiver burden.

Some of the greatest difficulties have reportedly arisen from the nature of the relationship. Modesty, for example, is a familial norm within Chinese society. In a series of sixteen semi-structured interviews with Hong Kong caregivers, O.M.H. Wong (2005) found that children might be reluctant or embarrassed to participate in activities requiring the intimate touching of their parents or seeing their parents naked. On their part, parents might feel uncomfortable or even shameful receiving intimate care, particularly when the caregiver is the opposite sex. Tasks associated with severe impairment such as diaper changing and clean-up after bodily malfunctions might also bring about feelings of repulsion. In this regard, C.-K. Cheung and Chow (2006) noted that informal caregivers experience more stress than professionals because they have less knowledge and spend more time performing tasks.

For family caregivers, managing stress brought on by the unpleasant aspects of caregiving can become complicated by exhaustion. MacKenzie and Holroyd (1996) interviewed ten Chinese families providing care for elderly relatives. Among the tasks they were required to undertake were feeding, toileting, bathing, cooking, changing diapers, lifting, washing, shopping, administering medications and offering companionship. In another study, some informal caregivers reported they were unlikely to receive adequate, if any, respite from these activities and were often sleep deprived (Luk 2002).

Add to this the financial burden. Luk (2002) interviewed thirty caregivers of dialysis patients and learned that some had to cut back on work; some changed from full time to part time and others quit work altogether. Diminished income can impede or eliminate the hiring of a professional caregiver or seeking respite (Holroyd and MacKenzie 1995). In addition to lost income, there are also likely to be expenses related to the care recipient such as doctor visits, medications and medical aids like walkers (Luk 2002).

Caregivers can also become isolated and lonely. Often, there is no time for a social life and in any event, they may be too fatigued to want one. Another disincentive to social contact, as Luk (2002) observed, are small houses like those in Hong Kong and Singapore, which can become crowded and messy. In addition to this, there is the potential for constant interruptions from care recipients requiring unrelenting attention. Finally, there are what K.-S. Yip (2004) called the 'burdens in management of problem behaviour', including dealing with mentally unstable care recipients with unpredictable, socially offensive, assaultive behaviour and mood swings.

Neither gender is exempt from the burden of caregiving. However, by far the great majority of family caregivers are women. Ngan and Wong (1996) articulately wrote about 'care injustice', referring to the practice of women being routinely assigned the role of hands-on caregiver to elderly people in the Chinese culture. According to them, this role is culturally assumed and executed without appreciation, acknowledgement or support from other family members. They summarised what they referred to as the 'community care drama' in Hong Kong:

> Firstly, it is taken for granted that the caregiving capacity in the community is adequate for long-term care. Secondly, the support networks for most families are not large and they are weakened by the split kinship networks between the communities of Hong Kong and mainland China. Thirdly, the caregiving load has reverted to women in the family so that community care is actually family care and care by women in reality. Worse still, normally it is one woman in a household acting as the sole caregiver. (Ngan and Wong 1996)

Caregivers who feel underappreciated, lack support or believe they are incapable of undertaking effective elder care (Cheung and Chow 2006) may still be forced to care for ailing relatives whose condition merits institutionalisation (Ho et al. 2009). This is essentially a no-win situation. If they decline to provide care they are likely to be blamed for the outcome; but if they do provide care and the patient's health becomes worse, they may also be blamed (Wong 2005). Regardless, if a woman is a member of a Chinese family, she is presumed to accept this responsibility to fulfil her kinship obligations (Holroyd 2001; Ng et al. 2002).

Ngan and Wong (1996) posited that care injustice could lead to a 'caring dilemma'. Caring dilemma results when the demands of caregiving become more associated with obligation than affection. Caregivers seek to be released, however guilt and obligation do not allow it. Those finding themselves in this position may feel trapped in what Ngan and Cheng (1992) referred to as a love-hate relationship with the care recipient. There is evidence to suggest that the longer care is administered, the greater amount of care provided and the greater the difficulty of care, the more negative the response to caregiving becomes (Holroyd 2003; Holroyd and Mackenzie 1995; Malhotra et al. 2012).

Domestic Helpers as Surrogate Daughters and Alternatives to Long-Term Care

Women's employment, smaller families, geographic distance, changing norms and an increasing number of elderly people living to extreme old age have necessitated alternative solutions to the traditional caregiving paradigm. In mainland China, domestic professionals (CDHs), members of the extended family or friends may be recruited to fill this role. In Hong Kong and Singapore, the widespread employment of foreign domestic helpers (FDHs) has become the norm. When the family or its domestic helper has been unable to cope, institutionalisation of elderly citizens has become a viable option.

Outsourced Care in Urban Mainland China

China's ageing problem is unique. There is a generational divide between families with children born before and after the One Child Policy; there is an urban-rural divide; and there is a floating population of migrants (and thus separated families) in a huge country. Each of these divisions have given rise to different issues, some of which the government has attempted to address, evidenced by the recent developments in pension schemes and health care reforms (Cai et al. 2012; Kornreich et al. 2012; Liu and Sun 2016; Xu and Wang 2015).

Care of the urban elderly in mainland China has increasingly been moving in the direction of home-based care supported by a variety of community services. Under this model, elders remain in their own homes where they receive help directly from the government or from private organisations supported in whole or part by the government through subsidies, tax breaks or service provision, and by families through funding (Shang and Wu 2011). The system, referred to as 'mixed care' or the 'multi-level framework', is generally available to those over age 60 with a local (urban) *Houku* (Chen and Han 2016; Shang and Wu 2011).

Shanghai was one of the first Chinese cities to adopt this model in furtherance of its '90–7-3' objective (keeping 90% of elders in their own homes, with 7% requiring community services and 3% needing institutionalisation).[6] The available services include personal care, day care, emergency support, meals, and lifelong learning delivered at community service centres or wellness centres. Following a needs assessment, some of the services (e.g., meals, ADL/IADL[7] assistance) can even be delivered to the elder's home (Chen and Han 2016).

The literature suggests that today many urban elderly in mainland China are living alone and most have become aware of the necessity of achieving some degree of financial independence. Elders lacking an urban *Houku*, or who are financially unable to avail themselves of the multi-level framework, also appear to have adapted to their circumstances by forming large, strong support networks among friends and associates (Cai et al. 2012; Ikels 1993; Whyte 2004; Zhang 2017).

In addition to this, urban mainland China has developed a household service industry (*jiazheng fuwu*), staffed by both Chinese domestic helpers (CDHs) and to a lesser extent, foreign domestic helpers (FDHs) who provide a variety of services on an hourly or full time, live-in basis. Almost entirely comprised of rural migrants and older laid-off urban workers, the chores these (mostly)[8] women undertake include what Wang and Wu called the 'three Cs': cleaning, cooking and care (Wang and Wu 2017; Zhang 2017).

Although the employment of paid caregivers has been growing in China, it has not yet reached the level of Hong Kong and Singapore. Nonetheless, CDHs share issues that are similar to FDHs, which are discussed below.

Foreign Domestic Helpers

In 2014, Singapore residents employed 218,300 foreign domestic helpers (Ministry of Manpower Singapore 2014), and there were 320,988 FDHs working in Hong Kong (Women and Men in Hong Kong 2014).[9] The overwhelming number of these workers was female, from the Philippines or Indonesia. Their backgrounds vary; however, many Filipinas have been educated and previously employed in teaching and other professions (Constable 1996). Some women have left their husbands and children behind in their countries of origin. Whatever their circumstances, migration in general, has generally been motivated by financial gain (Constable 1997).

FDHs are regulated by The Ministry of Manpower in Singapore (MOM) and the Immigration Department in Hong Kong.[10] In both venues employers and FDHs must meet certain criteria to enter the relationship. Among other things, FDHs must reside with their employer and may only work for one employer at a time. Training of FDHs is not required, but is recommended and some employment agencies in their home countries conduct optional courses for which prospective FDHs must apply and pay for themselves. These courses are general in nature and may or may not include skills training specific to elder care (Hong Kong Immigration Department 2016a; Ministry of Manpower Singapore 2017a; Yeoh and Huang 2010).

In Singapore, MOM imposes further restrictions, regarding country of origin, age, gender and education and additionally requires FDHs to undergo biannual sexual health and pregnancy checkups. Moreover, FDHs must be enrolled in a three day 'Settling in Programme' (SIP) before they can begin working (Ministry of Manpower Singapore 2017a) and employers must provide a bond and insurance for them.

FDHs are expressly excluded from Singapore's Employment Act (Ministry of Manpower Singapore 2017b). However, a 'checklist' for employers produced by MOM covers such things as well-being, salaries and work conditions to be agreed upon by the employer and employee. Since 2010, medical insurance must be provided and FDHs taking up employment after 1 January 2013 are entitled to one day off a week. From 2012, the employer and FDH must also agree upon safety standards and reduce them to writing, although there is no standard format for this. Nor is there a standard employment contract (Ministry of Manpower Singapore 2017c). Due to the subjective nature of the parties' understanding, in practice FDHs have few enforceable rights. Abuses, such as battery against FDHs within the scope of their duties, are governed by the Penal Code, amended in 1998 to strengthen penalties for crimes committed against them (Yeoh et al. 2004). Otherwise, FDHs have no special protection under the law.

In Hong Kong, FDHs are more highly regulated. Both they and their employers are subject to the Hong Kong government's employment ordinance and must execute the standard ID407 employment contract. These contracts include provisions for minimum wage, paid annual leave, statutory holidays, sick days and one rest day a week. The helper's duties are agreed upon and written into the contract and she or he must be given 'suitable accommodation … with reasonable privacy'. The medical bills of the FDH must be paid by the employer and the FDH is entitled to maternity leave (Hong Kong Immigration Department 2016b). FDHs in Hong Kong are also well organised and rely on NGOs and churches for support (Yeoh et al. 2004) in addition to the courts.

Upon completion of their last employment contract, FDHs in both Hong Kong and Singapore must immediately return to their home countries. Although residency through marriage to a citizen is possible, in Singapore an FDH may not marry a Singaporean without permission from the government. Moreover, FDHs are prohibited by law from being a party to the dissolution of a Singapore marriage (Gomes 2011). Immigration regulations regarding permanent residency were recently tested in the Hong Kong courts when two Filipina domestic workers sued to remain in the Special Administrative Region (SAR) after retirement. Following a favourable lower court ruling, the decision was overturned on appeal and in March 2013, it was upheld by Hong Kong's Court of Final Appeal (BBC World Asia, 25 March 2013). The women were required to return home.

Despite the regulations, problems and abuses by both employers and employees have been well documented. On their part, FDHs live with their employers, generally in small, confined spaces where living conditions can be less than desirable. As a practical matter this often means FDHs have little or no space of their own, no choice of where they sleep and no privacy. Some sleep in hallways and living rooms. However, even if they are given a room, FDHs may be unable to lock their door and thus be vulnerable to the sexual advances of employers in the night (Huang and Yeoh 2007).

Rights and obligations are asymmetrical. FDHs are often expected to be submissive and docile. They are expected to manage their emotions and behaviour at all times and are frequently given rules by which to conduct themselves in addition to their list of chores (Constable 1997; Huang and Yeoh 2007). At the same time, FDHs are expected to integrate themselves within the family structure, but paradoxically to remember they will never be 'one of them' (Huang and Yeoh 2007: 199). Regardless of education and background, status is demarcated. FDHs are generally treated as inferior (Constable 1996; Lan 2006; Wang and Wu 2017) and even morally suspect (Constable 1997). To reinforce their subordinate position within the household, FDHs may be subject to verbal or even physical abuse or disrespect of their property (Constable 1996). Reports of maid abuse, including punching, burning, slapping, shouting and being deprived of food are commonplace (Constable 1996; Yeoh and Huang 2010; Wang and Wu 2017).

Days can be long and exhausting and FDHs must live up to employers' expectations and standards for meals, housework and the provision of care, regardless of how subjective those are (Constable 1997; Huang and Yeoh 2007). While at work, every minute of the day may be accountable and is sometimes supervised. Sleep may be interrupted if care recipients are infants or elderly and disabled. If the helper is given a day off, curfews may be imposed even though FDHs are entitled to 24 consecutive hours off duty. Cultural and language difficulties must also be overcome and personal problems with family back home must be dealt with privately (Constable 1997).

Employers are frequently from the new middle class with little or no experience in managing servants. Married female employers may be threatened or jealous, forcing the domestic to wear a uniform or other imposed dress code to downgrade and de-feminise her appearance (Constable 1996). Constable (1997: 97) related a case in which an FDH, driving in from the airport with her employer on her first day in Hong Kong, was told she must only wear slacks, keep her shoulders and upper arms covered, wear no makeup, fingernail polish, jewellery or perfume. She was then taken to a barbershop where she was given a man's haircut.

Besides being neutralised as a sexual threat, FDHs must also carefully manage emotional bonds with those they are charged to care for. Lan (2006: 146) recounted the story of a Filipina FDH in Taiwan nearing the end of her employment contract. The children she was looking after told her they wanted to go back to the Philippines with her rather than stay in Taiwan with their biological mother.

The FDH experience has been characterised as 'emotionally demeaning and physically demanding' (Lau et al. 2009). These states are aggravated by the confinement of FDHs within the household together with what Yeoh et al. (2004: 15) described as 'mute bystanders'. Poor treatment and worse offences often go unreported by family members who have observed them. Trapped within the family home, FDHs have little freedom to seek help. Yeoh and Huang (2010) recorded the account of an FDH who had been molested by her employer and was reduced to throwing pieces of paper out the window on which she had written: 'please help me'. As the authors observed, it was not surprising then that incidences of abuse might repeatedly occur before they come to the attention of the authorities. FDHs might also remain silent out of fear that their contracts will be terminated and they will be sent home if they complain (Constable 1997; Yeoh and Huang 2010).

From the employer's viewpoint, FDHs have been accused of being selfish, impolite, too independent, immoral, impertinent, lacking in commitment and dedication and posing a sexual and moral threat to the community (Constable 1996: 458). Some have been blamed for allegedly stealing from their employers (Constable 1997). Other employers have claimed they were driven into a state of rage over their FDH's inability to carry out her duties in the manner and to the standard proscribed (Huang and Yeoh 2007).

Not all relationships between FDHs and their employers are negative. However, lack of trust and frustration has driven both sides to violence and worse. Yeoh and Huang (2010) described one incident in which an FDH injured her employer and two other cases resulting in the employer's death. Offences by FDHs have also regularly been recorded in the newspapers. For example, in 2013, the Singapore Straits Times reported on a maid jailed for banging her elderly dementia patient's head against the wall (Chong 2013). In addition, FDHs have been known to take their own lives. In March 2012, the Sun, a Hong Kong newspaper for Filipinos, wrote about two separate incidents in which workers jumped out of their employer's windows to their deaths (Pinay 2012).

Institutionalisation of Elderly Parents

Statistics on residential care are difficult to come by. To provide a general overview, at the end of 2010, there were 3.19 million beds for residential care in mainland China, with demand exceeding supply (Zhang et al. 2012). In 2011, roughly 3% of Singapore's over age 65 population lived in residential care (Statistics Singapore 2011), and in 2014, 1.05% of Hong Kong's over 65 population resided in elderly homes or institutions (Social Indicators of Hong Kong 2017b). Determinants of institutionalisation in these three locales have included mental problems and cognitive impairment, hypertension, Parkinson's disease, stroke, past fractures, poor vision and mobility problems, chronic pain, caregiver crisis and importantly, the unavailability of children. It has also been reported that three times as many women as men become institutionalised and the number of elderly people residing in care facilities increases with the age of the elder (Chen 2011; Tse et al. 2016; Wang et al. 2016; Woo et al. 1994; Zhan et al. 2006).

Among Chinese populations with a history of filial piety, institutionalisation has often been viewed as a last resort. In mainland China, until 1988 it was available only to elders with no children, income or relatives ('The three noes'; Zhan et al. 2008). Nonetheless, the stigma previously associated with residential care among the mainland Chinese has been dissipating, especially in urban areas. Although filial piety has certainly remained an influential determinant in the decision to institutionalise a parent, and some adult mainland children have continued to view residential care as unfilial (*buxiao*) (Chen 2011; Cheng et al. 2012), attitudes toward it have become increasingly redefined. The literature has even suggested that finding a residential care home with an excellent reputation and social environment and then paying for it is considered filial (*xiao*). Beyond that, once a parent has been institutionalised, the adult child's participation in care is crucial. Maintaining good relations with staff, supervising the quality of services and food, reporting parental abuse, frequently visiting, providing some instrumental and emotional care; helping elders with paperwork and policy matters, and even taking their laundry home (especially when parents are incontinent) all factor into the adjudication of whether an adult child is *xiao* or *buxiao* in mainland China (Cheng et al. 2012; Zhan et al. 2011).

When addressing their unavailability as a reason for institutionalising their parents, adult mainland children (both sons and daughters) have emphasised the practical side of things. Most often, this has been work, either by necessity or by choice (Zhan et al. 2006; Zhan et al. 2008; Zhan et al. 2006). Other reasons have included too many family responsibilities; the inability to care for a disabled parent at home; worry and guilt over leaving a parent at home alone during the day; the need for professional care and better care; and the cost effectiveness of institutional versus home care (Chen 2011; Zhan et al. 2006; Zhan et al. 2008; Zhan et al. 2006).

For their part, when the living conditions have been good, mainland elders have expressed broad acceptance of entering residential care. After relocating, institutionalised parents have reported better physical and emotional health and less loneliness (Zhan et al. 2006), although they have concurrently emphasised the importance of continuing to live near family and friends (Cheng et al. 2012). Although the findings have been mixed, some elderly parents have even said that entering residential care was their idea (Zhan et al. 2006).[11] Like their children, they have taken a practical approach, citing the unavailability of their children, especially daughters, loneliness at home and their own disability as reasons for entering care. The two reasons most often offered, however, have been wanting to repay their children for the help they provided during the elders' health crises and not wanting to burden their children with caregiving (Chen 2011; Cheng et al. 2012; Zhan et al. 2006; Zhan et al. 2008).

Sentiments toward institutionalisation in Singapore and Hong Kong have been both similar and different from mainland China. On one hand, more stress associated with caregiving has been observed in the city-states. The caregivers of elderly people, whether they have been FDHs or family members, have not only reported caregiver burden but caring dilemma, the love/hate relationship with the care recipient. In a study of 30 caregivers, Ngan and Cheng (1992) found 70% of those surveyed were irritable and 66.7% argued with their care recipient. Nearly 77% of the caregivers responded that caregiving was undertaken out of cultural obligation rather than love and concern and over 43% stated they had considered sending their care recipient to a nursing home.

Newspaper reports of adult children 'dumping' their elderly parents in hospitals and old age homes have also been abundant in both Hong Kong and Singapore. False names, changed addresses on identity cards and incorrect telephone numbers have been given to these facilities to hinder the return of elderly patients to their families (Khalik 2009; Moir 2012). So serious has this problem become in Singapore that one minister told the Straits Times that the law was being reviewed to allow third parties to sue children for maintenance if parents were unable to do so themselves (Khalik 2009).[12]

On the other hand, opinions of institutionalisation in Singapore and Hong Kong have been comparable to the mainland. For example, in a study of attitudes toward nursing home placement among three Hong Kong generations, Tang, Wu, Yeung and Yan (2009) found that middle aged and older respondents viewed residential care more favourably than their younger counterparts. However, unlike the mainland, they also discovered that filial piety was not a significant predictor of attitudes in any generation. The only significant predictor of the intention to institutionalise was a positive attitude toward it.

Several explanations have been offered for the generational differences. Older people, Tang et al. (2009) suggested, might be more well informed about the positive aspects of residential living and consistent with the mainland findings, want to consider the needs of their children. However, unlike the mainland studies, the elders surveyed by Tang et al. had not experienced residential care. Further, the middle-aged respondents of Tang et al. had been caring for their elderly parents, frequently balancing work, children and living in small spaces. The authors proposed that this group (like the mainland children and parents) might take a more practical approach, preferring to provide financial support for nursing home placement rather than attempting hands-on care. Referring to a study by Yeh, Johnson and Wang (2002), Tang et al. also noted that the duration of caregiving, caregiver burden and the relief experienced by caregivers following institutionalisation of care recipients, all intersected.

The totality of this points to a growing reliance on institutional care. To illustrate this, in his article on the proliferation of residential care in Hong Kong, S.-T. Cheng (1993: 451) explained that it would not have taken place but for the 'larger social environment [facilitating] the breakdown of the existing pattern of care and relationships'. According to him, these factors together with social security benefits offsetting the expense and financial incentives in the private sector have led to a 'booming elderly home industry' in Hong Kong (pp. 461, 464).

Likewise, eldercare in Singapore has been moving in the direction of more institutional care. Although the government still proclaims its intervention is a last resort, it has apparently recognised it cannot rely entirely on the family to care for its senior citizens. In 2000, the Singapore government established an 'Eldercare Fund' to help subsidise old age homes, and in 2006, the Ministry of Health (MOH) approved nearly half of its non-profit and about a fifth of its for-profit facilities for supplemental funding from 'Eldercare' (Rozario and Rosetti 2012).

Conclusion

Greater longevity and declining fertility portend a shortage of caregivers for the future. Singapore, Hong Kong and mainland China are now two generations into their past anti-natal policies with little or no success in reversing them. Younger generations are facing what the mainland

Chinese have described as '4-2-1' (Zhan 2004) and Salaff (1995) called the 'dependency squeeze': one child taking care of two parents and four grandparents.

Following years of upheaval and expansion and the development of urban, industrialised global economies, Singapore, Hong Kong and mainland China have witnessed the progression of universal education, a non-gendered educated working class and the emergence of women professionals. Together with public subsidised housing, internal and external migration and an increase in the number of nuclear families, the academic discourse suggests that these factors have contributed to the weakening or mutation of the traditional family structure and its underlying Confucian ethos.

Since Colonial times, the citizens of Hong Kong, Singapore and mainland China have relied on the ideological foundation of filial piety and their families for social support. This is not likely to change dramatically (Chan 1999; Lee 2000). However, the perception of children as 'old age insurance' is being reconfigured by both the younger and older generations. Social reorganisation and the re-interpretation of time-honoured values such as filial piety are spawning new attitudes. Adult children may be conflicted over what they feel they should do and what they are able to do (Holroyd 2001). Further, the pressures of modern society may impose limitations on their ability to provide hands-on support for their parents.

Daughters, upon whom the burden of caregiving has historically been placed, have made the greatest gains within the Chinese family over the past half-century. However, this has not relieved them of filial obligation. As their parents and possibly their in-laws have required an increasing amount of care, daughters have been confronted by the choice between work and family, experienced heightened stress, or been subjected to the demands of full time caregiving. Empirical evidence has shown that caregiving can be an arduous and unpleasant experience with detrimental health consequences for caregivers.

In mainland China, home care primarily falls within the domain of the family, spouse or Chinese domestic helper (CDH), with support from the government and private organisations. Conversely, the governments of Hong Kong and Singapore support one of the most visible indicators of modern familial norms: the pervasive employment of foreign domestic helpers (FDHs). These depersonalised individuals are hired to relieve working women from the burden of housework and caregiving. However, they encounter the same workload and stress their employers are attempting to escape from. Further, they live in a world of ambiguity within the family they are retained to serve, often in cramped conditions where employers can abuse them both mentally and physically. Employers also complain about FDHs and mistrust exists on both sides.

When caregiving becomes too troublesome, the institutionalisation of elderly relations has become a viable option. The governments and residents of Hong Kong, Singapore and mainland China largely continue to view this as a last resort. Nonetheless, filial norms are transitioning, and both elders and their children are coming to grips with the necessity and reality of residential care.

This is the background upon which this book is based and the environment in which the people whose stories are told have lived out their lives. In the next chapter the conceptual and theoretical framework of the book will be explained.

Notes

1. Interestingly, marriages between Hong Kong and mainland couples have been on the rise recently and the marriage rate has also been growing in Hong Kong.
2. Statistics for Muslim women in Singapore are administered under the Administration of Muslin Law Act. Their median age at first marriage in 2015 was 26.4.
3. Most of the available data on mainland China comes from its 2010 population census.
4. The People's Daily is the official newspaper of the Chinese government and the most widely circulated paper in China.
5. *Hukou* is a household registration system that in many respects binds Chinese citizens to the place they were born, and separates rural from urban workers in terms of the government benefits they are entitled to. The system is changing slowly.
6. Beijing has a similar structure: 90-6-4.

7. ADLs are activities of daily living; IADLs are instrumental activities of daily living.
8. Interestingly, about 13% of the mainland caregivers are men, as opposed to 1% in Hong Kong.
9. These are the most recent available statistics. Neither Singapore nor Hong Kong provides demographic information on foreign domestic helpers anymore.
10. They are currently unregulated in mainland China.
11. Although, there is some question of whether this is a 'Face' issue, with parents not wanting to bring shame on themselves or their children (Zhan et al. 2006).
12. This change appears to have been made. Under the Singapore Maintenance of Parent Act, 'If an aged parent resides with you, you or your organisation may also apply to the Tribunal for an order for payment from one or more of his children to defray the cost of maintaining the aged parent. However, you or your organisation must obtain approval from the Minister for Social and Family Development before applying to the Tribunal'.

References

BBC World Asia. (2013, March 25). Hong Kong court denies domestic workers residency. *BBC News China*. Retrieved online August 10, 2013, from www.bbc.co.uk/news/world-asia-china-21920811

Cai, F., Giles, J., O'Keefe, P., & Wang, D. (2012). *The elderly and old age support in rural China*. Washington, DC: The World Bank.

Chan, A. (1999). The role of formal versus informal support of the elderly in Singapore: Is there substitution? *Southeast Asian Journal of Social Science, 27*(2), 87–110.

Chan, A. C. M., & Lim, M. Y. (2004). Changes of filial piety in Chinese societies. *International Scope Review, 6*(11), 1–16.

Chan, S. S. C., Viswanath, K., Au, D. W. H., Ma, C. M. S., Lam, W. W. T., Fielding, R., Leung, G. M., & Lam, T.-H. (2011). Hong Kong Chinese community leaders' perspectives on family health, happiness and harmony: A qualitative study. *Health Education Research, 26*(4), 664–674.

Chen, L. (2011). Elderly residents' perspectives on filial piety and institutionalization in Shanghai. *Journal of Intergenerational Relationships, 9*(1), 53–68.

Chen, L., & Han, W.-J. (2016). Shanghai: Front-runner of community-based elder in China. *Journal of Aging & Social Policy, 28*(4), 292–307. https://doi.org/10.1080/08959420.2016.1151310.

Cheng, S.-T. (1993). The social context of Hong Kong's booming elderly home industry. *American Journal of Community Psychology, 21*(4), 449–467.

Cheng, S.-T., Chan, W., & Chan, A. M. (2008). Older people's realisation of generativity in a changing society: The case of Hong Kong. *Ageing and Society, 28*(5), 609–627.

Cheng, Y., Rosenberg, M. W., Wang, W., Yang, L., & Li, H. (2012). Access to residential care in Beijing, China: Making the decision to relocate to a residential care facility. *Ageing and Society, 32*, 1277–1299. https://doi.org/10.1017/So144686X11000870.

Cheung, C.-K., & Chow, E. O.-W. (2006). Spilling over strain between elders and their caregivers in Hong Kong. *International Journal of Aging and Human Development, 63*(1), 73–93.

Chiu, S. W. K., Choi, S. Y. P., & Kwok-fai, T. (2005). Getting ahead in the capitalist paradise: Migration from China and socioeconomic attainment in colonial Hong Kong. *International Migration Review, 39*(1), 203–227.

Chong, E. (2013, July 19). Myanmar maid jailed for abusing employer's mum who suffers from dementia. *Singapore Straits Times*. Retrieved online August 12, 2013, from www.straitstimes.com/.../myanmar-maid-jailed-abusing-employers-mum-who -suffers-dementia-2013071

Chow, N. (1991). Does filial piety exist under Chinese communism? *Journal of Aging and Social Policy, 3*(1/2), 209–225.

Constable, N. (1996). Jealousy, chastity, and abuse: Chinese maids and foreign helpers in Hong Kong. *Modern China, 22*(4), 448–479.

Constable, N. (1997). *Maid to order in Hong Kong; stories of migrant workers.* New York: Cornell University Press.

Croll, E. J. (1995). *Changing identities of Chinese women; rhetoric, experience and self-perception in twentieth-century China.* Hong Kong: Hong Kong University Press.

Croll, E. J. (2006). The intergenerational contract in the changing Asian family. *Oxford Development Studies, 34*(4), 473–491.

Dikötter, F. (2013). *The tragedy of liberation: A history of the Chinese revolution 1945–1957.* London: Bloomsbury Press.

Dikötter, F. (2016). *The cultural revolution: A people's history 1962–1976.* London: Bloomsbury Press.

Elman, B. A. (2013). The civil examination system in late imperial China, 1400–1900. *Frontiers of History in China, 8*(1), 32–50.

Evans, S. (2008). The introduction of English-language education in early colonial Hong Kong. *History of Education, 37*(3), 383–408.

Fenby, J. (2008). *History of modern China: The fall and rise of a great power 1850 to the present.* London: Penguin Books.

Fincher, L. H. (2014). *Leftover women.* London/New York: Zed Books.

Fong, P. E., & Lim, L. (1982). Foreign labour and economic development in Singapore. *International Migration Review, 16*(3), 548–576.

Gomes, C. (2011). Maid-in-Singapore: Representing and consuming foreign domestic workers in Singapore cinema. *Asian Ethnicity, 12*(2), 141–154.

Graham, E., Teo, P., Yeoh, B. S. A., & Levy, S. (2002). Reproducing the Asian family across generations: 'Tradition,' gender and expectations in Singapore. *Asia Pacific Population Journal, 17*(2), 60–86.

Hashimoto, A., & Ikels, C. (2005). Filial piety in changing Asian societies. In M. L. Johnson (Ed.), *The Cambridge handbook of age and ageing* (pp. 437–442). Cambridge: Cambridge University Press.

Ho, S. C., Chan, A., Woo, J., Chong, P., & Sham, A. (2009). Impact of caregiving on health and quality of life: A comparative population-based study of caregivers for elderly persons and non-caregivers. *Journals of Gerontology (Biological Sciences and Medical Sciences), 64A*(8), 873–879.

Holroyd, E. (2001). Hong Kong Chinese daughters' intergenerational caregiving obligations: A cultural model approach. *Social Science & Medicine, 53*(9), 1125–1134.

Holroyd, E. (2003). Hong Kong Chinese family caregiving: Cultural categories of bodily order and the location of self. *Qualitative Health Research, 13*(2), 158–170.

Holroyd, E. A., & Mackenzie, A. E. (1995). A review of the historical and social processes contributing to care and caregiving in Chinese families. *Journal of Advanced Nursing, 22*, 473–479.

Hu, Y. (2016). Impact of rural-to-urban migration on family and gender values in China. *Asian Population Studies, 12*(3), 251–272. https://doi.org/10.1080/17441730.2016.1169753.

Huang, S., & Yeoh, B. S. A. (2007). Emotional labour and transnational domestic work: The moving geographies of maid abuse in Singapore. *Mobilities, 2*(2), 195–217.

Ikels, C. (1993). Settling accounts: The intergenerational contract in an age of reform. In D. Davis & S. Harrell (Eds.), *Chinese families in the post-Mao era* (pp. 307–333). Berkeley: University of California Press.

Keay, J. (2009). *China, a history.* New York: Basic Books.

Khalik, S. (2009, August 17). Government may act against children who dump their elderly parents. *Singapore Straits Times*. http://news.asiaone.com/News/the+Straits+Times/Story/A1Story20090817-161452.html

Koh, E. M. L., & Tan, J. (2000). Favouritism and the changing value of children: A note on the Chinese middle class in Singapore. *Journal of Comparative Family Studies, 31*, 519–528.

Kornreich, Y., Veretinsky, I., & Potter, P. B. (2012). Consultation and deliberation in China: The making of China's health-care reform. *The China Journal, 68*, 176–203.

Lam, R. C. (2006). Contradictions between traditional Chinese values and the actual performance: A study of the caregiving roles of the modern sandwich generation in Hong Kong. *Journal of Comparative Family Studies, 37*(2), 299–318.

Lan, P.-C. (2006). *Global Cinderellas: Migrant domestics and newly rich employers in Taiwan*. Durham: Duke University Press.

Lau, P. W. L., Cheng, J. G. Y., Chow, D. L. Y., Ungvari, G. S., & Leung, C. M. (2009). Acute psychiatric disorders in foreign domestic workers in Hong Kong: A pilot study. *International Journal of Social Psychiatry, 55*(6), 569–576.

Law, W.-W. (2007). Schooling in Hong Kong. In G. Postiglione & J. Tan (Eds.), *Going to school in East Asia* (pp. 86–121). Westport: Greenwood Publishing.

Lee, W. K.-M. (2000). Women employment in colonial Hong Kong. *Journal of Contemporary Asia, 36*, 246–264.

Lee, W. K.-M., & Kwok, H.-K. (2005). Differences in expectations and patterns of informal support for older persons in Hong Kong: Modification to filial piety. *Ageing International, 30*, 188–206.

Lee, J., & Yip, N.-M. (2006). Public housing and family life in East Asia: Housing and social change in Hong Kong 1953–1990. *Journal of Family History, 31*, 66–82.

Li, D. (2004). Gender inequality in education in rural China. In T. Jie, Z. Bijun, & S. L. Mow (Eds.), *Holding up half the sky: Chinese women, past, present and future* (pp. 159–171). New York: Feminist Press of the City University of New York.

Li, M., & Bray, M. (2006). Social class and cross-border higher education: Mainland Chinese students in Hong Kong and Macau. *Journal of International Migration and Integration, 7*(4), 407–424.

Lieber, E., Nihura, K., & Mink, I. T. (2004). Filial piety, modernization, and the challenges of raising children for Chinese immigrants: Quantitative and qualitative evidence. *Ethos, 32*(3), 324–347.

Liu, T., & Sun, L. (2016). Pension reform in China. *Journal of Aging & Social Policy, 28*(1), 15–28.

Luk, W. S.-C. (2002). The home care experience as perceived by the caregivers of Chinese dialysis patients. *International Journal of Nursing Studies, 39*(3), 269–277.

MacKenzie, A. E., & Holroyd, E. E. (1996). An exploration of the carers' perceptions of caregiving and caring responsibilities in Chinese families. *Journal of Nursing Studies, 33*(1), 1–12.

Malhotra, C., Malhotra, R., Ostbye, T., Matchar, D., & Chan, A. (2012). Depressive symptoms among informal caregivers of older adults: Insights from the Singapore survey on informal caregiving. *International Psychogeriatrics, 24*(8), 1335–1346.

Mehta, K. (1999). Intergenerational exchanges: Qualitative evidence from Singapore. *Southeast Asian Journal of Social Science, 27*(2), 111–122.

Mehta, K., Osman, M. M., & Lee, A. E.-Y. (1995). Living arrangements of the elderly in Singapore: Cultural norms in transition. *Journal of Cross-Cultural Gerontology, 10*(1-2), 113–143.

Mingxia, C. (2004). The marriage law and the rights of Chinese women in marriage and the family. In T. Jie, Z. Bijun, & S. L. Mow (Eds.), *Holding up half the sky: Chinese women, past, present and future* (pp. 159–171). New York: Feminist Press of the City University of New York.

Moir, J. (2012, June 29). Families dump elderly in hospitals. *South China Morning Post.* www.scmp.com/article/119179/families-dump-elderly-hospitals

Mok, K. H. (2016). Massification of higher education, graduate employment and social mobility in the greater China region. *British Journal of Sociology of Education, 37*(1), 51–71. https://doi.org/10.1080/01425692.2015.1111751.

Ng, A. C. Y., Phillips, D. R., & Lee, W. K.-m. (2002). Persistence and challenges to filial piety and informal support of older persons in a modern Chinese society: A case study in Tuen Mun, Hong Kong. *Journal of Aging Studies, 16*(2), 135–153.

Ngan, R., & Cheng, I. C. K. (1992). The caring dilemma, stress and needs of carers for the Chinese frail elderly. *Hong Kong Journal of Gerontology, 6*(2), 34–41.

Ngan, R., & Wong, W. (1996). Injustice in family care of the Chinese elderly in Hong Kong. *Journal of Aging & Social Policy, 7*(2), 77–94.

Pereira, A. A. (2005). Religiosity and economic development in Singapore. *Journal of Contemporary Religion, 20*(2), 161–177.

Peterson, G. (2008). To be or not to be a refugee: The international politics of the Hong Kong refugee crisis, 1949–1955. *The Journal of Imperial and Commonwealth History, 36*(2), 171–195.

Pinay, B. (2012, Mid-March). *Two Filipinas thought to have jumped off employers' flat; Investigation on.* Sun Internet Edition. http://www.sunweb.com.hk/Story.asp?hdnStoryCode=7230&

Pong, S.-l. (1991). The effect of women's labor on family income inequality: The case of Hong Kong. *Economic Development and Cultural Change, 40*(1), 131–152.

Post, D. (2004). Family resources, gender, and immigration: Changing sources of Hong Kong educational inequality, 1971–2001. *Social Science Quarterly, 85*(5), 1238–1258.

Rajakru, D. (1996). The state, family and industrial development: The Singapore case. *Journal of Contemporary Asia, 26*(1), 3–27.

Rozario, P. A., & Rosetti, A. L. (2012). "Many helping hands": A review and analysis of long-term care policies, programs, and practices in Singapore. *Journal of Gerontological Social Work, 55*(7), 641–658.

Rudolph, J. (1998). Reconstructing collective identities: The Babas of Singapore. *Journal of Contemporary Asia, 28*(2), 203–232.

Salaff, J. W. (1976). Working daughters in the Hong Kong Chinese family: Female filial piety or a transformation in the family power structure? *Journal of Social History, 9*(4), 439–466.

Salaff, J. W. (1995). *Working daughters of Hong Kong: Filial piety or power in the family* (Rev ed.). New York: Columbia University Press.

Seng, L. K. (2009). Kampong, fire, nation: Towards a social history of postwar Singapore. *Journal of Southeast Asian Studies, 40*(3), 613–643.

Shang, X., & Wu, X. (2011). The care regime in China: Elder and child care. *Journal of Comparative Social Welfare, 27*(2), 123–131. https://doi.org/10.10 80/17486831.2011.567017.

Singapore Management University Social Sciences & Humanities. (2008). *The confucian filial duty to care for elderly parents* (Working Paper Series, Paper no. 02-2008, 1-26). Singapore: Williams, J., & Mooney, B.

Song, E. K. W. (2007). Ignoring "history from below": People's history in the historiography of Singapore. *History Compass, 5*(1), 11–25.

Tang, C. S.-K. (2009). The influence of family-work role experience and mastery of psychological health of Chinese employed mothers. *Journal of Health Psychology, 14*(8), 1207–1217.

Tang, C. S.-K., Wu, A. M. S., Yeung, D., & Yan, E. (2009). Attitudes and intention toward old age home placement: A study of young adult, middle-aged, and older Chinese. *Ageing International, 34*(4), 237–251.

Teo, P., Graham, E., Yeoh, B. S. A., & Levy, S. (2003). Values, change and intergenerational ties between two generations of women in Singapore. *Ageing and Society, 23*(3), 327–247.

Tse, M. M. Y., Lai, C., Lui, J. Y. W., Wong, E. K., & Yeung, S. Y. (2016). Frailty, pain and psychological variables among older adults living in Hong Kong nursing homes: Can we do better to address multimorbidities? *Journal of Psychiatric and Mental Health Nursing, 23*, 303–311.

Wang, P., Yap, P., Koh, G., Davies, J., Dalakoti, M., Fong, N.-P., Tiong, W. W., & Luo, N. (2016). Quality of life and related factors of nursing home residents in Singapore. *Health and Quality of Life Outcomes, 14*, 112–121. https://doi.org/10.1186/s12955-016-0503-x.

Wang, J., & Wu, B. (2017). Domestic helpers as frontline workers in China's home-based elder care: A systematic review. *Journal of Women & Aging*. https://doi.org/10.1080/08952841.2016.1187536.

Wanhua, M. (2004). The readjustment of China's higher education structure and women's higher education. In T. Jie, Z. Bijun, & S. L. Mow (Eds.), *Holding up half the sky: Chinese women, past, present and future* (pp. 159–171). New York: Feminist Press of the City University of New York.

Wen, Y., & Hanley, J. (2015). Rural-to-urban migration, family resilience, and policy framework for social support in China. *Asian Social Work and Policy Review, 9*, 18–28.

Whyte, M. K. (2004). Filial obligations in Chinese families: Paradoxes of modernization. In C. Ikels (Ed.), *Filial piety: Practice and discourse in contemporary East Asia* (pp. 106–127). Stanford: Stanford University Press.

Wong, A. K. (1981). Planned development, social stratification, and the sexual division of labor in Singapore. *Signs: Journal of Women in Culture and Society, 7*(2), 434–452.

Wong, T.-H. (2003). Education and state formation reconsidered: Chinese school identity in postwar Singapore. *Journal of Historical Sociology, 16*(2), 237–265.

Wong, O. M. H. (2005). Gender and intimate caregiving for the elderly in Hong Kong. *Journal of Aging Studies, 19*(3), 375–391.

Wong, O. M. H., & Chau, B. H. P. (2006). The evolving role of filial piety in eldercare in Hong Kong. *Asian Journal of Social Science, 34*(4), 600–617.

Woo, J., Ho, S. C., Lau, J., & Yuen, Y. K. (1994). Age and marital status are major factors associated with institutionalization in elderly Hong Kong Chinese. *Journal of Epidemiology and Community Health, 48*(3), 306–309.

Xu, G., & Wang, J. (2015). Primary health care, a concept to be fully understood and implemented in current China's health care reform. *Family Medicine and Community Health, 3*(3), 41–51.

Yan, E., Tang, C. S.-K., & Yeung, T. D. (2002). No safe haven: A review on elder abuse in Chinese families. *Trauma, Violence & Abuse, 3*(3), 167–180.

Yeh, S.-H., Johnson, M. A., & Wang, S.-T. (2002). The changes in caregiver burden following nursing home placement. *International Journal of Nursing Studies, 39*(6), 591–600.

Yeh, K.-H., Yi, C.-C., Tsao, W.-C., & Wan, P.-S. (2013). Filial piety in contemporary Chinese societies: A comparative study of Taiwan, Hong Kong and China. *International Sociology, 28*(3), 277–296. https://doi.org/10.1177/0268580913484345.

Yen, C.-H. (1981). Early Chinese clan organizations in Singapore and Malaya, 1819-1911. *Journal of Southeast Asian Studies, 12*(1), 62–92.

Yeoh, B. S. A., & Huang, S. (2010). Foreign domestic workers and home-based care for elders in Singapore. *Journal of Aging & Social Policy, 22*(1), 69–88.

Yeoh, B. S. A., Huang, S., & Devasahayam, T. W. (2004). Diasporic subjects in the nation: Foreign domestic workers, the reach of law and civil society in Singapore. *Asian Studies Review, 28*(1), 7–23.

Yin, L. C. (2003). Do traditional values still exist in modern Chinese societies? The case of Singapore and China. *Asia Europe Journal, 1*(1), 43–59.

Yip, K.-S. (2004). A critical review of family caregiving of mental health consumers in Hong Kong. *Journal of Family Social Work, 7*(3), 71–89.

Yip, P. S. F., & Lee, J. (2002). The impact of the changing marital structure on fertility of Hong Kong SAR. *Social Science & Medicine, 55*(12), 2159–2169.

Yongping, J. (2004). Employment and Chinese women under two systems. In T. Jie, Z. Bijun, & S. L. Mow (Eds.), *Holding up half the sky: Chinese women, past, present and future* (pp. 159–171). New York: Feminist Press of the City University of New York.

Young, A. (1992). A tale of two cities: Factor accumulation and technical change in Hong Kong and Singapore. *NBER Macroeconomics Annual, 7*, 13–54.

Yu, X. (2004). The status of Chinese women in marriage and family. In T. Jie, Z. Bijun, & S. L. Mow (Eds.), *Holding up half the sky: Chinese women, past, present and future* (pp. 159–171). New York: Feminist Press of the City University of New York.

Zhan, J. H. (2004). Socialization or social structure: Investigating predictors of attitudes toward filial responsibility among Chinese urban youth from one- and multiple-child families. *International Journal of Aging and Human Development, 59*(1), 105–124.

Zhan, H. J., Ba, G. L., Guan, X., & Bai, H.-g. (2006). Recent developments in institutional elder care in China. *Journal of Aging & Social Policy, 18*(2), 85–108.

Zhan, H. J., Liu, G., & Guam, X. (2006). Willingness and availability: Explaining new attitudes toward institutional elder care among Chinese elderly parents and their adult children. *Journal of Aging Studies, 20*, 279–290.

Zhan, H. J., Feng, X., & Luo, B. (2008). Placing elderly parents in institutions in urban China: A reinterpretation of filial piety. *Research on Aging, 30*(5), 543–571.

Zhan, H. J., Feng, Z., Chen, Z., & Feng, X. (2011). The role of the family in institutional long-term care: Cultural management of filial piety in China. *International Journal of Social Welfare, 20*, s121–s134. https://doi. org/10.1111/j.1468-2397.2011.00808.x.

Zhang, H. (2017). Recalibrating filial piety: Realigning the state, family and market interests in China. In G. Santos & S. Harrell (Eds.), *Transforming patriarchy: Chinese families in the twenty-first century* (pp. 234–250). Seattle/ London: University of Washington Press.

Zhang, L. J., Gu, P. Y., & Hu, G. (2008). A cognitive perspective of Singaporean primary school pupils use of reading strategies in learning to read English. *British Journal of Educational Psychology, 78*(2), 245–271.

Zhang, N. J., Guo, M., & Zheng, X. (2012). China: Awakening giant developing solutions to population aging. *The Gerontologist, 52*(5), 589–596.

Zhou, Y. (1997). Labor migration and returns to rural education in China. *American Journal of Agricultural Economies, 79*(4), 1278–1287.

Hong Kong

Hong Kong Census and Statistics Department, special administrative region. (2015, September 25). *Population projections 2015–2064.* http://www.censtatd.gov.hk/hkstat/sub/sp190.jsp?productCode=B1120015

Hong Kong Census and Statistics Department, special administrative region. (2017, May 19). *Statistics on domestic households.* https://www.censtatd.gov.hk/hkstat/sub/sp150.jsp?tableID=005&ID=0&productType=8

Hong Kong Housing Authority. Housing in Figures. (2016). https://www.housingauthority.gov.hk/en/common/pdf/about-us/publications-and-statistics/HIF.pdf

Hong Kong immigration department. (2016a). *Foreign domestic helpers.* http://www.immd.gov.hk/eng/faq/foreign-domestic-helpers.html#eligibility

Hong Kong immigration department. (2016b). *Practical guide for employment of foreign domestic helpers.* http://www.labour.gov.hk/eng/public/wcp/FDH guide.pdf

Hong Kong Monthly Digest of Statistics. (2015). *Marriage and divorce trends in Hong Kong.* https://www.censtatd.gov.hk/hkstat/sub/sp160.jsp?product Code=FA100055

Social indicators of Hong Kong. (2017a). http://www.socialindicators.org.hk/en/indicators/education/7.7

Social indicators of Hong Kong. (2017b). http://www.socialindicators.org.hk/en/indicators/elderly/31.12

Women and men in Hong Kong, key statistics. (2014). *Table 4.49, foreign domestic helpers by nationality and sex.* http://www.statistics.gov.hk/pub/B11303032014AN14B0100.pdf

Women and men in Hong Kong key statistics. (2016). *Labour force participation rate.* http://www.statistics.gov.hk/pub/B11303032016AN16B0100.pdf

Women and men in Hong Kong key statistics, Education. (2016). http://www.statistics.gov.hk/pub/B11303032016AN16B0100.pdf

Women and men in Hong Kong key statistics Marriage, fertility and family conditions. (2016). http://www.censtatd.gov.hk/hkstat/sub/sp180.jsp?product Code=B1130303

Mainland China

China Statistical Yearbook, Sect. 2-4. (2016). *National Bureau of statistics of China.* http://www.stats.gov.cn/tjsj/ndsj/2016/indexeh.htm

China Statistical Yearbook, Sect. 2-5. (2016). *National Bureau of statistics of China.* http://www.stats.gov.cn/tjsj/ndsj/2016/indexeh.htm

People's Daily Online. (2010, September 26). *Chinese delay average age of marriage, first child.* http://en.people.cn/90001/90782/7151025.html

People's Republic of China, Ministry of Education. (2017). http://www.moe.edu.cn/publicfiles/business/htmlfiles/moe/moe_2803/200907/49979.html

Women and Men in China, Facts and Figures. (2012). *National Bureau of statistics, tabulation on the 2010 population census of the People's Republic of China, 2012.* http://www.unicef.cn/en/uploadfile/2014/0109/20140109030938887.pdf

Singapore

Ministry of Education Singapore. (2017). *Compulsory education.* https://www.moe.gov.sg/education/education-system/compulsory-education

Ministry of Manpower. (2016a). *Labour force in Singapore.* http://stats.mom. gov.sg/iMAS_PdfLibrary/mrsd_2016LabourForce_survey_highlights.pdf

Ministry of Manpower. (2017a). *Work permit for FDW, eligibility and requirements.* http://www.mom.gov.sg/passes-and-permits/work-permit-for-foreign-domestic-worker/eligibility-and-requirements

Ministry of Manpower. (2017b). *Employment act, who it covers.* http://www. mom.gov.sg/employment-practices/employment-act/who-is-covered

Ministry of Manpower. (2017c). *Checklist for employers of FDWs.* http://www. mom.gov.sg/~/media/mom/documents/work-passes-and-permits/checklist-hiring-fdw-english.pdf?la=en

Ministry of Manpower, Singapore. (2014, June). http://www.mom.gov.sg/statistics-publications/others/statistics/Pages/ForeignWorkforceNumbers.aspx

Statistics Singapore. (2011/09). *The elderly in Singapore.* https://www.singstat. gov.sg/docs/default-source/default-document-library/publications/publications_and_papers/population_and_population_structure/ssnsep11-pg1-9. pdf

Statistics Singapore. (2016a). *Population trends.* http://www.singstat.gov.sg/publications/publications-and-papers/population-and-population-structure/population-trends

Statistics Singapore. (2016b). *Births and deaths, life tables 2015–2016.* http:// www.singstat.gov.sg/publications/publications-and-papers/population#births_and_deaths

Statistics Singapore. (2016c). *Marriages and divorce.* http://www.singstat.gov.sg/publications/publications-and-papers/marriages-and-divorces/marriages-and-divorces

Statistics Singapore. (2017a). *Education and literacy.* http://www.singstat.gov.sg/statistics/latest-data#20

Statistics Singapore. (2017b). *Households.* http://www.singstat.gov.sg/statistics/latest-data#22

Statistics Singapore. (2017c). *Households.* http://www.singstat.gov.sg/statistics/latest-data#22

Other

Central Intelligence Agency The World Factbook. (2016). https://www.cia.gov/library/publications/the-world-factbook/fields/2256.html

United Nations Department of Economic and Social Affairs Population Division. (2015). *World population ageing 2015*. Retrieved from http://www.un.org/en/development/desa/population/publications/pdf/ageing/WPA2015_Report.pdf

United Nations World Population Ageing 1950-2050. (2016). www.un.org/esa/population/publications/worldageing19502050/pdf/180singa.pdf

World Bank. (2016). *Population ages 65 and above (% of total)*. Retrieved from http://data.worldbank.org/indicator/SP.POP.65UP.TO.ZS

3

Core Perspectives and Theoretical Framework Underpinning Chinese Daughters' Support and Care of Elderly Parents

Introduction to the Conceptual and Theoretical Underpinnings

Two basic orienting assumptions underlying sociological theory are that: (1) history and structure impose order on society and that social reality exists separate and apart from what individuals want or do; or (2) the social order is the product of interaction between individuals and groups, with no existence apart from them. These perspectives are referred to as 'collective' (structuralist) or 'macro' and 'individualist' or 'micro' respectively (Appelrouth and Edles 2007). Arguably, there is no 'grand' sociological perspective that encompasses both societal level and small group or individual level aspects.

Traditional Chinese society and its values can be viewed from a macro level perspective whereby social patterns such as filial obligation originate from and benefit the society as a whole. In general, this perspective emphasises the interdependence of social institutions and their common interest in maintaining order. In contrast, the changes and contradictions in norms of filial responsibility and their enactments taking place in Asian societies today might be better explained through the theoretical

© The Author(s) 2018
P. O'Neill, *Urban Chinese Daughters*, St Antony's Series,
https://doi.org/10.1007/978-981-10-8699-1_3

lens of symbolic interactionism. This micro-level perspective focuses on the symbolic nature of human interaction; that is, how interpersonal interaction conveys meaning and promotes the socialisation of important cultural values and practices. In this book one can see the effect of young Chinese women being exposed to the changing opportunities and constraints of a wider world and through interactions with others, create new definitions of filial obligation and behaviour.

Within the interactionist framework, relevant conceptual models (filial obligation, reciprocity, affection) have been drawn on to make sense of what was observed in the interviews in terms of *why* these contemporary Chinese daughters have continued to provide support and care to elderly parents despite the competing demands of work and other family responsibilities. Arlie Hochschild's (1983) theory of emotion management has also been relied on, augmented by ideas from social exchange theory to understand *how* these daughters were able to accommodate or otherwise respond to the tensions involved in fulfilling their filial obligations and *why* they might have decided to seek alternatives to the direct caregiving of their elderly parents.

Negotiating Traditional Filial Obligations and Contemporary Norms

Traditional Chinese values, essentially synonymous with Confucianism and filial piety, have existed within Chinese communities for thousands of years. Originating primarily in rural society, the historical Chinese ethos was grounded in a sense of sameness, or what Durkheim might have called 'mechanical solidarity' (Appelrouth and Edles 2007). During the past half-century, Chinese cultural solidarity has largely metamorphosed into the inter-related and interdependent systems inherent in urbanising societies undergoing rapid industrialisation (Chilcott 1998). Nonetheless, some of the societal norms associated with the earlier structures and values, such as the subordination of the individual to the family, have remained (Allen 2010; Churton and Brown 2010; Clark 1972).

What has changed is the nature of action. In the past, individual free will outside the constraints of societal norms and values was minimal.

Although some traditional norms have continued to be internalised, in modern Chinese society individuals have been more likely to interact with each other and the outside world based on the meanings these things have for them rather than blindly accepting meanings that have been superimposed. These new meanings have themselves been derived from interaction among individuals and might have been managed and altered by the ways each one has interpreted what he or she has interacted with (Blumer 1969; Wallace and Wolf 2006). As a result, although traditional Chinese values have persisted, they might now mean different things to different people.

As discussed in the previous chapter, this transformation from a top down societally imposed understanding of normative behaviour to one that is more bottom up and individualistic is generally recognised as having evolved within Chinese society since the mid-twentieth century. Underpinning this transition has been the implementation of mandatory education, the availability of professional employment for women and new technologies, together with structural modifications to families and housing and both internal and external migration. As the women's stories told in this book illustrate, each of these changes has fostered social interactions beyond the confinement of kin networks and local communities, suggesting that the changes taking place in Chinese society, at least to the extent they are reflected in the lives of these women, can best be understood at a more micro-level through a symbolic interactionist framework.

Symbolic Interactionism

The descriptive words 'symbolic interactionism' have been attributed to one of its chief proponents, Herbert Blumer (1969), who together with George Herbert Mead (1863–1931), has generally been considered the intellectual forbearer of this theoretical approach. Drawing on Max Weber's action theory, emphasising interpretation and the subjective meaning individuals attach to human behaviour, Mead's major contribution has been the concept of 'self'. Mead viewed the self as being active and creative rather than passive and receptive, in addition to being dichotomous: The 'I' spontaneously responds to stimuli, whereas the 'me' adopts a perspective based on the attitudes of others that have been internalised. According to Mead, we interact with ourselves through internal conversations that allow us to rehearse our actions and organise our thoughts (Wallace and Wolf 2006). This 'self-interaction' then becomes the basis for 'role-taking'. In role taking one puts oneself in the position of others with whom one interacts, anticipating their actions and assessing oneself through the other's eyes (Turner and Stets 2005; Wallace and Wolf 2006). Mead also highlighted the importance of gestures, which he argued, become symbols once they are internalised by members of a community. In interactions, a common understanding regarding the meaning of gestures emerges among the participants (Wallace and Wolf 2006).

For symbolic interactionists, meaning is always the result of interaction and cannot exist apart from it. It is through the interpretative process of social action that meaning is created (Blumer 1969). Blumer specifically rejected the imposition of pre-existing roles and structures and argued that meaning is neither stationary nor defined by systems. He contended that interaction takes place between individuals not roles.

With meaning, interaction and interpretation at its core, Blumer (1969: 2) formalised and expanded Mead's theoretical perspective by defining what have widely been accepted as the three basic premises of symbolic interactionism: (1) That individuals act toward people, objects and all other things on the basis of the meanings these have for them; (2) That these meanings, themselves, are the result of social interaction between individuals; and (3) That the meanings of these 'things' are managed and modified on the basis of how they are interpreted by individuals as they come into contact with them.

Symbolic interactionism not only helps to explain how Chinese daughters negotiate the ideological terrain between traditional and contemporary norms of filial obligation; it also provides an overarching scheme within which to identify and investigate the conceptual discourses addressing why they continue to undertake traditional filial support and care despite their other role demands and expectations. From a theoretical perspective, symbolic interactionism is linked with the management of emotions and social exchange, both of which were relied on by many of the women in this book, as discussed in the subsequent chapters.

Conceptual and Theoretical Perspectives on the Support and Care of Elderly Parents

The current support and caregiving paradigm between Chinese daughters and their parents and in-laws can best be understood through a trio of analytic approaches. The first refers to the conceptual models of motivation underpinning why daughters provide support and care [*I have to/I want to*]. The second and third refer to theories that explain how daughters manage conflict and tension in the process of discharging filial obligations [*I should want to*] and why daughters may discontinue or decline to undertake practices of filial obligation [*I do not want to/I cannot*]. If shown in sequence, they would appear as in Fig. 3.1 below:

The remainder of this chapter discusses each of the key analytic categories that comprise the conceptual and theoretical foundation of this book.

Why Daughters Provide Support and Care: Motivations for Support and Caregiving

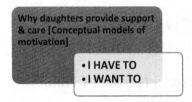

Image of structural/relational model of motivation

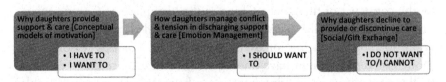

Fig. 3.1 Conceptual and theoretical perspectives of filial support and care

Numerous conceptual models have been developed in both the Asian and Western literature, to explain motivations for caregiving. These, however, can be grouped into two broad categories: structural norms of filial obligation and motivations deriving from positive personal relationships. Structural norms that equate to duty are embedded in a culture and are generally regarded as moral imperatives. They are involuntary in nature. One charged with a duty to provide care, for example, would feel that, '*I have to*'. Personal relationships, conversely, suggest voluntariness, a willingness to provide care out of, for example, affection, gratitude, altruism or feelings of reciprocity based on a mutual sense of what is fair or equal. These models are characterised by feelings of '*I want to*'.

Motivations stemming from structural norms and personal relationships can also intersect. For example, care for an elderly parent may be motivated by a belief in traditional Chinese values but also by love for the parent and gratitude for the sacrifices the parent has made. One of the difficulties in the past has been trying to ferret out the role of each model of motivation when they do overlap (Aboderin 2006).

In the sections below, the conceptual models underlying motivation for the support and care of elderly parents are discussed from the perspectives of both the Asian and the Western literature.

The Asian Perspective on Motivations for Support and Caregiving

Asian Motivations Based on Structural Norms of Filial Obligation ['I have to']

Within Asian cultures indoctrinated in Confucianism, structural norms of filial obligation are, and for many generations have been, underpinned by the construct of filial piety. China as the birthplace of Confucianism can look back on filial piety as a deeply embedded, society wide core moral ideology enduring for over two millennia. For this reason, even though filial piety might have undergone modification recently, conceptually some norms originating from it can be regarded as relatively stable in terms of the commitment of children to their parents. In the context of the Asian caregiving literature filial piety has invariably been the departure point for any discussion.

Filial Piety as Structural Support and Care Motivation Across Asia Historical events and cultural practices unique to their geographic locations are always going to imprint local customs and traditions on ideologies. Likewise, the pace of change in any society is bound to vary according to its circumstances. Where filial piety is concerned, comparisons between Asian countries highlighting the similarities and differences in their beliefs and practices have inevitably been made, even though the core idea has been essentially the same.

Comparing Korea, Japan and mainland China, for example, Sung (2000) found Confucian ethics, culture and tradition to be strong influences on filial support and care motivations everywhere. Responsibility, respect, sacrifice, harmony and the interdependence of family members were shared values. Differences were not found between cultures but within cultures where Sung noted inconsistencies in attitudes and behaviour. He observed that filial piety was becoming less structural and more relational, that parent-child relationships were moving from authoritarian to egalitarian based on 'reciprocal patterns of mutual respect between generations' and that obedience, the core value of filial behaviour, might be giving way to courtesy, companionship and compatibility (Sung 2001: 22).

In a comparative study of mainland China and Taiwan, Lin and Yi (2011) reported strong structural norms of filial obligation in both countries and the strength of filial norms to be positively associated with the amount of financial support provided by adult children to their parents. However, in Taiwan, higher income adult children, particularly daughters, were also more likely to provide emotional support and Taiwanese with strong filial norms were more likely to meet the health care demands of their parents. In contrast, mainland daughters were more likely to provide help with domestic chores to demonstrate filial behaviour.

Research performed in mainland China has affirmed the strength of filial piety as a central moral ideology. For example, in a study of caregivers and care recipients, W.L. Li, Long, Essex, Sui and Gao (2012), reported that both groups expected adult children to be responsible for the care of elderly parents and viewed filial piety as the best standard of care. However, other evidence from China has suggested that the influence of contemporary norms has been growing. From their three-city survey of 869 men and 932 women, Xie and Zhu (2009) concluded that the traditional family model no longer exists in urban China. In their sample daughters, particularly those who resided with their natal families, made more financial contributions to their parents than sons. Several factors were cited for this, including the obsolescence of arranged marriages, greater age at first marriage, lowered fertility, new housing arrangements, the ubiquitous education and employment of women and pensions. Additionally, the authors claimed that the financial contributions from all adult children were largely symbolic and in fact, a substantial number of urban Chinese parents gave money to their adult children rather than the reverse.

Lei (2013) also found downward financial transfers from urban Chinese parents. However, she asserted these contributions were made in exchange for instrumental and emotional support. In a survey of 10,000 households probing financial, instrumental and emotional support in rural and urban China, Lei examined the filial practices of both daughters and sons. In rural areas, she found that sons provided more financial support; however, there were no differences in the provision of emotional or instrumental support between daughters and sons. In urban areas, she found the financial contributions of sons and daughters to be similar, however, daughters provided more emotional and instrumental support than sons. Lei suggested her findings were an indication that the rural areas remained more traditional and the urban areas were more affected by modernisation.

The extent to which modernisation has undermined the traditional Chinese family, if at all, has been unclear. In a survey testing modernisation's effect on filial piety in six Chinese cities, C.K. Cheung and Kwan (2009) showed an association between higher levels of modernisation and lowered filial piety, particularly among adult children who moved away from their families to work and those with less education. However, although the more educated in their sample appeared to have been less influenced by modernisation and had more favourable attitudes toward filial piety than their uneducated counterparts, this did not raise the level of the monetary contributions they made to their parents, which was more dependent on available resources. Furthermore, the authors found age and gender differences: older adult children engaged in less filial behaviour than younger ones and daughters were more filial than sons. The age differences were explained by lack of opportunity because the older respondents were less likely to be living with their parents. Gender was explained based on socialisation into traditional roles. J.H. Zhan and Montgomery (2003), had previously advanced the gender role theory in the context of caregiving by asserting that women experienced intense social pressure to comply with traditional norms in a still patrifocal society.

Further indication of transitioning Asian filial norms was seen in Hsu, Lew-Ting, and Wu's (2014) Taiwanese study of age, period and cohort effects on parental support attitudes. Hsu et al., pointed to the decline of cohabitation as evidence of weakening filial obligation over time and a change in what was considered filial behaviour. They observed that although financial support was still expected, adult sons (and their wives) were no longer obliged to reside with his parents, or even to live within proximity of them, to demonstrate filial piety. Like C.K. Cheung and Kwan (2009), Hsu et al. also found an age effect, but for a different reason. In their study, respondents over 40 years of age were less likely to favour intergenerational households than those under 40. The authors suggested that the older respondents were more realistic about the burdens associated with caregiving.

As opposed to Taiwan, traditional filial norms have remained strong in Japan where neither sons (especially the eldest) nor their wives appear to have been relieved of caregiving responsibilities for his ageing parents. In a comparative study of Tokyo and Okinawa, K.S. Lee (2014) claimed that Japanese gender ideologies and expectations have continued to define women as innate nurturers and wives as the primary providers of care. Nevertheless, women were also reported to be experiencing conflict between traditional filial obligation to their in-laws and their own desires. This was expected to cause resentment, particularly when their natal families were left without care.

Unlike Japan, in Hong Kong and Singapore, the traditional bonds of mutual dependency no longer appear to be fundamentally, absolute. Like

Sung's (2000, 2001) three-country study, Ng et al. (2002) found that the relationship between Hong Kong parents and their children was becoming more reciprocal and less authoritarian. Likewise, Mehta and Ko (2004) observed that communication between generations in Singapore has become more egalitarian.

Other research conducted in Hong Kong has endorsed the reinterpretation of *xiao*. W.K.-M. Lee and Kwok (2005a) noted that filial obligation still acted as a motivation for parental support, but not in the strict Confucian sense. In their view, adult children no longer prioritised their parents over everything else or subscribed to absolute respect and obedience. It has also been suggested that *xiao* has been reduced to an economic model where filial obligation has become more closely aligned with financial, rather than emotional or instrumental support (Lee and Kwok 2005a; Ng et al. 2002). Chow (2006) reported that young people today take a 'practical approach' to filial piety. A great majority of those he surveyed wanted to make their elderly parents happy and to bring them honour. They were willing to provide money; however, most were unwilling to accept advice from their parents on such matters as careers and marriage and some were unwilling to receive any advice at all. Similarly, W.K.-M. Lee and Kwok (2005a) found that respondents were willing to provide instrumental support to ageing parents but less willing to become emotionally involved.

One particularly salient point Lam (2006) made was that elders have been expected to take care of themselves if they could and that caregiving has tended to cease upon recovery from illness or disability. This is congruent with the findings of W.K.-M. Lee and Kwok (2005a) who argued that elders who were financially and emotionally independent of their offspring had better relationships with them.

The pragmatism of Hong Kong residents has also been observed in Singapore, however with a different outcome. P. Teo, Mehta, Thang and Chan (2006: 90–91) explained that Singaporeans are socialised from birth into filial attitudes and behaviour. These values are not only transmitted by parents, but also (as discussed later) through social engineering, so that filial norms become deeply internalised. The authors asserted that adult daughters become 'convinced' that parental care is in their hands and that they have 'no choice' but to do it, thereby fulfilling gender expectations in a patriarchal society.

Yet the roots of filial piety might not run as deep as some have suggested. In a study of Singapore youth, E. Thomas (1990) found that identification of the concept was high among three age groups ranging from 12 to 17, but comprehension of what it meant fell to 51% for 15 year olds and 28% for 12 year olds. Moreover, when these groups were asked to make objective judgments regarding filial behaviour, none achieved scores above 56%.

More recently, Huat (2009) deduced that if filial piety was operationalised through marriage and childbirth, Singapore's dismal performance in these areas certainly did not suggest that the promotion of Confucian values was succeeding at all levels. In a broader context, Yin (2003) observed that although filial piety was an important value to Singapore Chinese, it must be viewed through the lens of a variegated and fluctuating society, which was still perceived as the most Western of all Asian countries.

Although consensus in Asia has been lacking on what filial piety has become, O.M.H. Wong and Chau (2006: 605) suggested there are some inviolable precepts that have endured. These are 'caring', 'not being rebellious', 'showing love', 'respect and support', 'displaying courtesy', 'continuing the family line', and 'concealing parents' blunders'. If this analysis is taken at face value, what is noticeable is the seemingly gratuitous rather than obligatory nature of the commitment itself in terms of its core beliefs. This will be discussed below.

Whatever the character of filial piety, one can see in the interactionist tradition how it has been personally interpreted and selectively adapted to meet the circumstances under which it has been applied (Lee and Kwok 2005a, b; Wong and Chau 2006). Consistent with the transitioning nature of modern Asian societies, attempts to define or reinterpret it in a modern context will therefore no doubt, continue to evolve according to the environments in which it survives (Teo et al. 2003).

It is not the intention of this book to resolve the many discrepant views of filial piety or even to identify them in their entirety. The objective is simply to explain what traditional filial piety once was and to advance the notion that its hierarchical and authoritarian nature may be experiencing renegotiation. Regardless of its multiple manifestations, filial piety is still integral to the caregiving discourse in the Asian context. It is viewed as a motivation, a historical standard against which to measure one's attitude and performance and a guidebook for discharging care (Wong and Chau 2006). It will be later shown how this relates to the current caregiving paradigm under discussion.

The Cultural Model Approach Holroyd (2001: 1127) like others, acknowledged that norms of filial obligation rarely act alone to induce caregiving. Nonetheless, she articulated how duty and caregiving could be conjoined in the minds of Chinese daughters. She called it the 'cultural model approach'. Within this theoretical framework, Holroyd asserted that women internalised 'what is considered "right"' and 'what ought to be done'. In her view, Confucian norms and government policy were the 'cultural models' driving these attitudes in the Chinese context.

According to Holroyd, the cultural model approach is grounded in the dyadic concept of personhood and self. She defined personhood as having a rightful place in the world. In the Confucian ideology, a 'right and proper person' belongs to an ordered hierarchy from family to state. For a filial Chinese daughter, being a right and proper person has historically meant subscribing to parentally transmitted generational and gender roles with their accompanying obligations and behavioural mandates. Caregiving, for example, has been part of the female domain.

In the Confucian sense, 'self' is subjugated to the obligations of personhood. Holroyd explained that this is internalised through the 'accumulated history' of knowing one's place in the hierarchy together with the responsibilities incumbent upon that status. These are then reinforced by social messages from the state, family and community, reminding women of gender stereotypes and expectations, further strengthened by guilt (Holroyd 2001).

In this way, Holroyd (2001: 1133) insisted, daughters convince themselves that caregiving is their duty, which no one will do if they do not and if they fail they will not only incur criticism from others but also defy their own sense of personhood. Therefore, she claimed, the obligation to care becomes a personal self-understanding, which it could be argued, might be central to all motivations for caregiving by Chinese daughters, whether based on structural norms, personal relationships, or a combination of both.

Asian Support and Caregiving Motivations Deriving from Personal Relationships ['I want to']

Lieber et al. (2004) observed that Confucian societies have always embraced altruistic ideals such as compassion, love, charity, magnanimity, benevolence and goodness. Moreover, they noted that filial piety has always been entwined with core Asian values such as harmony, personal relationships and Face,[1] what they called the 'social and moral' aspects of filial behaviour. The continuity of what might be called the emotional and altruistic aspects of Confucian values has helped to explain why family bonds and values have remained strong. Affection, for example, has been posited to be one principle of traditional filial piety that has carried over into contemporary norms (Wong and Chau 2006).

Like affection, reciprocity in the traditional Chinese context has been rooted in filial piety: parents are obligated to provide a reasonable upbringing for their children who in turn must take care of their parents in old age. In the past, this model might have taken the form of inheritance and power earned by adult sons through *xiao* (Lee and Kwok 2005a). However, Croll (1995: 482–483) suggested that the word '*yang-dao*', meaning support, service and caring, represents a new paradigm based more on 'need, voluntarism and mutual appreciation, gratitude and affection', rather than on piety or obedience. Ng et al. (2002: 141) called this new construct a 'network of responsibilities and obligations'. The rationale for this new interpretation, they contended, was role ambiguity resulting from the financial independence and greater knowledge of young adults, depriving elders of the means of their traditional authority.

Because this new model endorses mutuality and equitable exchange (or reciprocity) instead of traditional filial piety and irredeemable obligation, it may extend the contributions of parents well into their children's adulthood. There has been some agreement among Asian scholars that old age support must now be earned (Chou et al. 2004). Some have argued that the more parents bring to the contemporary exchange, the greater likelihood of strengthening the adult child's sense of filial responsibility (Lee and Kwok 2005b; Ng et al. 2002). Possibly to incentivise children to provide care when needed, younger healthy parents have offered baby-sitting, domestic labour and money to their adult children (Chou et al. 2004). In return, children have provided financial assistance to parents or employed domestic helpers to become companions or aides for them. Verbrugge and Chan (2008) found that the more financial support Singaporean elders received from their children, the more services they offered in return. The employment of a helper, however, was perceived as being potentially problematic if she deprived ageing parents of the opportunity to build up credits in the exchange role.

The Convoy Model Borrowing from the Western literature, K.-L. Chou (2009: 228) introduced the 'convoy of social support', or 'convoy model' as a reciprocal arrangement among Chinese family members. Parents build up a 'support bank' of money and time when their children are young. For example, they might pay for their children's education and help with their homework. This could be viewed as a loan to be repaid later, with the amount of repayment in proportion to the amount given. Chou examined the convoy model in relation to the number of children in a family and claimed there was a ceiling effect on upward transfers. He interpreted this to mean that smaller family size due to lower fertility might not have as much financial impact as some have predicted. He also found Chinese filial norms to be strong.

Social Exchange As a motivation for caregiving, social exchange in the Western literature has been characterised as a reciprocal arrangement based on the costs and benefits each party has received from the other. Hong and Liu (2000) suggested that this characterisation is inadequate in the Asian context because culture should be factored into the exchange. Specifically, they asserted that one must consider the communal and interdependent nature of Asian families in addition to filial piety, which together shape the expectations and perceptions of caregivers. In this manner, the authors argued, the needs of the care recipients outweigh the importance of maximising rewards and minimising costs. Caregivers they urged, might engage in filial behaviour even when it is not needed, simply as a gesture of filiality without any expectation of reward.

Asian Support and Caregiving Motivation Derived from Combined Structural and Relational Norms ['I have to and I want to']

In reviewing the Chinese caregiving literature, it is difficult to find contemporary situations in which obligation or relationships alone motivate adult children to support or care for their ageing parents. For example, in O.M.H. Wong's (2000) study of adult children caregivers, both daughters and daughters-in-law alternatively cited affection, structural obligation, unwillingness of others to care, family structure and position, availability of time, higher income and women's work as reasons for caregiving.

Holroyd's (2003) study of Beijing and Hong Kong caregivers, similarly demonstrated how both structural and relational norms were driving support and care motivations and how culture was implicated. Holroyd claimed the motivations of her Beijing caregivers were more strongly linked with Confucian ideals such as gratitude for one's birth and the sacrifices of one's parents, a structural perspective, whereas gratitude emanating from her Hong Kong caregivers arose more from self-interest such as the investment of parents in their education, a relational perspective. In either case, Holroyd noted the presence of a generational shift in values, from a model based strictly on duty and control to one that reflected more affection, gratitude and reciprocity. Likewise, Ng et al. (2002) posited that caregiving motivated by duty might now simply be an amalgam of social norms and intergenerational expectations. Normative obligation in the traditional sense, they maintained, has been eroded and is currently based more on reciprocity than obligation.

Conceptualising a more complex multivariate model of reasons for parent care, W.K.-M. Lee and Kwok (2005a, b) described the contemporary motivation for caregiving in the Asian setting as a combination of traditional and modified filial piety and social exchange. These were then moderated by the quality of the parent-child relationship and structural impediments such as economic independence of the young, education, migration and the erosion of parental power. Lee and Kwok argued that reciprocity was stronger than duty and support was also dependent on love, gratitude and sympathy. Further, they observed that the support adult children were willing to provide to their parents was ultimately based on personal choice.

The combination of structural and relational norms motivating adult children to provide support and care for their parents has become a distinguishing feature in the Asian caregiving literature. If filial obligation has been the starting point, relationships have been driving caregiving forward.

Asian Daughters and Daughters-in-Law In their study of urban mainland China, J.H. Zhan and Montgomery (2003) observed that daughters were providing nearly as much instrumental support for their own parents as daughters-in-law and were additionally contributing financial support almost equal to sons. Further, in their sample, more than 40% of the older parent respondents were living with daughters, rather than sons. Although some of this might have been attributed to low fertility and migration, the fact that it was happening at all was indicative of a normative shift.

Separate research in China and Japan has offered some insight into why more daughters and fewer daughters-in-law might be providing parental care. In a study of informal Chinese caregivers O.M.H. Wong (2000) reported that the daughters-in-law in her sample performed caregiving for their husband's parents as a way of helping their husbands, not out of affection, gratitude or even duty toward their in-laws. Because they lacked this filial connection, most daughters-in-law were unwilling to provide more than financial or instrumental support for in-laws. In contrast, Wong found, daughters to be motivated by both filial obligation and reciprocity for their own parents. Interestingly, she also suggested that daughters-in-laws' lack of feeling for their husband's parents could actually result in less caregiver burden and stress than that experienced by daughters who genuinely care about their parents.

In a Japanese study, Long, Campbell and Nishimura (2014) found that among their respondents, the daughters-in-law said they had no choice of whether to provide care for their in-laws. They viewed this as a moral obligation and normative extension of their domestic role, but complained that family members took them for granted. Long et al. (2014: 3) cited a popular Japanese saying originating in the twentieth century: 'Never marry an eldest son'. This maxim was said to be derived from the comments of daughters-in-law pertaining to the history of unhappy relations with their husband's family. The grievances recounted by Long et al., included lack of appreciation, being treated as an outsider as a new bride, interference from the husband's siblings and criticism from the husband's mother, all of which could result in longstanding feelings of resentment, bitterness and anger. Therefore, the authors asserted, more educated and self-sufficient Japanese women with greater bargaining power might refuse to live with in-laws or negotiate conditions under which they were willing to provide elder care for them.

A different situation was said to exist with Japanese daughters, who might volunteer to become caregivers of their elderly parents. Like O.M.H. Wong (2000), Long et al. (2014), found that daughters' filial obligation most likely originated in feelings of affection, reciprocity and gratitude, including the desire to pay back parents for their previous kindness and sacrifice. Daughters-in-law received no such benefits from their in-laws; their husbands did. Thus, Long et al. suggested that gratitude and reciprocity for in-laws were unlikely to occur.

The daughters in the study of Long et al. (2014: 15) expressed no need to be appreciated, but instead said caring for their mothers, was a 'natural thing'. Daughters-in-law expressed guilt over being unable to take care of their own mothers. Both daughters and daughters-in-law related the desire to fulfil social expectations by being a 'good' role model. It was, however, the personal history each caregiver had with her care recipients that determined how she actually felt about the support and care she was asked to provide. According to K.S. Lee (2014), personal history is why mothers and daughters prefer the company of one another as opposed to those who are unrelated to them by blood.

How Asian Governments Manipulate the Conceptual Discourse Underlying Caregiving Motivations to Preserve Norms of Filial Obligation

Much has been written about how structural impediments such as geographic distance, employment and contemporary norms influenced by modern society, have modified the nature of traditional filial obligation.

Perhaps to counterbalance some of the effects these changes have had on Asian families, the governments of many Asian countries have implemented legislation, policies and other procedures intended to preserve traditional filial obligation associated with Confucian cultural norms.

How Government Policies and Legislation Influence Support and Caregiving Motivations in Asia

Over countless generations, filial piety has been woven into the fabric of East Asian society, underpinning family support systems. Since the end of the Second World War, however, traditional norms have been juxtaposed with new policies brought about by, in some cases, changes to the nature of governance, (e.g., China, Japan) and in all cases, situational developments (e.g., the decline of intergenerational housing) resulting from urbanisation, industrialisation and modernisation (Izuhara 2010). In attempting to preserve norms of filial obligation, some governments of traditionally Confucian countries have taken a two or three prong approach: Articulating public policy, enacting legislation and in some cases engaging in social engineering.

Hong Kong, for example, has relied on the moral imperatives underlying filial piety without legislating it (Ghy and Woo 2009; Lee 2014; Lei 2013; Sung 2000). Its 'family first' policy has officially endorsed the family as the primary support of elderly parents (Chan 2011; Holroyd 2001), however, ironically, while advocating for a 'caring and harmonious society' predicated on happy and harmonious families (Chan et al. 2011; Nip 2010: 72) the government has done little to advance these objectives in actual practice.

Unlike Hong Kong, filial piety has been legislated in other Asian countries, both directly and implicitly. For example, the laws of the Republic of Korea do not expressly require adult children to support their parents. However, under the Basic Livelihood Security Act (1999) elders and others living below the minimum cost of living only become eligible when the 'person liable for supporting' them (defined as a 'lineal relation') has no ability to do so (Office of the High Commissioner on Human Rights 2009). Taiwan has similar provisions under its 'Senior Citizens Welfare Act' (Republic of China, Taiwan 2012).

In contrast, Japan's filial obligation laws are explicit. Prior to the Second World War, adult children were required under the 1898 Meiji Civil Code to support their parents even before their nuclear families (Rickles-Jordan 2007). Although this was abolished by Japan's 1947 Constitution, the support of elderly parents has continued under the new Constitution and Civil Code, Article 877 imposing reciprocal support obligations on parents and children. Additionally, Japan's 'Law for the Welfare of Elderly Persons' mandates that adult children who live with their parents, or who lived with their parents prior to institutionalising them, be financially responsible for them (Moskowitz 2002).

The government of Singapore has also legislated filial obligation, through its Maintenance of Parents Act of 1995. Under the Act's provisions all adult children regardless of gender are required to provide financial support to their parents if need can be demonstrated (Singapore Attorney General's Chambers, Maintenance of Parents Act 1996). As can be seen in the statement of Tarmugi Abdullah, Acting Minister for Community Development before the Act was passed, love and moral obligation have been combined in the rationale underpinning the law:

> But it is wrong to expect Government to assume the responsibility of children to at least maintain their parents when they are able to do it, out of love, out of moral duty. Government will, in fact, only exacerbate the problem of abandoned parents should it relieve children of this responsibility. (Parliament of Singapore 1994: 270, Cited in Rozario and Hong 2011: 614)

Like Japan, Article 49 of China's constitution imposes reciprocal obligations on children and their parents (Chou 2011). Like Singapore, moral obligation is featured in China's 'Law of the People's Republic of China on Protection of the Rights and Interests of the Elderly' (1996). Chapter II of the law, entitled 'Maintenance and support by families', compels grown children to comfort and look after their parents, cater to their special needs, pay their medical expenses and arrange for proper housing. Conversely, it prohibits children from seizing the personal and real property of their parents without express permissions.

On 1 July 2013, a new 'Elderly Rights Law' expanded filial obligation in China to include the 'spiritual needs' of one's parents and a duty to visit them, although it failed to specify the frequency of these visitations or take into consideration the distances between family members in a large country. As a result, the new law has been criticised, even though it is still enforceable through fines and detention (Hatton 2013).

In support of the policies and laws promoting filial piety and family caregiving, the governments of many Asian countries have been slow to develop social welfare programmes that would lessen the burden on families. In Hong Kong, for example, most programmes designed to provide relief for families have not emanated from the government but from a loose network of NGOs, community care and support services, churches and charities. The government's reluctance to supersede these agencies as the direct primary provider of services has been evidenced by the subsidies it has provided to many of them (Chan 2011; Nip 2010).

Japan, Taiwan and Korea now provide Long-Term Care (LTC) Insurance and/or other programmes for elderly people (Fu 2008; Kim and Han 2013; Long et al. 2014; Yoon et al. 2000). Singapore and China (including Hong Kong) have taken steps to provide nominal pensions and health care to elders. However, it is expected that considerable time will pass before the family is relieved of its responsibility as the primary caregiver of ageing parents and the government is no longer viewed as the 'last resort' for eldercare in Asia.

Filial Piety by Contract Reforms have taken place in mainland China since 1949, initiating pensions, creating then disbanding collectives, changing marriage and inheritance laws, limiting family size and allowing migration. Together with the decline of intergenerational households, these are purported to have gradually deprived many Chinese elders of their traditionally high family status and leverage and to have jeopardised the old age security previously guaranteed by their children and living arrangements (Chou 2011; Hashimoto and Ikels 2005). Perhaps in response to this, in the 1980s, the Family Support Agreement (FSA) was conceived of and implemented in the Chinese countryside. Spreading throughout the rural areas, by 2005, 13 million Chinese villagers were purported to have entered into such agreements and some FSAs had even begun to emerge in the cities (Chou 2011).

The FSA is a contractual relationship between adult children and their parents in which the children's obligations are defined and agreed to. The terms of these agreements may range from financial and material support alone to include such things as emotional support, caregiving, farm labour, health care, long term care and funeral expenses (Chou 2011). FSAs are voluntary. However, local governments, the central government, the Chinese constitution and elder laws have all encouraged and supported them. Local governments have offered guidelines on how the agreements should be structured, and the central government has promoted them through its 'resolution of the state council on strengthening senior services'. In furtherance of this, the government has used a 'carrot and stick approach', publicly praising those who have been filial and rebuking those who have not. In addition, parents have been authorised to sue children who have breached these agreements (Chou 2011: 7).

Social Engineering Driving Family Support and Care Motivation in Asia The Chinese government did not create the FSA. However, its support for it is one example of how filial piety can be socially engineered. Other Asian countries have similarly strived to incentivise families to support their ageing members. For example, in Korea, corporations have awarded filial piety prizes. Korea and Japan have implemented Respect for the Elderly Day and Elderly Week (Sung 2000). Taiwan has offered subsidies to families who care for their parents (Republic of China, Taiwan 2012). Japan has provided tax deductions and has additionally supported the housing industry in creating elder friendly homes; offered loans to caregivers who are willing to remodel their homes to accommodate elderly parents; and given tax benefits to day-care centres and businesses promoting health care. In Japan, it has been possible to rent a family to provide care if one has no immediate family of one's own to do it. In addition, Japan has created a new pension plan for women, enabling them to leave the workforce to care for children or elderly parents (Moskowitz 2002).

These efforts are notable. However, a more sophisticated approach to social engineering has been conceived by the government of Singapore, who has orchestrated its elder care policies to advance its other policy objectives. Although Singapore has often been described as a confluence of East and West there is substantial evidence to suggest that filial piety and Confucian values have been used as 'an important ideological tool' and an 'asset to promote economic development and modernisation' (Kuah 1990: 375).

From the time Singapore achieved nationhood in 1965, its government has systematically endeavoured to forge a national identity with uniquely 'Singaporean' values centred on the family. Since the 1980s it has promoted Confucian ethics to offset influences from the West, justify its social welfare policies and reinforce its authority. Under the guise of civic responsibility and moral education in a multi-ethnic population Confucian values, for example, have been integrated into the school curriculum. Additionally, the 'public awareness programme on ageing' and the 'parent education programme' have been implemented in the school system as a means of bolstering filial piety among the young (Kuah 1990; Rozario and Rosetti 2012).

On another level, the Housing Development Board has developed a variety of schemes to incentivise adult children to live with or near their parents (Housing Development Board 2016). Many such schemes have offered grants, loans, reduced down-payments, 'wait list' priority and larger flats (Teo et al. 2003), directed at strengthening the family and ensuring that it remains the primary caregiver of elderly parents.

In Singapore, the family has been idealised by promoting familism and family values as exemplified by the following quote from the Ministry of Community Development and Sports (MCYS):

> The family is an important institution. It brings fulfilment to our lives and is our anchor in this fast-paced, ever-changing environment. Families serve as an important pillar of support for the nation. At the individual level, families are the primary source of emotional, social and financial support. At the national level, they contribute to social stability and national cohesiveness as they help develop socially responsible individuals and deepen the bond Singaporeans have with our country. (Ministry of Community Development and Sports 2003, cited in Teo 2010: 339)

In campaigns, policies and the speeches of its leadership, the Singapore government has promoted the model family as being a young, heterosexual, educated, employed married couple with children living as a nuclear unit in a Housing Development Board (HDB) flat. Elderly Singaporeans have been portrayed as 'pioneers' of the country and adult children have been expected to bring them into their homes and care for them when they become frail. Until then, ageing parents have been encouraged to help their children with childcare (Teo 2010).

Policies have been established to influence and shape norms, particularly those concerning marriage, child bearing and elder care decisions. For example, the tax code provides a S$9000 per dependent exemption for adult children who have supported and lived with their parents, in-laws, grandparents or grandparents-in-law during the taxable year, or a S$4500 per dependent exemption if support has been provided but the parties live apart[2] (Inland Revenue Authority of Singapore 2017; Rozario and Rosetti 2012). Under the Central Provident Fund (CPF) Housing Grant Scheme, adult children who purchase flats with their parents, live with their parents or within two kilometres of their parents are eligible to receive up to S$20,000 in grant money toward the purchase (Housing and Development Board 2017). The government has additionally regulated the salaries of foreign domestic helpers (FDHs) to keep them low (Teo 2010) and has provided concessions for caregivers. If an FDH has been employed to care for an elderly parent, under the foreign domestic worker levy concession, aged person scheme, the foreign maid levy is reduced by S$60 month (Ministry of Manpower 2017; Rozario and Rosetti 2012).

By shifting the financial burden for elderly parents from the state to the family, many benefits have accrued to the government. As the last resort for its elderly citizens, the state has not dissipated its wealth through social security programmes. When it has intervened, it has appeared to be altruistic and philanthropic. It has preserved its status as a non-welfare state and taxes have been kept low thereby maintaining Singapore's economic competitiveness (Rozario and Rosetti 2012).

In following this course, the government has also achieved its other objective of promoting a Singaporean identity. There has been a 'Singapore way' of doing things that has followed an orderly pattern aimed at preserving the family. This Confucian approach to governance has been portrayed as 'unique and superior' to liberal democracy in which the West has been characterised as materialistic and individualistic (Rozario and Hong 2011; Tan 2003: 763). Pride has been taken in Singapore's government-endorsed practice of filial piety with the whole of Singaporean values being viewed as protecting tradition despite modernisation (Teo 2010: 343).

Work-Life-Balance As part of its social engineering agenda, for the past several years, Singapore has actively promoted *Work-Life-Balance*. In 2007, its Ministry of Community Development, Youth and Sports (MCYS) issued a press release proclaiming the success of its inaugural work-life study which headlined: 'Confirms positive benefits of work-life harmony to individuals and businesses'. The lead paragraph advised:

> Singaporeans who achieve work-life harmony are more likely to enjoy their work, have better family relationships and enjoy a better quality of life, according to an inaugural National work-life Harmony Study jointly commissioned by the Ministry of Community Development, Youth and Sports (MCYS) and the National Family Council (NFC)... Another key finding of the study was the positive correlation between an employee's work-life harmony and employee engagement and retention, as well as an organisation's productivity and its bottom line. (Ministry of Community Development, Youth and Sports, Singapore 2007)

The release went on to say that MCYS, together with the Ministry of Manpower (MOM), would work with employers to initiate work-life programmes and to 'promote an environment that values flexibility and performance' over time spent in the office (Ministry of Community Development, Youth and Sports, Singapore 2007). It concluded with a list of 'work-life initiatives' including S$10 million in funding to support them, an award scheme for compliant employers, seminars, conferences and media exposure for exemplary enterprises. A four-part documentary aired on television to disseminate the information.

MOM currently maintains a website devoted to work-life harmony, with strategies for achieving it (Ministry of Manpower 2016); and in fact, the programme has had some success. In 2013, the Singapore Business Review announced that Singapore's *Work-Life-Balance* was the third best in Asia (Singapore Business Review, 22 June 2013). Conversely, Hong Kong's *Work-Life-Balance* has been called the worst in Asia (Yu 2015). The government has sponsored no work-life programmes, nor promoted the concept in any official way. The only effort to advance *Work-Life Balance* since 2008 appears to have come from Community Business, a membership based NGO that has sponsored a 'Work-Life-Balance Week' in addition to conducting case studies and creating a guidebook (Hong Kong Community Business Online n.d.).

Apart from this grassroots effort, Hong Kong, unlike Singapore, has recently been described by community leaders as having a 'workaholic culture' that has kept its citizens in a 'perpetual state of stress' (Chan et al. 2011: 669). Citing a report by Chung, Pang and Tong (2010) of over 2.6 million employees with a fixed working week, R.K.H. Chan (2011) observed that 28.4% worked 8–10 hours a day and 5.8% worked more than 10 hours a day. In an even more recent analysis, K.L. Chou and Cheung (2013) reported 25.8% of Hong Kong employees worked more than 50 hours a week, 63% worked unpaid overtime, 52% worked late hours and 37% reported having no time to spend with family. Further, in an investigation of 50 married, female professionals, Lo (2003) found that even though they were working long hours their husbands were still unwilling to share household responsibilities. Nor have their employers implemented family-friendly policies. The result has been widespread exhaustion and burn out.

Hong Kong recently instituted some remedial measures to rectify work-life conflict for government employees and in 2006 it passed an employment ordinance addressing issues such as maternity leave, respite, holidays and a five-day working week (Chou and Cheung 2013). Nonetheless, even with these improvements, S.S.C. Chan et al. (2011: 671) subsequently described the Special Administrative Region (SAR) as 'neither family-oriented nor friendly as a whole'. In fact, according to them, 'the current working policy hinders the promotion of a family-friendly working environment'. K.L. Chou and Cheung (2013) claimed the reason for this was resistance from the owners of small and medium size companies that constitute 98% of Hong Kong's business community.

Work-Life-Balance in mainland China has been similar to Hong Kong. That is to say, virtually non-existent. However, the mainland's approach to the subject is philosophically distinct from both Hong Kong and Singapore. In the mainland, work-life conflicts, including long hours, interruptions to time off, excessive travel and other demanding conditions have tended to be accepted as a natural part of life, or at least as part of China's ongoing push toward modernisation and a higher standard of living for its citizens (Xiao and Cooke 2012). Additionally, the mainland has remained for the most part a collectivist society in which the well-being of the family, not the individual is the goal. Work has been a means to that end, and whatever dimensions it has taken or sacrifices it has required, they are likely to have been viewed as fulfilling one's duty for the benefit of the family unit (Zhang et al. 2013). As part of this, rigid gender expectations have continued to exist. Even when both husband and wife are working, and even if the wife makes more money, men are still considered to be the 'breadwinners'. Thus, even though women constitute over 38% of China's workforce (Xiao and Cooke 2012), supporting their husbands and extended family comprises their primary role, and they are expected to fulfil it for the happiness of all (Choi 2008; Qian and Qian 2015; Zhang et al. 2013). As an extension of this construct, employers and the government are unlikely to be sympathetic to women's multiple roles or view their work-life conflict as being a corporate responsibility (Foster and Ren 2015).

The extent to which the divergent approaches to family support and caregiving have been reflected in intergenerational exchanges and care are discussed in later chapters.

Contribution of the Western Literature to Understanding Asian Caregiving Motivations

Although this is a study of Chinese women, considering the Western perspectives on caregiving motivations in addition to the Asian perspectives helps to broaden our understanding beyond filial piety and give definition to transitioning norms that otherwise might evade explanation. Some crossover may also exist between caregiving motivations in Western and Asian countries, particularly those with a history of familism (Jang et al. 2012). However, despite some similarities between the familistic and patriarchal norms of Confucian Asia and, for example, the Mediterranean countries, it does not necessarily mean that they ascribe the same meanings and interpretations to attitudes and behaviour. Shared history, knowledge, cultural norms and values among the citizens of a given country can be strong influences, working at both the individual and societal levels (Brant et al. 2009; Suanet et al. 2012). For this reason, the Western literature is intentionally treated separately, except where it is deemed appropriate to do otherwise.

Western Motivations Based on Structural Norms of Filial Obligation ['I have to']

Subtle differences exist between the Western and Asian perspectives of structural norms of filial obligation. Unlike Asian countries with long histories of Confucianism, Western society is culturally heterogeneous and both individualism and the family structure vary by country and sub-cultures within countries.

Structural norms of filial obligation have been conceptualised in the Western literature as an attitudinal approach to parental caregiving. Attitudes concerning the rights and needs of ageing parents and the appropriate social roles assigned to their adult children have been defined by societal standards and expectations (Cicirelli 1993; Del Corso and Lenz 2013; Stein et al. 1998). Internalisation of what have been called socially responsible behavioural norms, often attributed to the Judeo-Christian heritage in the West, (e.g., honour your father and mother), has been said to occur through early childhood socialisation (Cicirelli 1993). This would likely have been operationalised through the transmission of acceptable or expected values and behaviour or through social learning and role modelling (Hess and Waring 1978). The expected outcome, it has been argued, is an indelible and fully integrated sense of duty owed by children to parents.

Some expressions of how duty is manifested in later life have been seen in the results of Wallhagen and Strawbridge's (1995: 560) study of 100 American adult caregivers. Among the 15 caregivers motivated by duty, the responses included remarks such as: 'Yes, it's a responsibility'; It is 'a duty we owe them'; 'Family obligation...I wouldn't live with myself if I didn't'; and 'It has been too easy in our society to put away our parents and forget them'. For the 28 caregivers citing family values as their motivation for caregiving, their justifications included: 'Our value system from family and faith supports caregiving'; 'Values inculcated in me [of] family obligation'; 'The Bible says so-as far as you are able'; 'I come from an Italian background-close family'; '...the way I was raised-the country (Columbia) that I come from. It is the way of living there'. To these comments, Walker, Pratt, Shin and Jones (1990) added that the duty to provide care might have originated with children being socialised into nurturing roles or the belief that if a child did not take care of his or her parent, no one would.

Expanding on the concept of filial obligation, or what has been called normative solidarity, Silverstein, Parrott and Bengtson (1995) found that normatively prescribed obligation to parents, (conforming to the concept of duty discussed above), has been an important predictor of upward flowing intergenerational support.

Finally, the structural nature of filial obligation has implied that there are consequences for failing to live up to societal expectations. Thus, fear of underperforming the appropriate filial behaviour has been posited to act as a social control implemented through self-judgment and reaction to the opinions of others (Aronson 1990; Hess and Waring 1978).

Western Motivations Deriving from Personal Relationships ['I want to']

The personal relational approach to motivations for caregiving, which has been predominant in Western theorising, has emphasised the importance of negotiated commitments within families with respect to what they are willing and unwilling to do for one another (Finch and Mason 1993; Stein et al. 1998). This approach is multifaceted and has very often involved the combination and overlapping of disparate concepts. In the discussion that follows, the core concepts, as they relate to the motivation to care for elderly parents, are presented together with some of the ways these relational sources of obligation overlap.

Affection Affection among family members has been described as an emotional state based on love, positive feelings, closeness, security and intimacy (Cicirelli 1993; Silverstein and Bengtson 1997), and it has appeared as one of the most robust motivations for caregiving in the Western literature. Children who have stronger affection for parents have been portrayed as being more likely to have increased contacts, provide greater social support and be more committed to them over the life span (Horowitz and Shindelman 1983; Silverstein, et al. 1995). Parrott and Bengtson (1999) found that past affection between parents and children could predict emotional support for both mothers and fathers and financial support to mothers. Likewise, Horowitz and Shindelman found a relationship between the strength of affection and the amount of care provided in addition to the ability to handle the stress and burden of caregiving. Affection has been widely reported to motivate daughters in particular, whereas sons have tended to be motivated by structural norms of filial obligation (Silverstein et al. 1995; Walker et al. 1990).

A few variations of the affection model have developed over the years. The 'friendship model' combines affection with reciprocity and suggests that anything done for parents by adult children should be motivated by their current 'friendship' and given voluntarily (Dixon 1995; Stuifbergen and Van Delden 2011). The 'special goods' model claims that the things each party does for the other occur solely because of the relationship. It is premised on the belief that the relationship between a parent and child is unique and mutually beneficial (Keller 2006; Stuifbergen and Van Delden 2011). The 'attachment' model is reliant on the emotional bond between the child and mother in infancy and adheres to the idea that this creates a desire in the adult child to be with the parent (Cicirelli 1983, 1993).

Gratitude and Reciprocity Norms of reciprocity have also served to motivate filial behaviour. Reciprocity begins with the assumption that adult children owe their parents for the sacrifices the parents have made for them in the past. This relates to a child's 'gift of life' and upbringing: providing a home, food, education and so forth. It encompasses all the burdens parents have endured and the special consideration they have given to their children's needs to nurture them into successful adulthood. In return, when parents become old, frail and dependent, *fairness and equity* require children to repay them by being cognisant of their needs and providing them with support and care (Stuifbergen and Van Delden 2011; Wicclair 1990).

Repayment however is not always a simple matter. Keller (2006) and Wicclair (1990), for example, bifurcated reciprocity into debt and gratitude. Debt, they argued, is akin to a fixed sum to be repaid, whereas gratitude carries with it no duty to repay or criteria for repayment. Berman (1987: 25) posited that parent-child reciprocity is imbalanced from the beginning. Gifts such as the education given to children engender what Berman called an 'irredeemable obligation' that can never be repaid.

The concept of 'lagged reciprocity' offers an elaboration of the classic reciprocity model by incorporating a life course perspective (Silverstein et al. 2002). Borrowing from the field of economics, lagged reciprocity has been separated into two subcategories of exchange that add the element of life course timing: (1) the *return on investment* model and (2) the *insurance policy* model. In return on investment, the idea is that parents' sacrifices and nurturing on behalf of young children are returned as a matter of right when children reach adulthood. In the insurance model, childhood transfers are repaid when parents are most in need. In both, the earlier investment is viewed as earned and is repaid in roughly an equivalent value to what was given. As can be seen, these models have elements of exchange because both are driven by parents' self-interest.

The concept of 'negotiated responsibilities' is another variant of reciprocity (Finch and Mason 1993) in which it is assumed that there are no fixed rules when it comes to negotiated reciprocity among family members, only guidelines. Responsibilities do not exist solely because of the kinship relationship, but rather are created between family members as active participants. Because they are negotiated rather than superimposed, the commitments tend to be stronger and more enduring in addition to being fluid and diverse. Because they are negotiated over the life course and in the context of what has gone before, achieving balance between dependence and independence is a principle objective. Due to the indissoluble nature of the relationship, a moral element is also overlaid onto family negotiations, with one's reputation, or standing within the family and one's self-identity undergoing reconstruction during each negotiation. From this perspective, morality is implicated in all kinship negotiations. It defines the terms of the negotiations and determines the legitimacy of each person's negotiating position. It also determines how the parties are perceived by the outcome. If one's moral identity is at risk it may influence whether one remains in or abandons a negotiated exchange (Finch and Mason 1993).

Altruism and Need Altruism is another source of support and care motivation. It has been defined as 'giving to others with the most need and the least ability to repay' where there is 'no ostensible resource benefit to the provider' (Silverstein et al. 2012: 1250). However, Silverstein et al. (2002) also noted that 'pure altruism' does not exist. They suggested there are two explanations for selfless demonstrations of support for elderly parents: The altruistic caregiver is either *selfish but faced with exclusion* from inheritance (rational choice exchange) or receives a *'warm glow of satisfaction'* from good deeds. Stuifbergen and Val Delden (2011) also noted that responding to parental need is emotional, based on the parents' vulnerability and concern for their well-being.

Western Support and Caregiving Motivation Derived from Combined Structural and Relational Norms ['I have to and I want to']

An affection-obligatory model offers another understanding of caregiving motivations. As discussed, affection is a strong motivator for providing care. However, affection and structural norms of obligation are not mutually exclusive. Walker et al. (1990) reported that one-fifth of the mother-daughter dyads in their study experienced combined discretionary-obligatory motives. Horowitz et al. (1983: 15) found that 51% of their respondents mentioned affection as a reason for caregiving and 58% cited structural norms of obligation. They concluded that 'most often, however, obligation and affection went hand-in-hand'. Finley, Roberts and Banahan (1988) found that female respondents who had strong affection for their mothers were also resolute in their attitudes of filial obligation toward them. Neither higher education, role conflict nor greater income significantly affected these feelings.

Limitations on Caregiving Motivations

Filial Belief Verses Filial Behaviour

Transitioning Chinese norms have raised the question of whether filial attitudes have continued to translate into filial behaviour. However, the answer has been inconclusive. Lam (2006) suggested a chasm might exist between professed allegiance to *xiao* and actual conduct. In a study of sandwich generation caregivers, caught between the needs of children and parents, he asserted that Hong Kong respondents had internalised filial piety. Their failure to act in accordance with their filial beliefs was explained by such determinants as work, family income and the quality of relationships with family care recipients.

Some adult children have expressed filial attitudes but have only been willing to provide financial, not emotional or instrumental support (Chappell and Funk 2012). Some have professed filial beliefs but have subsequently expected ageing parents to take care of themselves, perhaps with help from a spouse or a domestic helper (Lam 2006). Others have perceived attitude as being only one element driving support (Chen et al. 2007). Adding to this discourse, Finch and Mason (1993) contended that attitude might be irrelevant in explaining why individuals provide support for family members. Taking a symbolic interactionist approach, they argued that what was important was how one's actions were interpreted by others and the meanings conveyed, not the belief in one's head.

Structural or Situational Impediments

Structural impediments limit the ability to provide caregiving by making performance practically difficult if not impossible, generating role conflict and affecting the quality of the relationship between grown children and their parents. Factors such as living arrangements, employment, education and the quality of parental relationships influence filial behaviour (Chappell and Funk 2012). These impediments are discussed in Chap. 2 (Chan 1999; Lee and Kwok 2005a; Ng et al. 2002).

Lack of Affection as Negative Motivation

Parents' unsympathetic attitudes, disagreeable behaviour and poor communication skills when their children are young can induce negative consequences once the children are grown. Whitbeck, Simons and Conger (1991) found that adults who perceived rejection from their parents during childhood were less inclined toward closeness and affectual solidarity with them when the latter became elderly. They were less likely to feel concern over their parents' well-being and more likely to experience relationship strain (Whitbeck et al. 1994). According to Parrott and Bengtson (1999) this could affect the parent-child relationship up to 20 years.

Conditionality

Conditionality has been linked with the concept of reciprocity and the idea that one has a duty to repay one's parents for a good and proper upbringing. However, if one's childhood has been characterised by deliberate parental neglect, abuse or the failure of a parent to fulfil expected normative obligations, the reciprocal obligation owed to the offending parent when one has reached adulthood could be excused (Aboderin 2006).

How Emotion Work Moderates Conflict and Tension in Fulfilling Filial Obligation

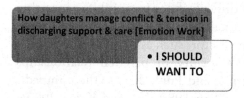

Image of managing conflict and tension (emotion work)

Theoretical ideas about the management of emotions have been associated with the sociology of emotion, which emerged as a distinct field of empirical inquiry in the 1970s. Writing recently about the sociology of emotions, sociologists Jonathan Turner and Jan Stets (2005) opined that it was incomprehensible why it took so long to emerge as a discipline:

> Emotions pervade every aspect of human experience and all social relations … Emotions are the 'glue' binding people together and generating commitments to large-scale social and cultural structures; in fact, emotions are what make social structures and systems of cultural symbols viable. Conversely, emotions are also what can drive people apart and push them to tear down social structures and to challenge cultural traditions. Thus, experience, behaviour, interaction and organisation are connected to the mobilisation and expression of emotions. (Turner and Stets 2005: 1)

Mainstream sociological theories such as symbolic interactionism, dramaturgy and social exchange all have elements of emotion in them. For symbolic interactionists, positive and negative emotions in one's interactions with others serve to confirm or disaffirm one's perception of self and how one should relate to others. Similarly, for dramaturgists who analogise behaviour to theatrical performance, emotions interplay with cultural beliefs and rules of proper behaviour to determine the appropriate ways to portray oneself. For social exchange theorists both costs and rewards are accompanied by emotions and ultimately it is the emotional component that drives choice as well as change (Turner and Stets 2005).

American sociologist, Arlie Hochschild (1983) developed the theory of emotion work, drawing from the aforementioned theories and other fields. According to Hochschild, the core idea of emotion work builds on the space between what we actually feel and what we believe we *should* feel or *try* to feel.

In her book, *The Managed Heart*, Hochschild (1983: 21) wrote that feeling was a sense, the same as hearing or seeing. From the emotional content, we take in and put out we learn how to view the world. Hochschild suggested that in our private lives we have probably always managed our emotions and that doing so is 'fundamental to civilised living'. However, in modern society we are also called upon to manage emotion at work. Thus, she organised emotions into two parts. The first falls under the umbrella of what she called our 'private emotional system'. The other is what she called 'emotional labour'. Both consist of framing rules, feeling rules, display rules, emotion work, rule reminders and interpersonal exchange. The difference is context. Hochschild distinguished between them:

> I use the term *emotional labour* to mean the management of feeling to create a publicly facial and bodily display; emotional labour is sold for a wage and therefore has *exchange value*. I use the synonymous term *emotion work* or *emotion management* to refer to these same acts in a private context where they have *use value*. (Hochschild 1983: 7, fn; *Emphasis added*)

In this book, the private emotional system, or *emotion work*, is explored. Emotion work differs from emotional labour to the extent that cultural norms, as opposed to employers, determine the rules by which emotion is felt and expressed. The recipients of the caregiving effort are likely to be family and friends rather than customers, and the display is private not public. The discussion below is framed in the context of private *emotion work*. First, the key concepts of the theory of emotion work are described.

Emotion Work Defined and Explained

In the following chapters, the discussions of when and how emotion work is undertaken make frequent reference to the core emotion management techniques set forth below.

Framing Rules Hochschild (1979: 566) defined framing rules as 'rules according to which we ascribe definitions and meanings to situations'. It is how we interpret things. Framing rules may be broad, such as cultural norms or practices within cultural norms that have been widely accepted within a society or group. Traditional Chinese values for example, could be framing rules. Framing rules may be specific or even individual, that is, how one person interprets cultural norms in the context of their own experience. Framing rules can also be redefined when the context or circumstances change.

Feeling Rules Hochschild (1979: 566) said that feeling rules are 'guidelines for the assessments of fits and misfits between feeling and situation'. According to her, feeling rules and framing rules are 'back to back and mutually imply each other'. Feeling rules represent what we *should* feel in view of the interpretation framing rules have given to a situation (Hochschild 1983).

What we should feel is often taught to us as children and gradually internalised so that these messages become integrated into our personal values. As a result, what we feel and how we act on those feelings should be synchronised with cultural norms and expectations (Hochschild 1983). Feeling rules also determine the strength of the emotion we should feel in a given situation and the length of time we should feel it; and helps us decide whether the appropriate emotion should be positive or negative (Turner and Stets 2005). As Hochschild (1979) observed, it creates a worry-free zone where our emotions are safe from criticism or guilt.

In Hochschild's (1983: 57) words, we know feeling rules exist when we experience a discrepancy between what we *do* feel and what we believe we should feel. We know we are applying feeling rules when we and others view our emotional behaviour in relation to what is acceptable under the circumstances and how we and others, feel about it.

Feelings can be situated or held over a long duration during which we may want to change them but are unable to. Hochschild (1983: 56, 68–72) specifically examined this in the context of the family. She pointed out that parent-child relationships are often fraught with feelings of love-hate and that framing rules tell us what the appropriate 'mix' of these feelings should be. When we experience the discrepancy between what we feel, or have a right to feel, that causes us to perform emotion work. As Hochschild articulated, feeling rules establish 'the sense of entitlement or obligation that govern emotional exchanges'.

Display Rules Display is the outward expression reflecting inward emotion. Display rules are 'the rights and obligations' that accompany this outward display (Hochschild 1983: 60). If one's inner feeling and outward appearance are in harmony then the display is authentic. If there is a discrepancy between what one *actually* feels and thinks and what one *should* feel and think, the display is considered 'wrong'. Where the discrepancy is between what one *actually* feels or thinks and what one *appears* to feel and think, the display is defined as 'false'.

Emotion Work Hochschild (1979: 561, 562) described emotion work as 'the act of trying to change the degree or quality of an emotion or feeling'. It is how we *try* to bridge the gap between what we *do* feel and what we believe we *should* feel. Hochschild emphasised that emotion work refers to the effort that is expended, the 'act of trying', not the success of the effort.

Emotion work has been divided into two categories, what Hochschild (1979: 561) called 'evocation' and 'suppression'. In the first, effort is applied to induce or 'shape' a feeling that is not initially present. In the second, effort is made to suppress or prevent unwanted feelings. These techniques can be applied in conjunction with or separate from the core approaches to emotion management: surface acting and deep acting.

In surface acting, Hochschild (1983: 37) reported, it is the 'body, not the soul that is the tool of the trade'. It is the part of emotion work that attempts to project the proper facial and bodily display to match expectations of what others think they should be. As she explained, we 'pretend to feel what we do not'. Surface acting does not attempt to change feeling: 'In surface acting we deceive others about what we really feel, but we do not deceive ourselves' (Hochschild 1983: 33).

In contrast, deep acting attempts to alter what we feel. Hochschild drew from the Stanislavski Method in which the actor attempts to develop genuine feelings that he or she really believes. This can be done in two ways, through exhortation or trained imagination.

Through exhortation we order our feelings to change by directly manipulating them to induce or prevent feeling. We give ourselves commands like 'stop feeling sad' or 'I must feel happy'. However, we do not attempt to access our deep inner resources or emotional memory in doing so. According to Hochschild, it is only when we draw on our imaginations that we are really doing method acting.

As Hochschild (1983) wrote in the *Managed Heart*, Stanislavski told his actors not to try to create a feeling, but to 'become' the character. To do this, the actor must imagine or relive events or settings from his or her own past and experience the feelings that accompanied them. If done successfully, the actor feels 'as if' the image of the past is occurring in real time and the feelings authentically reproduce themselves in the present.

So too, in deep acting the private individual attempts to recreate a state of mind by invoking or suppressing emotions and images from the past. For example, an adult child might remember the love he or she felt when a parent was attentive or performed a kindly gesture. In so doing feelings of gratitude, pity or other emotions could be replicated in the present to support the desired manifestation of the emotion in a heartfelt way. Conversely, one might try to suppress beatings from parents or parents' negative personality traits to conjure up feelings of warmth for them.

Rule Reminders Rule reminders reinforce or prompt us to change our feelings by making us stop and examine the appropriateness of them. Often rule reminders come in the form of comments or gestures from others: scolding language, teasing, smiles, or scowls (Hochschild 1979: 564). Alternatively, they may come from within, through feelings of guilt or shame. Either way, rule reminders tell us whether we are complying with normative expectations.

Theoretical Advancement

Since 1983, a significant body of work has grown out of the theory of emotion work. It has been used to understand the dynamics and circumstances of people's daily lives and how individuals interact with one another on an emotional level. For example, Cahill and Eggleston (1994) used Hochschild's theory to show how wheelchair users managed their emotions in interactions with people reacting to their disabilities. Pierce (1995) used the theory to explore gender and role differences in law firms. In her article on how nurses offered emotion work as a 'gift' to their patients, beyond the emotional labour they did for their jobs, Bolton (2000: 584) described how they masked their 'feelings of abhorrence' in certain situations to achieve a positive display for the benefit of the patients' families.

Emotional labour in particular has been extensively tested. Steinberg and Figart (1999: 22) wrote that Hochschild's theory of emotions had 'blossomed' and 'stood the test of time'. Scholars, who have explored and expanded the theory, have 'grounded and shaped our understanding of what it means' in the workplace to 'induce or suppress feeling' or to produce the 'proper state of mind in others'. In the Chinese context, emotional labour was recently explored by F. Cheung and Wu (2013) who were interested in the ways surface and deep acting affected successful ageing in the Hong Kong workplace. Their findings suggested that deep acting had positive benefits in the work environment, but surface acting did not.

In contrast to emotional labour, past research on private emotion work has been strongly associated with families, the division of household labour and *Work-Life-Balance*. In '*The Second Shift*' Hochschild (1989) examined gender ideologies in the context of balancing family and work, showing how couples performed emotion work to reinforce their idealised concepts of what marriage should be.

In other American literature on emotion work, Wharton and Erickson (1993: 469) suggested that within the family context, women have been 'the primary providers of socioemotional support'. As such, they have not only been expected to manage their own emotions but to be responsible for the emotional well-being of other family members. According to the authors, an 'on-going attentiveness' to emotional display has been required to achieve this.

Erickson (1993, 2005: 349) also stated that 'being the family's emotional caretaker' is often perceived as something women 'are', a role stereotype such as 'women are nurturers', as opposed to something women 'do', like housework or a job. This further suggests that emotion work is effortless or invisible and likely to be exacerbated by a woman's internalisation of the expectation to care. Erickson described emotion work done for the well-being of others as 'shadow labour'. But, she added, the inability to recognise emotion work should not foster the notion that it does not exist. Nurturing behaviour must be 'managed, focused and directed so as to communicate the appropriate and intended emotion'.

DeVault (1999) wrote about how women perform family emotion work to suppress anger, disappointment and frustration while advocating for other family members. Erickson (2005) also explored the relationship between emotion work, gender and household labour, suggesting that emotion work is implicated in projecting attitudes and support behaviour that are gender appropriate.

Since the turn of the millennium, more research on emotion work has been directed at the ways in which caregivers of acutely ill and cognitively impaired family members have relied on it in providing care. In a study of cancer patients' informal carers, C. Thomas, Morris and Harman (2002: 537) found that managing emotions was 'crucial'. Caregivers performed emotion work to generate a positive environment for their care recipients; they performed emotion work on themselves to remain strong, to refrain from succumbing to their own emotions and to prevent depression; and they performed emotion work to feel they had some control over the difficult situations they were in.

In other research on cancer carers, Olsen (2011: 906) found that caregivers performed emotion work not only to control their own emotions, but also to encourage care recipients to conform to what was determined to be appropriate feeling rules. This included the endorsement of proper display rules for being a good patient. Being positive, brave and stoic were contrasted with bad patient attitudes and behaviour such as giving up hope and being uncooperative. One of Olsen's respondents even commented that, '90% of caregiving is emotion work'.

In a more recent study of dementia caregivers, Simpson and Acton (2013) tested the effects of emotion work in four areas: managing feelings, weighing options, being parental and ensuring emotional well-being. Caregivers performed emotion work to hide their true feelings (particularly irritation) from the care recipients, avoid projecting their feelings onto others and to suppress or override negative emotions. They used it to determine how to respond to the erratic behaviour of the care recipients and to adjust the care relationship from a more egalitarian to a less egalitarian model. Finally, they did emotion work to promote the well-being of the care recipient. According to the authors, all of this was strongly motivated by feeling rules of what it means to be a good caregiver.

Addressing Tension: The Importance of Emotion Work to Understanding Caregiving Women

Being a 'good caregiver' has been a prominent theme, not only in the caregiving literature but among the women in this book. Conceptually, it is a framing rule, defined by individual interpretation. As discussed, framing rules are reinforced by rule reminders, which are strongly advised by self-image and guilt.

Guilt

Over two decades ago, Jane Aronson (1990: 70, 72) wrote about Canadian women caregivers, observing that they were pressured to conform to gender stereotypes of domesticity by aligning 'their personal realities with prevailing ideologies' [framing rules]. Failure to live up to internalised social norms, she claimed, could negatively impact a woman's concept of selfhood and bring about feelings of shame and guilt:

> Guilt can be understood as the incorporation of prevailing moral codes, in this instance, the shared assumptions about obligation and caregiving. It signals their internalisation in such an effective way that they are levelled against the self, producing a kind of estranged self-criticism. (Aronson 1990: 73)

According to Aronson, tension and conflict are created when women 'strive to balance...between responsiveness to competing others and responsiveness to themselves, between self-enhancement and self-denial' (Aronson 1990: 72). Caregivers, she urged, suppress their own feelings and needs to release themselves from guilt. In emphasising the role of guilt and shame in driving caregiving forward, she asserted:

> In summary, the feelings--guilt and shame--associated with women's concerns at not living up to socially approved ideas about giving and receiving care reflect their profound internalisation of cultural prescriptions. Their incorporation and the resulting self-criticism and self-control represent highly effective-and invisible –forms of social control. Motivated to reduce feelings of guilt and shame, women implicitly suppress assertion of their own needs, so that the broad pattern of care of old people goes unchallenged-rather, it is sustained and reproduced. (Aronson 1990: 76)

Aronson's findings can be seen in Holroyd's (2001) cultural model, which similarly relied on internalised cultural norms reinforced by feelings of guilt.

Self-image

In between Aronson (1990) and Holroyd (2001), Hazel Mac Rae (1998) studied family caregivers of Alzheimer's patients who, she said were often conflicted between feelings of love and anger. In the Chinese context, this has been called 'caring dilemma' (Ngan and Wong 1996). Caregivers perform emotion work to control their tempers by suppressing, invoking and adjusting emotions, attempting to conform to feeling rules of what a 'good caregiver' should be (Mac Rae 1998; Simpson and Acton 2013). Difficulty with or failure to control negative emotions, Mac Rae claimed, induces feelings of guilt, resentment and shame. She asserted that maintaining a positive image of oneself is essential to one's self-identity. Thus, caregivers are highly motivated to develop emotions that are acceptable to them.

In Mac Rae's (1998) research, caregivers implemented strategies for controlling their emotions such as blaming the disease and not the patient. Others adopted avoidance strategies through both physical separation and silence. Over time, however, the strain of trying to present the appropriate display and pushing down emotions had potentially adverse effects. One of Mac Rae's respondents said she could understand why elder abuse takes place. Citing prior research on the negative consequences of surface acting, Mac Rae speculated that if emotion work becomes too difficult, one's ability to feel may be lost, or one may become ill from stress and exhaustion. In any event, something is likely to change. Hochschild (1983: 90) was also mindful of this. In her words:

> Over the long run display comes to assume a certain relation to feeling...a separation of display and feeling is hard to keep up over long periods. A principle of *emotive dissonance* analogous to cognitive dissonance, is at work. Maintaining a difference between feeling and feigning over the long run leads to strain. We try to reduce this strain by pulling the two closer together either by changing what we feel or by changing what we feign.

Caregiver Identity Theory

If emotion work attempts to bridge the gap between what one feels and what one's framing rules and feeling rules prescribe one *should* feel, 'caregiver identity theory' attempts to bridge the gap between how one views one's role as a caregiver and what that role actually is. This appears to be an expansion of Hochschild's core principles (Montgomery and Kosloski 2009).

In 'caregiver identity theory' the caregiver role originates with the existing relationship between the parties and is driven by cultural norms and values personal to one's family [i.e., framing rules]. As the needs of the care recipient and the demands on the caregiver become greater, the relationship begins to change, potentially creating a discrepancy between what the caregiver envisions his or her caregiving role to be [the 'identity standard'] and what the role actually is. Montgomery and Kosloski (2009: 49, 50) claimed this discrepancy could cause such discomfort that caregivers would become highly motivated to seek relief and 'restore congruence'. This could be accomplished in three ways: a change in behaviour (e.g., educating oneself to accept the situation or obtaining outside relief from, for example, an FDH); a change in one's self-appraisal (e.g., how one perceives one's behaviour); or a change in one's identity standard (e.g., a new set of rules redefining the appropriate caregiver behaviour).

The objective of what might be called 'behaviour work' was to harmonise the existing identity standard with actual caregiving activities so the relationship became tolerable for the caregiver and arguably so that it would continue. It is worthy to note that Montgomery and Kosloski progressed the caregiving relationship through five stages, during which caregivers committed increasingly more time, energy and resources to the care recipients. The final stage was characterised by exchange in which primary caregiving was discharged by a third party and the original caregiver returned to his or her initial identity standard. Such an exchange would seem to indicate an inability to restore congruence. The potential for guilt and the implications for self-image could also be observed because it is likely these drove the discomfort experienced through incongruence.

Emotion Work in the Chinese Context

The duty to provide caregiving for family members is often instilled in Chinese daughters as a framing rule from early childhood. Feeling rules under which caregiving is conducted prescribe the avoidance of conflict and direct confrontation (Sullivan 2005). Women are expected to administer care and gift emotional support to the family with the right attitude and display. Holroyd (2001) suggested that Chinese women both internalise the obligation to care and judge themselves by their ability to care, self-imposing guilt if they fail. She also found that 'personhood', a form of self-image, is what is at stake.

These cultural mandates, kin expectations, self-imposed guilt and the need to protect one's self-image, can work together to create tension and conflicting emotions between one's own needs and filial obligation, with potentially negative consequences such as caring dilemma. Thus, how emotions are managed in the caregiving process may not only affect the caregiver's ability to continue in the relationship but the quality and duration of care.

Emotional labour has previously been written about in the Chinese context (Cheung and Wu 2013). However, there appears to have been no literature in which emotion work performed by Asian caregivers has been studied. What one finds are discourses on various coping strategies suggesting that a rudimentary form of emotion work exists, but is unrecognised as such. For example, T.C. Cheng, Ip and Kwok (2013) noted in their study of Chinese caregivers, that those who controlled their emotions by forgiving care recipients' behavioural problems reduced their own caregiver burden, provided the disruptive behaviour did not become too extreme. The authors did not explain how forgiveness was generated; however, some degree of surface acting or deep acting might have been expected.

In other research T.C. Cheng, Lam, Kwok, Ng and Fung (2013) explored the effects of self-efficacy in caregiving of family members with Alzheimer's disease. Self-efficacy was examined in three contexts: controlling negative thoughts, controlling care recipients' behavioural problems and controlling respite decisions. The authors found that Chinese family caregivers who exhibited greater self-efficacy in controlling their negative thoughts experienced lower caregiver burden and more personal growth than the other two controls, suggesting how important controlling one's thoughts and emotions are to caregiving.

As part of their investigation into a 'coping with caregiving' programme in Hong Kong, Au et al. (2010: 258) studied the effectiveness of *cognitive-behavioural therapy* (CBT) as a means of teaching Chinese caregivers 'how to assess and modify the negative thoughts induced by the caregiving role'. One of their goals in using CBT was to teach the caregivers how to change their 'unhelpful' thoughts before they manifested into negative behaviour. This is similar to the stated objectives of emotion work.

In the tradition of symbolic interactionism and the broader Asian context, S.W.-C. Chan (2010) observed that the ways in which caregivers interpret the behaviour of their care recipients, in addition to their caregiving responsibilities, might be determinative of how they cope. Culture, she added, provides the framework for such interpretations. Chan referred to the influence of Confucianism, Buddhism and Taoism in Asian countries, which she suggested predisposed caregivers to fatalistic views of caregiving. In support of this, she pointed to research conducted in Hong Kong in which Hong Kong Chinese accepted events in their lives as 'heaven's will'. This was a framing rule. It ascribed meaning to the situation. Chan (2010: 472) stated that acceptance of this 'cultural conceptualisation' enabled caregivers to endure caregiving hardships free of guilt. If what one felt, however, in the context of this framing rule, was not acceptance but for example, doubt, emotion work would likely to have been needed to achieve the desired result.

The subject matter of each of these studies, although not identified as emotion work, has suggested ways in which individuals can change their outlook and emotional content to tolerate the circumstances they are in. This is discussed in the context of emotion work in the chapters that follow.

Interpersonal ('Gift') Exchange and Chinese Families

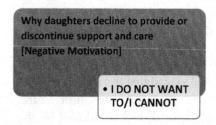

Image of negative model of motivation

Feelings can be experienced alone; however, according to Hochschild (1983) they are most often experienced in exchanges with others. She observed:

> Feeling rules are standards used in emotional conversation to determine what is rightly owed and owing in the currency of feeling. Through them, we tell what is 'due' in each relation, each role. (Hochschild 1983: 18)

Hochschild (1983) described this as 'bowing from the heart' or *gift exchange*. Feeling rules determine what one owes to another and what the other expects to receive. Conversely, feeling rules determine what is owed in return. Hochschild remarked that we all keep a mental ledger of debits and credits. The depth of the bond between parties to an exchange and the equality or disparity of their status and gender are influential in determining what and how much may be owed.

Exchange is the ultimate manifestation of the private emotional system. The practice of managing emotions is likely to occur in every person every day in one form or another. However, it is particularly so within the family, where bonds are strong, relationships are long, complex and changing and there are inequalities based on age and gender.

Social exchange has been addressed in the Asian literature in the caregiving context, with different outcomes. For example, in a study of Hong Kong caregivers of dialysis patients, role conflict was found where caregivers were employed or taking care of more than one family member. Caregiver burden existed; however, internalised cultural 'guidelines', strongly informed by duty, imposed negative stigma and guilt as disincentives to institutionalising care recipients. As a result, patients remained at home and the caregiving relationship remained intact. Nonetheless, the relationship was out of balance. Caregiver burnout and caring dilemma were major themes (Luk 2002).

In another study, Hong Kong caregivers of mentally ill relatives were required to manage the family member's disruptive behaviour, often in public, thereby risking humiliation; take on the disabled family member's responsibilities; and argue with other family members over the course that caregiving should take. This was in addition to providing care. The authors found that by continuing the relationship, the respondents lost their temper with the care recipients, some experienced financial strain and others developed ill health (Ip and Mackenzie 1998). Again, the relationships were out of balance, evidenced by caregiver burden being expressed outwardly in the form of anger and inwardly in worse caregiver health.

A third study compared primary caregivers with non-caregivers. Worse health and poor quality of life, depression, weight loss and anxiety were associated with those who remained in the caregiving relationship (Ho et al. 2009).

These studies represent the negative extremes of caregiving. However, similar scenarios have frequently been seen in the literature and they have been exemplary to the extent they have demonstrated how difficult caregiving can be. In these cases, parents can no longer contribute to the exchange. To keep the relationship in balance, it has been posited that structural norms of obligation and relational norms of affection and reciprocity must be relied on. The strength of these norms could determine the outcome of the exchange, because once it is out of balance, according to exchange theorists, the relationship should shift (Brody 1985). With parents currently living into extreme old age in Asia and the adult children in the family still designated as the primary caregivers, the question arises as to how much these caregivers will be able to endure. Because this is the first generation facing this issue on a wide scale and in light of changing norms of filial obligation and lifestyles, the outcome is anything but certain.

Emotion Work Expanded and Criticised

Interest in Hochschild's theory over the past 34 years has contributed to its expansion in significant ways. Tools to measure it empirically have been deployed (Kruml and Geddes 2000). Four new categories of emotional labour have been introduced to demonstrate how employees could become skilled actors whose emotions were not necessarily transmuted into the 'flat lifeless landscape' of their employer (Bolton and Boyd 2003: 304). The concept of 'citizen regimes' has been created to link emotion work with social policy (Tonkens 2012).

Nonetheless, emotion work has also been criticised. Bolton and Boyd (2003) argued that Hochschild overemphasised the difference between emotional labour and emotion work and incorrectly equated the two. They also criticised the theory for being too rigid, particularly with regard to the transmutation of feelings. Tonkens (2012) pointed out that Hochschild's work failed to explain the relationship between concepts and did not consider them in the wider context. She further alleged that emotion management had seldom been explored beyond the gendered division of labour and *Work-Life-Balance*. Finally, Tonkens observed that a theoretical gap existed, in that Hochschild did not show how individual emotions, social interactions and macro-processes such as globalisation were related.

Conclusion

This chapter aimed to introduce the conceptual and theoretical framework of this book. The overarching framework of symbolic interactionism helped to explain how norms of filial obligation are enacted and how they change; the conceptual models underpinning the motivation to provide support and care; Hochschild's (1983) theory of emotion management showing how emotions are controlled during the provision of care in the face of conflicting demands and feelings; and Hochschild's related concept of gift exchange, clarifying why caregiving may be discontinued.

Traditional Chinese society is collectivistic in its orientation and structure and social order is maintained through institutions rather than individual interaction, although traditional norms of filial obligation are in a state of transition. Symbolic interactionism offers one way to understand how these normative changes may affect the willingness and ability of Chinese women to support and care for their elderly parents: It emphasises the ways individuals interact with one another on the basis of the meanings things have for them and how these are interpreted to create new meanings. Thus, this theory helps to explain how individuals give meaning to and experience the structures of education, employment, living conditions and altered family forms and their impact on contemporary norms and values.

In this regard, the conceptual and theoretical bases for caregiving were broken down into three analytic components: (1) Why daughters provide care, using normative and relational models of motivation characterised as '*I have to*' and '*I want to*'; (2) How daughters manage conflict and tension in discharging care, applying the theory of emotion management portrayed as '*I should want to*'; and (3) Why daughters decline to provide care or discontinue caregiving, drawing from social exchange theory and the idea of 'gift exchange', represented as '*I do not want to/I cannot*'.

Structural norms of filial obligation ['*I have to*'] consist of socially acceptable behavioural norms transmitted through role modelling or teachings internalised in childhood. These manifest as duty and are tied to normative expectations and guilt. In the Asian context, structural norms are strongly associated with contemporary interpretations of filial piety and reinforced by government policy. The 'cultural model approach' is linked with the Confucian notion that the self is subjugated to the obligations of personhood, informed by gender and generational roles.

A personal relational approach to motivations ['*I want to*'] originates with filial piety in the Asian context. However, it is widely believed that the altruistic and emotional aspects of it are primarily what remain. Additionally, Asian relational norms are believed to be strongly influenced by contemporary norms, which are less obligatory and more voluntary and egalitarian in nature than traditional filial piety. *Yangdao*, (not *xiao*), is the distinguishing feature based on what has been referred to as a 'network of responsibilities and obligations' (Ng et al. 2002: 141).

Borrowing from the Western literature, the convoy model subscribes to the concept of a 'support bank' into which parents make deposits when their children are young and withdraw from in their old age. Social exchange is also implicated in Asian relational norms. However, some contend it must be adapted to the collective nature of Asian families. The Asian literature embraces no one particular relational model. Reciprocity and affection are most often combined with structural norms, especially modified versions of filial piety. This is particularly apparent in studies of daughters and daughters-in-law, who no longer strictly accept traditional norms of filial obligation.

Despite changes in the nature of filial support and caregiving motivations, government policies, incentives, laws and social engineering still aim to encourage and in some cases require, adult children to care for elderly parents, particularly in Singapore. One of the emerging instruments from these government endeavours has been the Family Support Agreement, which has gained widespread popularity in the rural areas of mainland China. Taking a different approach, Singapore supports a programme of *Work-Life-Balance*.

Unlike Asia, Western concepts underpinning motivations of support and care are dominated by affection and reciprocity. Reciprocity can refer to a debt, where a fixed sum is to be repaid and to gratitude, where the lack of duty to repay can result in irredeemable obligation. The life course approach of lagged reciprocity is likewise bifurcated: as a return on investment and as an insurance policy, where delayed repayment of childhood investment is deemed earned. Negotiated responsibilities are also reciprocal, but based on guidelines, not rules. They are driven by one's moral identity and the desire to balance independence with dependence within the family context.

Affection is the strongest motivator for caregiving in the Western literature, which can also be combined with reciprocity. Other models growing out of affection are the friendship model, the special goods model and attachment. Altruism, encompassing need, is defined as giving without the expectation of receiving a benefit. However, it may be motivated by self-interest or a 'warm glow'.

There are limitations to caregiving motivations. Studies on the gap between filial belief and filial behaviour have yielded mixed results. However, Finch and Mason (1993) argued that the attitude vs. behaviour debate is irrelevant. According to them, the only thing that matters is whether one's actions are viewed positively by others. Negative motivation, or lack of affection, can act as a disincentive to providing support and care ['*I do not want to/I cannot*']. Likewise, conditionality involves the idea that if parents have not fulfilled obligations to their children, children's reciprocal obligations might be excused. Finally, structural impediments such as smaller living quarters and female employment may make parent care impractical or impossible.

Chinese women caregivers are arguably bound, to some extent by the traditional norms of filial obligation they have internalised, aligned with their sense of self, then linked with guilt when they fail to live up to socially expected norms of behaviour. Arlie Hochschild's theory of emotion management suggests that in our interactions with others we attempt to conform our emotions to social expectations ['*I should want to*']. Difficulties arise when what we believe we *should* feel is distinct from what we *actually* feel. To bridge this gap we do emotion work. We can create a proper display through surface acting or try to change what we feel through deep acting. A derivation of emotion management can be found in the 'caregiver identity theory' in which caregivers try to bridge the gap between what the caregiver believes her role to be and what it actually is.

Whereas emotional labour has been studied in Asia, emotion work in the private sense has not. Nonetheless, research into self-efficacy and cognitive-behavioural therapy has provided some insight into behaviour that might be considered emotion work but has not been acknowledged as such.

Hochschild also asserted that individuals maintain a mental ledger of what is owed and what is expected in their relationships with others. This is a version of social exchange, what she refers to as 'gift exchange'. Like classical exchange theory, when the ledger becomes imbalanced, a change in the relationship or circumstances may result [*I do not want to/I cannot*]. With this framework in place, the typology of support and care is now examined.

Notes

1. The concept of "Face" in the Asian culture is roughly equivalent to self-respect, or respect for and from others. Embarrassment (loss of Face) is something to be avoided at all costs.
2. There are conditions to this. The dependent must reside in Singapore; at least S$2000 must have been spent on the dependent's upkeep; the dependent's income is less than S$4000; and the dependent is at least 55 years of age.

References

Aboderin, I. (2006). *Intergenerational support and old age in Africa*. New Brunswick: Transaction Publishers.

Allen, K. (2010). *Classical sociological theory* (2nd ed.). Los Angeles: Pine Forge Press.

Appelrouth, S., & Edles, L. D. (2007). *Sociological theory in the contemporary era*. Los Angeles: Pine Forge Press.

Aronson, J. (1990). Women's perspectives on informal care of the elderly: Public ideology and personal experience of giving and receiving care. *Ageing and Society, 10*(1), 61–84.

Au, A., Li, S., Leung, P., Pan, P.-C., Thompson, L., & Gallagher-Thompson, D. (2010). The coping with caregiving group program for Chinese caregivers of patients with Alzheimer's disease in Hong Kong. *Patient Education and Counselling, 78,* 256–260.

Berman, H. J. (1987). Adult children and their parents: Irredeemable obligation and irreparable loss. *Journal of Gerontological Social Work, 10*(1-2), 21–34.

Blumer, H. (1969). *Symbolic interactionism: Perspective & method.* Berkeley: University of California Press.

Bolton, S. C. (2000). Who cares? Offering emotion work as a 'gift' in the nursing labour process. *Journal of Advanced Nursing, 32*(8), 580–586.

Bolton, S. C., & Boyd, C. (2003). Trolley dolly or skilled emotion manager? Moving on from Hochschild's managed heart. *Work, Employment & Society, 17,* 289–308.

Brant, M., Haberkern, K., & Szydlik, M. (2009). Intergenerational help and care in Europe. *European Sociological Review, 25*(5), 585–601.

Brody, E. M. (1985). Parent care as a normative family stress. *The Gerontologist, 25*(1), 19–29.

Cahill, S., & Eggleston, R. (1994). Managing emotions in public: The case of wheelchair users. *Social Psychology Quarterly, 57,* 300–312.

Chan, A. (1999). The role of formal versus informal support of the elderly in Singapore: Is there substitution? *Southeast Asian Journal of Social Science, 27*(2), 87–110.

Chan, S. W.-C. (2010). Family caregiving in dementia: The Asian perspective of a global problem. *Dementia and Geriatric Cognitive Disorders, 30,* 469–478.

Chan, R. K. H. (2011). Patterns and paths of child care and elder care in Hong Kong. *Journal of Comparative Social Welfare, 27*(2), 155–164.

Chan, S. S. C., Viswanath, K., Au, D. W. H., Ma, C. M. S., Lam, W. W. T., Fielding, R., Leung, G. M., & Lam, T.-H. (2011). Hong Kong Chinese community leaders' perspectives on family health, happiness and harmony: A qualitative study. *Health Education Research, 26*(4), 664–674.

Chappell, N. L., & Funk, L. (2012). Filial responsibility: Does it matter for care-giving behaviours? *Ageing and Society, 32*(7), 1128–1146.

Chen, S. X., Bond, M. H., & Tang, D. (2007). Decomposing filial piety into filial attitudes and filial enactments. *Asian Journal of Social Psychology, 10*(4), 213–223.

Cheng, T. C., Ip, I. N., & Kwok, T. (2013). Caregiver forgiveness is associated with less burden and potentially harmful behaviours. *Aging & Mental Health, 17*(8), 930–934.

Cheng, T. C., Lam, L. C. W., Kwok, T., Ng, N. S. S., & Fung, A. W. T. (2013). Self-efficacy is associated with less burden and more gains from behavioural problems of Alzheimer's disease in Hong Kong Chinese caregivers. *The Gerontologist, 53*, 71–80.

Cheung, C.-K., & Kwan, A. Y.-H. (2009). The erosion of filial piety by modernisation in Chinese cities. *Aging and Society, 29*, 179–198.

Cheung, F., & Wu, A. M. S. (2013). Emotional labour and successful ageing in the workplace among older Chinese employees. *Ageing and Society, 33*(6), 1036–1051.

Chilcott, J. H. (1998). Structural functionalism as a heuristic device. *Anthropology & Education Quarterly, 29*(1), 103–111.

Choi, J. (2008). Work and family demands and life stress among Chinese employees: The mediating effect of work-family conflict. *The International Journal of Resource Management, 19*(5), 878–895.

Chou, K.-L. (2009). Number of children and upstream intergenerational financial transfers: Evidence from Hong Kong. *Journal of Gerontology: Social Sciences, 65B*, 227–235.

Chou, R. J.-A. (2011). Filial piety by contract? The emergence, implementation, and implications of the "family support agreement" in China. *The Gerontologist, 51*, 3–16.

Chou, K.-L., & Cheung, C. K. (2013). Family-friendly policies in the workplace and their effect on work-life conflicts in Hong Kong. *The International Journal of Human Resource Management, 24*, 3872–3885.

Chou, K.-L., Chow, N. W. S., & Chi, I. (2004). Preventing economic hardship among Chinese elderly in Hong Kong. *Journal of Aging & Social Policy, 16*(4), 79–97.

Chow, N. (2006). The practice of filial piety and its impact on long term care policies for elderly people in Asian Chinese communities. *Asian Journal of Gerontology & Geriatrics, 1*(1), 31–35.

Chung, T. Y. R., Pang, K. L. K., & Tong, Y. W. J. (2010). *Work-life balance survey of the Hong Kong working population 2010.* (Tech. Rep.). Hong Kong: The University of Hong Kong Public Opinion Programme.

Churton, M., & Brown, A. (2010). *Theory and method* (2nd ed.). Basingstoke: Palgrave Macmillan.

Cicirelli, V. G. (1983). Adult children's attachment and helping behavior to elderly parents: A path model. *Journal of Marriage and the Family, 45*(4), 815–825.

Cicirelli, V. G. (1993). Attachment and obligation as daughters' motives for caregiving behavior and subsequent effect on subjective burden. *Psychology and Aging, 8*(2), 144–155.

Clark, T. N. (1972). Structural-functionalism, exchange theory, and the new political economy: Institutionalization as a theoretical linkage. *Social Inquiry*, *42*(3–4), 275–298.

Croll, E. J. (1995). *Changing identities of Chinese women; rhetoric, experience and self-perception in twentieth-century China*. Hong Kong: Hong Kong University Press.

DeVault, M. L. (1999). Comfort and struggle: Emotion work in family life. *Annals of the American Academy of Political and Social Science, 56*, 52–63.

Del Corso, A., & Lanz, M. (2013). Felt obligation and the family life cycle: A study on intergenerational relationships. *International Journal of Psychology, 48*, 1196–1200.

Dixon, N. (1995). The friendship model of filial obligation. *Journal of Applied Philosophy, 12*(1), 77–87.

Erickson, R. J. (1993). Reconceptualizing family work: The effect of emotion work on perceptions of marital quality. *Journal of Marriage and Family, 55*(4), 888–900.

Erickson, R. J. (2005). Why emotion work mattes: Sex, gender, and the division of household labour. *Journal of Marriage and the Family, 67*(2), 337–351.

Finch, J., & Mason, J. (1993). *Negotiating family responsibilities*. Abingdon: Routledge.

Finley, N. J., Roberts, M. D., & Banahan, B. F. (1988). Motivators and inhibitors of attitudes of filial obligation toward aging parents. *The Gerontologist, 28*(1), 73–78.

Foster, D., & Ren, X. (2015). Work-family conflict and the commodification of women's employment in three Chinese airlines. *The International Journal of Resource Management, 26*(12), 1568–1585. https://doi.org/10.1080/095851 92.2014.949621.

Fu, T.-h. (2014). Do state benefits impact on intergenerational family support? The case of Taiwan. In S. Harper (Ed.), *Critical Readings on Ageing in Asia* (pp. 1419–1432). Reprinted from Intergenerational Relationships (2008) *6*(3), 339–354.

Ghy, T., & Woo, J. (2009). Elder care: Is legislation of family responsibility the solution? *Asian Journal of Gerontology and Geriatrics, 4*(2), 72–75.

Hashimoto, A., & Ikels, C. (2005). Filial piety in changing Asian societies. In M. L. Johnson (Ed.), *The Cambridge handbook of age and ageing* (pp. 437–442). Cambridge: Cambridge University Press.

Hatton, C. (2013). New China law says children 'must visit parents'. *BBC News*.www.bbc.co.uk/news/world-asia-china

Hess, B. B., & Waring, J. M. (1978). Changing patterns of aging and family bonds in later life. *The Family Coordinator, 27*(4), 301–314.

Ho, S. C., Chan, A., Woo, J., Chong, P., & Sham, A. (2009). Impact of caregiving on health and quality of life: A comparative population-based study of caregivers for elderly persons and non-caregivers. *Journals of Gerontology (Biological Sciences and Medical Sciences), 64A*(8), 873–879.

Hochschild, A. R. (1979). Emotion work, feeling rules and social structure. *American Journal of Sociology, 85*(3), 551–575.

Hochschild, A. (1983, 2012). *The managed heart: Commercialization of human feeling*. Berkeley: University of California Press.

Hochschild, A. R. (with Machung, A.). (1989, 2012). *The second shift: Working families and the revolution at home*. New York: Viking Penguin, Inc.

Holroyd, E. (2001). Hong Kong Chinese daughters' intergenerational caregiving obligations: A cultural model approach. *Social Science & Medicine, 53*(9), 1125–1134.

Holroyd, E. (2003). Chinese family obligations toward chronically ill elderly members: Comparing caregivers in Beijing and Hong Kong. *Qualitative Health Research, 13*(3), 302–318.

Hong, Y.-H., & Liu, W. T. (2000). The social psychological perspective of elderly care. In W. T. Liu & H. Kendig (Eds.), *Who should care for the elderly* (pp. 165–179). Singapore: Singapore University Press.

Hong Kong Community Business Online. *Work-Life Balance*. http://www.communitybusiness.org/focus_areas/WLB.htm

Horowitz, A., & Shindelman, L. W. (1983). Reciprocity and affection. *Journal of Gerontological Social Work, 5*(3), 5–20.

Housing Development Board. (2017). Living with/near parent or married child. http://www.hdb.gov.sg/cs/infoweb/residential/buying-a-flat/resale/living-with-near-parents-or-married-child

Hsu, H.-C., Lew-Ting, C.-Y., & Wu, S.-C. (2014). Age, period, and cohort effects on the attitude toward supporting parents in Taiwan. In S. Harper (Ed.), *Critical readings on ageing in Asia* (pp. 1373–1390). Leiden: Brill. Reprinted from *The Gerontologist* (2001) *41(6),* 742–750.

Huat, C. B. (2009). Being Chinese under official multiculturalism in Singapore. *Asian Ethnicity, 10*(3), 239–250.

Inland Revenue Authority of Singapore. (2017). Parent relief. https://www.iras.gov.sg/IRASHome/Individuals/Locals/Working-Out-Your-Taxes/Deductions-for-Individuals/Parent-Relief-/-Handicapped-Parent-Relief/

Ip, G. S. H., & Mackenzie, A. E. (1998). Caring for relatives with serious mental illness at home: The experiences of family carers in Hong Kong. *Archives of Psychiatric Nursing, 12*(5), 288–294.

Izuhara, M. (2010). Housing, wealth and family reciprocity in East Asia. In M. Izuhara (Ed.), *Ageing and intergenerational relations* (pp. 77–94). Bristol: Policy Press.

Jang, S.-N., Avendano, M., & Kawachi, I. (2012). Informal caregiving patterns in Korea and European countries: A cross-national comparison. *Asian Nursing Research, 6*(1), 19–26.

Keller, S. (2006). Four theories of filial duty. *The Philosophical Quarterly, 56*(223), 254–274.

Kim, T.-H., & Han, S.-Y. (2013). Family life of older Koreans. In J.-N. Bae, J.-M. Kyung, Y.-K. Roh, J.-C. Sung, & Y.-H. Won (Eds.), *Ageing in Korea, today and tomorrow* (pp. 68–93). Seoul: Federation of Korean Gerontological Societies.

Kruml, S. M., & Geddes, D. (2000). Exploring the dimensions of emotional labour: The heart of Hochschild's work. *Management and Communication Quarterly, 14*, 8–49.

Kuah, K.-E. (1990). Confucian ideology and social engineering in Singapore. *Journal of Contemporary Asia, 20*(3), 371–383.

Lam, R. C. (2006). Contradictions between traditional Chinese values and the actual performance: A study of the caregiving roles of the modern sandwich generation in Hong Kong. *Journal of Comparative Family Studies, 37*(2), 299–318.

Law of the People's Republic of China on Protection of The Rights and Interests of the Elderly, Chapter II: Maintenance and support by families. (1996). Retrieved online September 14, 2014, from http://www.china.org.cn/english/government/207403.htm

Lee, K. S. (2014). Gender, care work, and the complexity of family membership in Japan. In S. Harper (Ed.), *Critical readings on ageing in Asia* (pp. 853–876). Leiden: Brill. Reprinted from *Gender & Society* (2010) 24(5), 647–671.

Lee, W. K.-M., & Kwok, H.-K. (2005a). Differences in expectations and patterns of informal support for older persons in Hong Kong: Modification to filial piety. *Ageing International, 30*, 188–206.

Lee, W. K.-M., & Kwok, H.-k. (2005b). Older women and family care in Hong Kong: Differences in filial expectation and practices. *Journal of Women and Aging, 17*(1-2), 129–150.

Lei, L. (2013). Sons, daughters and intergenerational support in China. *Chinese Sociological Review, 45*(3), 26–52.

Li, L. W., Long, Y., Essex, E. L., Sui, Y., & Gao, L. (2012). Elderly Chinese and their family caregivers' perceptions of good care: A qualitative study in Shandong, China. *Journal of Gerontological Social Work, 55*(7), 609–625.

Lieber, E., Nihura, K., & Mink, I. T. (2004). Filial piety, modernization, and the challenges of raising children for Chinese immigrants: Quantitative and qualitative evidence. *Ethos, 32*(3), 324–347.

Lin, J.-P., & Yi, C.-C. (2011). Filial norms and intergenerational support to aging parents in China and Taiwan [special issue]. *International Journal of Social Welfare, 20*(Supp.s1), S109–S120.

Lo, S. (2003). Perceptions of work-family conflict among married female professionals in Hong Kong. *Personnel Review, 32*(3), 376–390.

Long, S. O., Campbell, R., & Nishimura, C. (2014). Does it matter who cares? A comparison of daughters versus daughters-in-law in Japanese elder care. In S. Harper (Ed.), *Critical readings on ageing in Asia* (pp. 1373–1390). Leiden: Brill. Reprinted from *Social Science Japan Journal* (2009) *12(1)*, 1–21.

Luk, W. S.-C. (2002). The home care experience as perceived by the caregivers of Chinese dialysis patients. *International Journal of Nursing Studies, 39*(3), 269–277.

Mac Rae, H. (1998). Managing feelings: Caregiving as emotion work. *Research on Aging, 20*(1), 137–160.

Mehta, K. K., & Ko, H. (2004). Filial piety revisited in the context of modernizing Asian societies. *Geriatrics and Gerontology International, 4*(Supp. 4), S77–S78.

Ministry of Community Development, Youth and Sports, Singapore. (2007). Inaugural study confirms positive benefits of work-life harmony to individuals and business: MCYS Media Release No. 43/2007: app.msf.gov.sg/portals/0/summary/publication/43-20071.pdf

Montgomery, R. J. V., & Kosloski, K. (2009). Caregiving as a process of changing identity: Implications for caregiver support. *Generations: Journal of the American Society on Aging, 33*(1), 47–52.

Moskowitz, S. (2002). Adult children and indigent parents: Intergenerational responsibilities in international perspective. *86 Marquette Law Review 401*.

Ng, A. C. Y., Phillips, D. R., & Lee, W. K.-m. (2002). Persistence and challenges to filial piety and informal support of older persons in a modern Chinese society: A case study in Tuen Mun, Hong Kong. *Journal of Aging Studies, 16*(2), 135–153.

Ngan, R., & Wong, W. (1996). Injustice in family care of the Chinese elderly in Hong Kong. *Journal of Aging & Social Policy, 7*(2), 77–94.

Nip, P. T. K. (2010). Social welfare development in Hong Kong. Changes and challenges in building a caring and harmonious society. *Asia Pacific Journal of Social Work and Development, 20*(1), 65–81.

Office of the High Commissioner on Human Rights. (2009). *Responses to the office of the United Nations High Commissioner for Human Rights.*www.ohchr. org/Documents/Issues/EPoverty/casher/Korea.pdf

Olsen, R. E. (2011). Managing hope, denial or temporal anomie? Informal cancer carers' accounts of spouses' cancer diagnoses. *Social Science & Medicine, 73*(6), 904–911.

Parliament of Singapore. (1994, July 25–27) Maintenance of Parents Bill – Second Reading. Parliamentary Debates Singapore: Official Report. Singapore: Singapore National Printers. In P. A. Rozario & S.-I. Hong (2011) Doing it 'right' by your parents in Singapore: A political economy examination of the maintenance of parents act of 1995. *Critical Social Policy, 31*(4), 607–627.

Parrott, T. M., & Bengtson, V. L. (1999). The effects of earlier intergenerational affection, normative expectations, and family conflict on contemporary exchanges of help and support. *Research on Aging, 21*(1), 73–105.

Pierce, J. L. (1995). *Gender trials: Emotional lives in contemporary law firms.* Berkeley: University of California Press.

Qian, Y., & Qian, Z. (2015). Work, family and gendered happiness among married people in urban China. *Social Indicators Research, 121*, 61–74. https:// doi.org/10.1007/s11205-014-0623-9.

Republic of China (Taiwan) Ministry of the Interior. (2012). *Senior citizens welfare act.* http://www.moi.gov.tw/english/english_law/law_detail. aspx?sn=180

Rickles-Jordan, A. (2007). Filial responsibility: A survey across time and oceans. *Marquette Elder's Advisor, 9*(1), 183–204.

Rozario, P. A., & Hong, S.-l. (2011). Doing it "right" by your parents in Singapore: A political economy examination of the Maintenance of parents act of 1995. *Critical Social Policy, 31*(4), 607–627.

Rozario, P. A., & Rosetti, A. L. (2012). "Many helping hands": A review and analysis of long-term care policies, programs, and practices in Singapore. *Journal of Gerontological Social Work, 55*(7), 641–658.

Silverstein, M., & Bengtson, V. L. (1997). Intergenerational solidarity and the structure of adult child-parent relationships in American families. *American Journal of Sociology, 103*(2), 429–460.

Silverstein, M., Parrott, T. M., & Bengtson, V. L. (1995). Factors that predispose middle-aged sons and daughters to provide social support to older parents. *Journal of Marriage and the Family, 57*(2), 465–476.

Silverstein, M., Conroy, S. J., Wang, H., Giarrusso, R., & Bengtson, V. L. (2002). Reciprocity in parent-child relations over the adult life course. *Journals of Gerontology: Social Sciences, 57B*(1), S3–S13.

Silverstein, M., Conroy, S. J., & Gans, D. (2012). Beyond solidarity, reciprocity and altruism: Moral capital as a unifying concept of intergenerational support for older people. *Ageing and Society, 32*(7), 1246–1262.

Simpson, C., & Acton, G. (2013). Emotion work in family caregiving for persons with dementia. *Issues in Mental Health Nursing, 34*(1), 52–58.

Singapore Attorney General's Chambers. Maintenance of Parents Act, Chapter 167B, original enactment: Act 35 of 1995; revised edition 1996: Singapore statutes online: statutes.agc.gov.sg/.../cgi_getdata.pl?actno...MAINTENANCE%20 OF% 20PARENTS%20ACT%0A

Singapore Business Review. (2013, June 22). *Singapore offers third best work-life balance in Asia.* http://sbr.com.sg/economy/news/singapore-offers-third-best-work-life-balance-in-asia

Stein, C. H., Wemmerus, V. A., Ward, M., Gaines, M. E., Freeberg, A. L., & Jewell, T. C. (1998). Because they're my parents: An intergenerational study of felt obligation and parental caregiving. *Journal of Marriage and the Family, 60*(3), 611–622.

Steinberg, R. J., & Figart, D. M. (1999). Emotional labour since the managed heart. *Annals of the American Academy of Political and Social Science, 561*, 8–26.

Stuifbergen, M. C., & Van Delden, J. J. M. (2011). Filial obligations to elderly parents: A duty to care? *Medicine Health Care and Philosophy, 14*(1), 63–71.

Suanet, B., Van Groenou, M. B., & Van Tilburg, T. (2012). Informal and formal home-care use among older adults in Europe: Can cross-national differences be explained by societal context and composition? *Ageing and Society, 32*(3), 491–515.

Sullivan, P. L. (2005). Culture, divorce, and family mediation in Hong Kong. *Family Court Review, 43*(1), 109–123.

Sung, K.-t. (2000). An Asian perspective on aging east and west: Filial piety and changing families. In V. L. Bengtson, K.-D. Kim, G. C. Myers, & K.-S. Eun (Eds.), *Aging in east and west: Families, states and the elderly* (pp. 41–58). New York: Springer Publishing Co.

Sung, K.-t. (2001). Elder respect: Exploration of ideals and forms in East Asia. *Journal of Aging Studies, 15*(1), 13–26.

Tan, E. K. B. (2003). Re-engaging Chineseness: Political, economic and cultural imperatives of nation-building in Singapore. *The China Quarterly, 175*, 751–774.

Teo, Y. (2010). Shaping the Singapore family, producing the state and society [special issue]. *Economy and Society, 39*(3), 337–359.

Teo, P., Graham, E., Yeoh, B. S. A., & Levy, S. (2003). Values, change and intergenerational ties between two generations of women in Singapore. *Ageing and Society, 23*(3), 327–247.

Teo, P., Mehta, K., Thang, L. L., & Chan, A. (2006). *Ageing in Singapore, service needs and the state.* Oxford: Routledge.

Thomas, E. (1990). Filial piety, social change and Singapore youth. *Journal of Moral Education, 19*(3), 192–205.

Thomas, C., Morris, S. M., & Harman, J. C. (2002). Companions through cancer: The care given by informal carers in cancer contexts. *Social Science & Medicine, 54*(4), 529–544.

Tonkens, E. (2012). Working with Arlie Hochschild: Connecting feelings to social change. *Social Politics, 19*(2), 194–218.

Turner, J. H., & Stets, J. E. (2005). *The sociology of emotions.* New York: Cambridge University Press.

Verbrugge, L. M., & Chan, A. (2008). Giving help in return: Family reciprocity by older Singaporeans. *Ageing & Society, 28*(1), 5–34.

Walker, A. J., Pratt, C. C., Shin, H.-Y., & Jones, L. L. (1990). Motives for parental caregiving and relationship quality. *Family Relations, 39*(1), 51–56.

Wallace, R. A., & Wolf, A. (2006). *Contemporary sociological theory; expanding the classical tradition* (6th ed.). Princeton: Pearson/Prentice Hall.

Wallhagen, M. I., & Strawbridge, W. J. (1995). My parent-not myself: Contrasting themes in family care. *Journal of Aging and Health, 7*(4), 552–572.

Wharton, A., & Erickson, R. J. (1993). Managing emotions on the job and at home: Understanding the consequences of multiple emotional roles. *The Academy of Management Review, 19*(3), 457–486.

Whitbeck, L. B., Simons, R. L., & Conger, R. D. (1991). The effects of early family relationships on contemporary relationships and assistance patterns between adult children and their parents. *Journals of Gerontology, Social Sciences, 46*(6(Supp. 6)), S330–S337.

Whitbeck, L., Hoyt, D. R., & Huck, S. M. (1994). Early family relationships, intergenerational solidarity, and support provided to parents by their adult children. *Journal of Gerontology, Social Sciences, 49*(4(Supp. 2)), S85–S94.

Wicclair, M. R. (1990). Caring for frail elderly parents: Past parental sacrifices and the obligations of adult children. *Social Theory and Practice, 16*(2), 163–189.

Wong, O. M. H. (2000). Children and children-in-law as primary caregivers: Issues and perspectives. In W. T. Liu & H. Kendig (Eds.), *Who should care for the elderly* (pp. 297–321). Singapore: Singapore University Press.

Wong, O. M. H., & Chau, B. H. P. (2006). The evolving role of filial piety in eldercare in Hong Kong. *Asian Journal of Social Science, 34*(4), 600–617.

Xiao, Y. & Cooke, F.L. (2012) Work-life balance in China? Social policy, employer strategy nd individual coping mechanisms. Asia Pacific Journal of Human Resources, 50, 6-22, DOI: 19.1111/j.1744-7941.2011.00005.x.

Xie, Y., & Zhu, H. (2009). Do sons or daughters give more money to parents in urban China? *Journal of Marriage and the Family, 71*(1), 174–186.

Yin, L. C. (2003). Do traditional values still exist in modern Chinese societies? The case of Singapore and China. *Asia Europe Journal, 1*(1), 43–59.

Yoon, G., Eun, K.-S., & Park, K.-S. (2000). Korea: Demographic trends, socio-cultural contexts, and public policy. In V. L. Bengtson, K.-S. Eun, K.-D. Kim, & G. C. Myers (Eds.), *Aging in east and west; families, states and the elderly* (pp. 121–137). New York: Springer Publishing.

Yu, A. (2015, June 16). Hongkongers have worst work-life balance in Asia-Pacific as 77pc take calls on holiday. *South China Morning Post.* http://www.scmp.com/news/hong-kong/economy/article/1822705/hongkongers-have-worst-work-life-balance-asia-pacific-77pc

Zhan, J. H., & Montgomery, R. J. V. (2003). Gender and elder care in China: The influence of filial piety and structural constraints. *Gender and Society, 17*(2), 209–229.

Zhang, M., Foley, S., & Yang, B. (2013). Work-family conflict among Chinese married couples: Testing spillover and crossover effects. *The International Journal of Resource Management, 24*(17), 3213–3231. https://doi.org/10.1080/09585192.2013.763849.

Singapore

Housing Development Board. (2016). *Living with/near parent or married child.* http://www.hdb.gov.sg/cs/infoweb/residential/buying-a-flat/resale/living-with-near-parents-or-married-child

Ministry of Manpower. (2016b). *Strategies for work-life harmony.* http://www.mom.gov.sg/employment-practices/good-work-practices/work-life-strategies

Ministry of Manpower. (2017d). *Levy concession for a foreign domestic worker.* http://www.mom.gov.sg/passes-and-permits/work-permit-for-foreign-domestic-worker/foreign-domestic-worker-levy/levy-concession#for-aged-persons

4

The Typology of Support and Care™

Context and Trends in Which the Research Puzzle Is Embedded

> My generation, oh I think my generation is really [the] transition genera-
> tion… The traditional Asian women…are mostly at home. [They] are
> mostly very submissive and may not have [a] career, while we are [a] very
> educated group. Most of us would want to have something [to] fulfil our
> career aspirations and at the same time, we are still very oriented towards
> being the person that cares for the home and…the family. (Jun)[1]

The women in this book straddled the traditional norms of their parents and the high tech, globalised, materialistically driven world of their
children. As Chinese daughters in the Baby Boom and Gen X[2] generations, they forged a unique identity 'in-between' these two disparate cultures, and they were acutely aware of their status as the link between
them.

For centuries, until the end of the Second World War, most Chinese
women in Asia lived within a collective, hierarchical system in which they
had no power or choice. Confined primarily to the home, they were

© The Author(s) 2018
P. O'Neill, *Urban Chinese Daughters*, St Antony's Series,
https://doi.org/10.1007/978-981-10-8699-1_4

judged by their domestic skills and the ability to comply with the conditions under which they lived. Most mothers of the Baby Boomer women in this book were described by their daughters as enduring lives dominated by poverty, discrimination, lack of education and dependency. Following marriage, they were responsible for the family and the household. If they worked at all it was at menial jobs or the family business to earn extra money for the family. According to some of the daughters, their fathers were frequently absent and sometimes abusive or adulterous. Mothers who were widowed, abandoned or part of a polygamous family often raised children alone. Probably due to the hardship and responsibility that characterised their lives, the mothers, as reported by their daughters, though submissive were disciplined and strong.

In their daughters' words, as mothers raised their families, most transmitted traditional Chinese values to their children by setting an example, providing verbal cues and directly instructing them. The importance of family was highly emphasised together with such filial norms as respect and obedience, and values such as honesty and thrift. However, as conditions changed in the second half of the twentieth century, opening up opportunities for women, the daughters born to these women said they were encouraged to pursue education and employment. While retaining many of their parents' values, independence and self-sufficiency became integrated into their cultural ethos. Education and professional employment began to drive change.

As the daughters in this book navigated the educational process, many of them learned how to think for themselves and were exposed to the world outside the home. Self-confidence, pride and belief in their abilities frequently replaced feelings of inferiority and submissiveness. When they entered the workforce with academic qualifications, already vested with a strong work ethic from the home, most did well. Financial independence resulted, engendering greater bargaining power with their families and prospective marriage partners. Some of the daughters reported they were even treated like sons by their parents.

Most of the daughters admitted to some outside influence, especially those from the Gen X generation. Many had been exposed to the 'West' through school, work, travel or the media. Singapore and Hong Kong in fact were frequently characterised as the most 'westernised' societies in Asia. Nonetheless, the daughters universally remarked that they were still very 'Chinese' in their thinking. This was probably due to the reinforcement of Asian values in the home and elsewhere, in addition to sporadic or mixed exposure to both Asian and 'Western' cultures.

The resulting values of the daughters were an amalgam of old and new. Among them it was mostly love for and devotion to the family at the core of their personal ideologies. Commitment to family, however, did not mean what it once did. Although the daughters in this book said they valued their families, they also claimed to value themselves. They described themselves as being independent, self-sufficient and capable. How they prioritised their own needs and desires with those of their families, according to them, was determined by the circumstances under which different situations arose.

The Chinese daughters in this book appeared to trust their own judgment. However, many had become Christian, turning to God for moral instruction. Christian and Chinese values were facilely integrated, and issues concerning traditional Chinese religious practices such as ancestor worship were resolved respectfully with parents. The only area of potential conflict was whether God or one's parents had the final moral authority.

The relationship with their parents was also pivotal to understanding how they navigated the practical side of everyday life. Although most unmarried daughters still lived with their parents, many of the married daughters did not permanently reside with their parents or parents-in-law as adults.[3] The daughters, especially the Gen X daughters, stated that they were reluctant to live with in-laws and were supported in this by their husbands. They were, however, willing to live with their own parents, depending on the need and feasibility of doing so. Many daughters in Hong Kong and Singapore said they were choosing not to marry because they were financially self-sufficient. They were looking for partnership and were unwilling to sacrifice their independence without it. Divorce had lost most of its stigma for them, although some of the Baby Boomers remained in unsatisfactory marital relationships out of duty.

Family was also at the centre of the work-life paradigm. All the daughters in this book were working or had worked, and the potential for conflict between children, work and parents was substantial. Nonetheless, most asserted that they managed these competing demands successfully. Many Singaporeans practiced *Work-Life-Balance* where work hours were fewer and flexible. In contrast, the mainland and Hong Kong daughters were more likely to maintain a full work schedule in addition to their family commitments, enduring greater stress.

Because family was still important to these daughters, effort was made to incorporate traditional cultural practices into their modern lifestyles. However, nearly all of them said they did not believe the next generation would observe the same core values. Some in Hong Kong and Singapore described Generation Y as being self-centred and selfish, lacking respect and valuing money over family. According to them, the younger generation was more apt to ask what others would do for them than the reverse. Virtually none of the daughters interviewed for this book expected their children to care for them in old age, and they worried that it would be more difficult for parents in the future to transmit family values to their children.

The interaction between the values transmitted to the daughters and the practicalities of the world in which they lived produced an eccentric reinterpretation of traditional Chinese ideology. The old values were still present and always in the background. The daughters conveyed that they saw them in their parents and they understood the culture of their ancestors. The new values were observed in their children and the world around them. These women knew they were navigating between norms. They said so; and they knew why. The stories they told suggested that although they have remained committed to family, education and employment have given them new opportunities, freedom and independence. They strongly related that they were unwilling to give up either one.

This is the foundation for the discussion comprising the remainder of this book: why these daughters were still willing to care for their elderly parents despite the demands of their busy lives; what they were willing to do; and at what point, if any, it might all be too much.

Introduction to the Typology of Support and Care

The word 'caregiving' has routinely been used to describe the combined social and cultural practices in which one person provides help to another who is in need. However, within the overarching framework of culturally defined intergenerational exchanges, its abstruse and complex nature has defied a 'one size fits all' approach even to describe the small number of interactions taking place in this book. From the process of interviewing the daughters and analysing the stories they told, it was clear that 'caregiving' meant different things depending on how filial obligation was interpreted in light of contemporary cultural norms. For example, for some caregiving was understood as face-to-face or telephone conversations between children and parents or in-laws (hereinafter referred to collectively as 'parents' unless otherwise designated) or providing parents with financial support. Others said caregiving involved sacrifice during times of emergencies. Caregiving was often defined in terms of emotional or instrumental support over the long-term. However, hiring a domestic helper (FDH/CDH) to care for a parent or even institutionalising a parent in a nursing home could satisfy one's filial caregiving obligation if the circumstances prescribed it. Whether support was emotional, financial, instrumental or a combination of all three, the opinions were diverse, and the transitional nature of the two generations of women in this book no doubt contributed to the lack of consensus.

Yet despite the multiplicity of opinions and practices reflected in the daughters' narratives, patterns did emerge, making it possible to characterise the network of filial attitudes and behaviour emerging from the interviews. The patterns can be grouped into four distinct types or stages of filial obligation: *support, temporary care, caregiving* and *outsourced care.* Their sequence is shown below in Fig. 4.1, reflecting the increasing intensity of support and care offered to elderly parents: from support provided to younger healthier parents to emergencies and temporary care and then hands-on long-term care at home for elderly and disabled parents. The first three stages of the typology investigate support and care from the

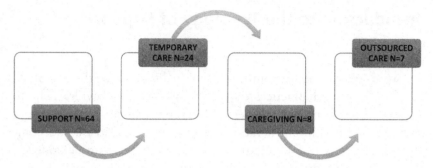

Fig. 4.1 The typology of support and care and number of daughters providing support or caregiving at each stage

daughters' perspective. The fourth stage, outsourced care, takes a broader approach, examining the implications of employing domestic helpers as surrogate caregivers in addition to institutionalising parents and in-laws. Together these four stages or types comprise the typology of support and care emerging from the interviews with the 64 women in the main sample.

As seen in Fig. 4.1, all of the daughters are included at the first stage of the typology. However, as support transitions into temporary care and then caregiving and outsourced care, the number currently providing care, or who have provided care, grows smaller. Part of the reason for this is most likely because when parents progress from overall youth, independence and good health at the support stage into requiring more time and attention, daughters may be less willing or unable to provide it, driven by their changing roles, reinterpretation of traditional Chinese cultural norms or circumstances.

It is the purpose of this chapter to establish the *framework* within which to understand and explain: (1) the characteristics of each stage of the typology; (2) the differences between each stage of the typology; (3) the motivations behind support and caregiving at each stage of the typology; (4) how tensions and conflicts involved in discharging support and care are resolved at each stage of the typology; and (5) what happens when contemporary Chinese daughters are unwilling or unable to provide care at the end of the typology.

Explaining the Stages of the Typology Through the Accounts of Chinese Daughters and Their Domestic Helpers

Having established the stages of support and care and their place within the typology, the daughters' own accounts help to define and explain each of them. Throughout this and subsequent chapters, statements are quoted and short stories are told to annotate specific points. Longer narratives, tied to the typology, provide deeper understanding of the topics under investigation and are also used to gain insight into the attitudes and behaviour of the individual Chinese daughters.

Moving through the typology it is important to remember that the narratives and comments of the daughters only represent a snapshot in time. Unlike a longitudinal study, the typology does not follow the progression of the daughters from one stage of care to another, but rather, portrays the current and previous experiences of the respondents at a given point in time and stage of support or care.

Support

As will be noted, at the first stage of the typology, the word 'care' does not appear. Although the daughters consistently referred to their activities and exchanges with healthy parents as 'care', or 'caregiving' the word 'support' better describes their behaviour. At this level, the parents for the most part lived alone, sometimes with a domestic helper and did not require assistance with the activities of daily living (ADLs). A complete list of the support provided to parents by their daughters appears below in Table 4.1.

The investment of time and effort required at this stage of the typology was unlikely to substantially interfere with the daughter's day-to-day life. Thus, it should not be surprising that every daughter in this study provided at least one form of support to a parent at some time in her adult life. By far the most common forms of support were visiting or having meals with parents, speaking on the telephone and providing financial assistance. Among the daughters who had living parents at the time of their interview, 83% of those from Hong Kong, 78% from Singapore and

Table 4.1 Support activities provided to healthier parents

Financial assistance 1× a month +	Supervising parents' medications
Regular telephone calls, as often as 1× a week +	Renovating parent's home to make elder friendly
Visiting regularly, as often as 1× a week +	Driving parents to medical appointments
Living in same household, assisting w/chores + some meals together	Hiring FDH to live w/parents in their own home
Assisting w/banking, grocery shopping, errands	Supervising FDH caring for parents in their own home
Taking trips	Organising siblings to help w/parents
Regular meals together, as often as 1× a week +	

44% from the mainland visited or dined with their family at least once a week. The lower percentage of face to face contact by mainland daughters can be explained by the greater distances between theirs' and their parents' homes. In Hong Kong and Singapore, 72% and 96% respectively provided monetary support at least once a month. Mainland daughters made financial contributions on birthdays, holidays or when needed (e.g., house repairs). They pointed out that their parents had pensions or other children to help with their support, or that their parents were still working and did not need the money. In all three locations, if daughters were living with their parents, they paid the household expenses.

Huizhong, a Singaporean Baby Boomer, explained the support she provided. Other daughters were similar:

> On a weekday…I will go and visit my mother first and normally we will talk, sometimes watch TV… From there, I will… either…go home or … drop by my mother-in-law's place…. Then on a weekend, I will have [a] meal with my mother. (Huizhong)

Very often weekend meals were family affairs, as Meili, a Hong Kong Baby Boomer described:

> Nearly every week my family will…take a tea together…I only [go] about [every] two [weeks] because [it] always is a dinner or lunch….and then sometimes [we] go somewhere. But…every week [we] can have a gathering. (Meili)

Visits and meals were supplemented by regular telephone contact, particularly with one's own parents. This was viewed by the daughters as emotional support, as seen from Xiaoli:

> I call them more often than before.... Because they do not have more energy to make friends, to talk with others, to do a lot of things. They just sometimes stay home alone. So, I think they need more persons to care, and the government cannot do the thing [provide emotional support]. (Xiaoli, mainland Gen X)

Monetary subsidies most often came from the daughter's pay cheque, not her husband's (if she was married). Like the mainland, in Hong Kong and Singapore support could be enhanced by donations from other siblings, and additional financial contributions were provided during festivals and birthdays or depended on circumstances and need.

Based on what the daughters said, the types of support were linked to the decline of intergenerational households, the number of these women who were working and the geographic distances separating family members. As other research has found, the high percentage of financial contributions suggest it might have been a substitute for the regular interaction of living together (Lin Yi 2011) combined with the high cost of living, particularly in Hong Kong and Singapore. Likewise, family meals were a way of maintaining closeness not only among parents and children but also among siblings.

Temporary Care

Temporary care is the second stage of the typology. It refers to situations, in this case lasting six months or less, in which there is a family crisis or emergency involving a parent. A parent may suddenly be taken ill, have some temporary cognitive impairment or be in an accident. In such a case, he or she may be hospitalised or at some point returned to his/her own home or to one of the children's homes to recuperate. The emphasis at this stage is on the transitory nature of care, although it can also be intense. The variation in intensity is attributed to the type of illness, the size of the family and the number of those able or willing to help, in addition to the employment status of the primary caregiver and the length of care.

Homecare among these daughters was not shared with siblings. Based on the circumstances, most often the families made a collective decision regarding the location where care was to be administered and the designation of the caregiver. Alternatively, some daughters voluntarily took it upon themselves to provide temporary care for reasons that are discussed in Chap. 6. Among the women interviewed, it was always the daughter or daughter-in-law, not the son administering temporary care.

Whether the parent was hospitalised or at home, that person's care and recuperation was the principle goal of the family, and during these times, the daughter's life revolved entirely around the needs of the family. Te', a 34-year-old Singaporean, for example, related how some years ago, her father had a mental breakdown lasting two months. Recalling the incident and its aftermath, she described how the 'family was in…chaos' and she did not have 'a lot of time to think'. She had to visit her father at the hospital, regularly interface with the doctors, control her mother who was depressed and threatening to commit suicide and manage her brother who 'didn't handle it very well because he couldn't accept it'. She added that her brother suggested they 'send the father to an old folks' home and just leave him there'. Te' wound up having to take a month off from her job to oversee all of this.

Unlike Te', Yan, a 50-year-old woman from Kunming, was unable to take time off work when her mother was hospitalised with an illness. Remembering how exhausted she was, Yan noted how she and her sister, together with Yan's housekeeper, took shifts at the hospital, while Yan's husband cooked the meals she brought there. For four months Yan spent Monday through Friday mornings with her mother, then worked in the afternoons and evenings, often 8 to 10 hours. Some nights she slept at the hospital. When her sister took over on the weekends, Yan caught up on work. Recalling this time, her only comment was that she was, 'very, very tired', and it was 'very, very hard'.

Te's and Yan's responses to their family crises were similar to other daughters' management styles in family emergencies. Aside from duty, love and gratitude, these women were trained from childhood to be

Table 4.2 Activities of temporary care

Temporary care in hospital	Temporary care in home
Preparing & bringing food for parent to eat in hospital, feeding parent	Respondent living in parent's home during parent's recovery- providing hands- on care
Visiting parent in hospital or nursing home every day, all day or several times a day-even if working	Parent living in respondent's home during recovery- respondent providing hands-on care
Sometimes more than one parent in hospital at a time – may have to shuttle between hospitals	Respondent living in parent's home during parent's recovery – supervising and assisting FDH who provides hands-on care
Interfacing with medical staff	Parent living in respondent's home during recovery – FDH providing hands-on care with supervision and assistance from respondent
Taking charge of care and medical decision making	Driving parent to and from hospital & Doctor's office for follow up
Cleaning and massaging parent	Supervising and paying for medications
Pay for hospital, doctors and medications	Cook parent's favourite foods or supervise FDH to do it
Drive other parent to hospital	Support other parent and siblings emotionally; if final illness, prepare for death
Donate blood	Dealing with parent's demands and bad temper
	Rush to hospital if parent relapses

responsible. As adults, they were disciplined, restrained and authoritative. Moreover, as Te' demonstrated, they frequently held the family together.

In addition to assuming command, other tasks undertaken by the daughters while providing temporary care are shown in Table 4.2.

Caregiving

The third stage of the typology is caregiving. Within the typology, caregiving is defined as hands-on instrumental care provided over an extended period of time (>6 months) in one's own home where both the caregiver

Table 4.3 Activities of caregiving

Hands-on care of parent in one's own home, with or without a helper
Assist with dressing, feeding, transferring, bathing, washing of parent
Housework, meal preparation, grocery shopping
Manage medications
Toileting, diaper changing, body and home clean-up following incontinence accidents
Spending time together, e.g., watching TV
Deal with erratic and aggressive behaviour
Train and communicate with the domestic helper
Intervene, arbitrate between the domestic helper and the parent
Substitute for the domestic helper on her day off
Take to day-care centre [the domestic helper remains with the parent]
Renovate house to accommodate parents' disabilities
Manage parents' money

and care recipient reside. Daughters provide care alone or with the assistance of a domestic helper, with caregiving incorporating the management of all collateral emotional and financial needs of the care recipient. *The emphasis in this third stage of the typology is on the daughter.* What motivates her to provide caregiving; how caregiving affects her; and how she manages it.

The activities of the caregiving daughters interviewed for this book are shown in Table 4.3. Among the eight daughters who were self-described caregivers, six had domestic helpers who were the primary caregivers of parents in the daughter's home.

Niu's situation provides a glimpse into the nature of caregiving and how it changes. Both Niu, and her sister were unmarried and had lived with their family their entire lives. Since their father had died approximately ten years prior to her interview, Niu and her sister had cared for their mother, whose dementia had progressively grown worse. During this time both sisters continued to work outside the home.

In the early stages of their mother's dementia, care was minimal. The mother attended day-care three days a week, with Niu accompanying her in the morning and Niu's sister picking her up in the afternoon. Niu's sister did the weekday cooking and washing and stayed home with her mother on the days she did not attend day-care. Niu did the cooking on weekends and the ironing. Eventually they hired a part time FDH to clean the house three days a week.

Eleven months before Niu's interview the sisters employed a full time FDH. She helped with food preparation and ensured their mother ate while the sisters were at work. She cleaned the house and did the laundry. Niu described how the FDH cared for her mother:

> She helps...with showering, because the fact is she can't [do it herself]. [She] makes sure that she [is] dressed up...The doctor told us: let her do as many things as possible on her own.... The maid will be her bodyguard to make sure that she doesn't trip and fall down. So the maid will be watching her. (Niu)

Niu's mother's condition had recently deteriorated, requiring all three women to bathe her and change her diapers. The mother had begun to repeat herself, which Niu said she found irritating. Niu described the care of her mother as a team effort, which for the time being would continue in the home. However, given that the mother's condition was deteriorating, new choices would have to be made between discontinuing full time employment or institutionalising their mother. This is a dilemma that will almost certainly face Chinese daughters in the future, if they choose not to marry and remain at home as the primary providers of financial, instrumental and emotional support to ageing parents, or more importantly, if they are the only child.

Outsourced Care

When caregiving becomes too difficult or impossible or a daughter does not want to do it, either initially or following a term as a caregiver, it has become culturally acceptable to hire a domestic helper. The helper then assumes the instrumental aspects of the daughter's filial obligation. If at some point the helper becomes inadequate, a growing option is to institutionalise the parent. *In this fourth and final stage of the typology the emphasis is on the domestic helper*, and specifically the foreign domestic helper (FDH).

Seven daughters included in this stage of the typology institutionalised a parent, and while the parent was in the nursing home or hospital continued to provide care for him or her, either alone or with assistance from a domestic helper. Three of these women also provided caregiving at home prior to institutionalising their parent and are included in the third stage of the typology.

From the interviews with the daughters and the FDHs, one can see certain patterns emerging once a helper becomes involved with parent care. In Chap. 8, this behaviour is explored in detail. Here, the activities of Lola, a caregiving FDH are briefly described to illustrate outsourced care and its effect on the parent-daughter relationship.

At the time of her interview, Lola was a 53-year-old Filipina who had worked for three Hong Kong families over 19 years. In her second family, she cared for the daughter's mother in the family home, sleeping in the same room with her. Lola bathed, dressed and changed the grandmother's urine catheter, administered her medications, took her blood pressure, and massaged her legs during the night, interrupting her own sleep. She stated that the daughter checked on her mother for 10 minutes in the morning before leaving for work. Upon returning from work at 19:00 the daughter retreated to her bedroom until dinner. The entire family dined together, but after dinner each retired to their own room. On Sunday the family, including the grandmother, went out for lunch.

In Lola's third family, the daughter also worked. Initially, the grandmother, who had mild dementia, lived alone and Lola cleaned her house once a week. Later, when she became ill, for several months Lola arrived at her home at 9:00 and spent all day with her. She assisted with bathing, toileting, grooming, transfers and walking; she cooked, cleaned, watched television with the grandmother, then put her to bed before walking back to her employer's home around 20:00. In the beginning, Lola's employer, the daughter, visited her mother for an hour a week. This changed to 30–60 minutes twice a week after the grandmother became ill, according to Lola.

Lola reported that the grandmother was very unhappy and angry. She told Lola that she could not understand why her daughter would not take care of her. Lola recalled how the grandmother cried every day and said about her daughter that it was 'always money'. She told Lola 'you are good, you take care of me…my own daughter did not take care of me'… 'My daughter is no good'.

Table 4.4 Elements of outsourced care

Issues between respondents and domestic helpers
Domestic helper doing emotion work
Helper's relationship and caregiving activities with respondent's parents
Daughter assistance with institutionalised parent, including food preparation and feeding
If more than one party institutionalised, daughter and/or helper may shuttle between them
Effect of a domestic helper on the daughter-parent relationship

The grandmother was eventually institutionalised. For the first year, Lola brought her food and visited her at least once a week. The daughter, prohibited her from going more often because the grandmother would ask to be brought home. At first the daughter visited once or twice a week on her way to work, however, these visitations eventually dwindled to once a month, with Lola accompanying her to the nursing home. Eventually, the family moved to the United States, leaving the grandmother in the nursing home in Hong Kong, and Lola's employment was terminated. The elements of outsourced care are shown in Table 4.4.

Explaining the Key Analytic Categories Driving Support and Care Through the Daughters' Own Stories

Establishing a typology through stages or types of support and care helps us understand how it changes as parental health gradually deteriorates. However, alone it cannot answer the research questions proposed in the first chapter. In Chap. 3, a review of the theoretical and conceptual norms appearing in the contemporary caregiving literature generated three broad analytical categories for the purpose of explaining *why* the Chinese daughters in this study provided support and care to their parents ['*I have to/I want to*'], *how* they managed conflict and tension in the process of providing support and care ['*I should want to*'] and *why* they might have declined to undertake or discontinue the filial practices embedded in their culture ['*I do not want to/I cannot*']. The reader will recall it as follows:

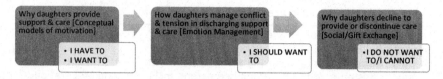

Image representing the three analytical categories

In this section, the daughters' own narratives illustrate each of the analytical categories. While following the narratives presented in this chapter and throughout the remainder of the book, it should be kept in mind that the daughters were not asked to break down their motivations and coping strategies by categories or stages. The typology was developed later, during the analysis of the interview data. In their interviews, the daughters were invited to discuss their motivations and coping strategies at length. In most cases these were complex. However, the analysis revealed that at each stage of the typology, common elements of normative motivation and coping strategies were present.

Structural and Relational Filial Norms of Motivation

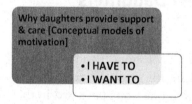

Image of structural/relational model of motivation

Structural Motivation ['I have to']

Bo, the eldest of three daughters, did not recall her childhood enthusiastically. Among other things, for six years her nuclear family shared their home with a maternal aunt and her family. Bo and her sisters were compared unfavourably with their male cousin and blamed when something went wrong. She said this went 'into my heart subtly', making her feel inferior, and she felt betrayed by her mother for not protecting her. Bo also perceived her mother's preferential treatment of her youngest sister and said it challenged her self-worth. Her strongest complaint, however, was her mother's neglect of the nuclear family. According to Bo, her mother spent more time with her own siblings and social circle than with her husband and daughters. Watching her father struggle to support the family while her mother socialised created 'a lot of grievances' in Bo. She expounded, 'I dislike my mom [because] she cares for herself too much'. Offering several examples, Bo concluded that her mother was irresponsible.

Bo did not feel loved by her mother, but she did by her father. She remembered when he gave her all his savings for a trip to America, even though he had never taken a plane trip himself. Bo's father had died, but during his lifetime they were close. She admired him for 'working hard and never giving up'. He was also a strong influence on moulding her values, teaching her honesty, integrity and virtue through his own example. She related this story:

> My father…was taken care of by a relative even though I know that he was ill treated by [her]…. That relative [lived] in Macao and she eventually got the stroke. …Every few months my father will bring me to go to that old lady … Even though that lady…didn't treat him well…he said…she gave me a shelter to stay. So, I have to pay [her] back. I think for [an] entire ten years he kept on travelling to Macao to visit that lady. Even the children of that lady didn't take care of her. But, my father will visit [her] very frequently. (Bo)

During her interview, Bo maintained, the relationship with her mother was still 'very distant', although she claimed since her father's death she had 'more sympathetic feelings' towards her. She attributed the mitigation of her animosity to a number of factors, including her mother's grief over her father's death and her help with Bo's children.

Bo explained that she and her sisters dined with their mother every two weeks and supplemented their mother's income. Bo did this 'because of [the] family value', which she defined as duty learned from her father.

She said she wanted to follow her father's example, and did so for her mother, but she added that it was 'more like a duty, rather than love', ingrained from birth: 'I think it's a duty, yeah…definitely it is a duty'. When she envisioned what could lie ahead she used 'rationality to overcome her [negative] feelings' toward her duty:

> I will try to make a meaning of fulfilling this duty. And, make myself feel comfortable and at ease with my decision. I will definitely think that this is something not enjoyable. But, when you do some tough job as a duty, and if you…fulfil your duty, then I will console myself by saying oh, you really do a good job, and that sort of satisfaction can compensate the stress, the burden, caused by the caregiving. (Bo)

Relational Motivation ['I want to']

From the beginning of her interview, Chunhua remarked that she had always felt 'a lot of love from our parents'. Growing up in Kunming as the oldest of five children, she remarked that her family had always been close and her parents were very kind. Describing them, she said:

> They really love us. They care about us. So, even until today we are still very close, and actually we almost get together once a month, my brothers, my sisters and my parents. We always try to find some time… and very often we go back to my parents' home to eat together. (Chunhua)

Chunhua recalled how, when she was a child, her family 'did not have much money to go to the theatre or to have a lot of entertainment', so her father played his musical instrument while the children sat together, sang, danced and laughed. She added that, 'actually it was quite unforgettable in my memory'. She also reported that her father 'worked very hard to support us', and how even on a tight budget, her parents supported her dreams. As she described it:

> Actually, in such a big family, if I choose to take some vocational training I would work earlier and ease the family burden. But, because I was doing very good at school…my parents really supported me to fulfil my dreams so I could go to university to finish my education. (Chunhua)

Chunhua was grateful for her education, and was also grateful to her parents for guiding her 'to be a good person'. She said she learned from her parents' example and by watching them, and remarked how her parents' 'attitude and behaviour' influenced her.

When I asked Chunhua if she also felt a duty to her parents, she replied that she did not see it 'as a duty but it's really kind of love'. She went on to explain how duty grows out of love and gratitude. In her words, 'it's difficult to really separate because you know this kind of love is accumulated'. She then elaborated on her experience with her parents and why she loved them:

> Since we were young, they always encourage us, especially [when] you have a challenge you have struggling; So, whenever we have this kind of thing, they try to understand, and also try to support as much as they can to accompany us through that period. Sometimes you know, they can't do much. But, that kind of support, you still feel the warmth. (Chunhua)

Chunhua reported that her parents continued to help all of their children, even in the latter's adulthood, thereby prolonging the unity of a still close family. On her part, it was important to Chunhua 'to improve the quality of [her parents'] life'. Besides eating and spending time together, maintaining telephone contact and traveling, she explained that she and her brother and sisters, were already planning for their parents old age. In her words, 'we know there will be a time coming they will not be able to take care of themselves'. According to her, she and her siblings would do 'whatever we can to support them'.

Combined Motivation [Structural and Relational] Norms of Filial Obligation ['I have to and I want to']

Huiqing was the oldest child in her family and had six siblings. Speaking about her parents, she explained that, 'I wasn't close to anyone of them.... They had so many children to look after.... Mom was always busy doing housework, busy just taking care of our physical needs and then, if not, she will be working with my dad in the shop'. According to Huiqing, her parents did not 'sit us down and explain things to us'. Rather, a 'whole package' of Chinese values was learned by 'just watching them, how they looked after their own parents... and how they... also looked after...the siblings and their families...so that was more modelling, rather than teaching'.

Huiqing described her father as a violent, angry man who verbally abused his wife and physically abused his children. Her mother was portrayed as emotionally inaccessible and unsupportive. Nonetheless, although she was not close to her parents and 'didn't like the way my parents raised me', Huiqing said they had fulfilled their obligations to her and she was grateful, particularly for her education. These mixed feelings manifested in combined structural and relational motivation for providing support and care. When asked about this, Huiqing first replied that she wanted to repay her parents for meeting her physical needs and educating her, which was 'more duty than love'. Of her father, she said he 'did so much for me, it's the least I can do for him'. Later this was amended to: 'With my dad it was more duty. With my mom *now* it's more love'.

Huiqing had not tested her feelings for her mother, but she had for her father. In carrying out her duty during the last three months of his life, she took him to the hospital nearly every day. Huiqing related, 'the emotional part was just killing me'. Her father's difficult behaviour got on her nerves and she was angry. She said she internalised everything. Although she had been through assertiveness training, she 'couldn't confront the issues with my dad at all'. She had 'mini-explosions...whenever there was just a little bit of pressure', but never at him. She said she felt guilty over her anger and prayed that God would take it away. She cried a lot, and when she went home to her nuclear family she said she 'got quite hysterical in front of my husband'.

Huiqing's conflicted emotional state and mixed motivations are common, and instructive. Core ideological elements of obedience and respect, plus the 'moral values' of integrity and responsibility were inculcated and internalised at an early age for redemption later on. Gratitude for the economic investment made in Huiqing's education was also internalised. Internalised commitment and a sense of obligation to parents can drive adult children to fulfil their duty to meet parents' needs regardless of whether the relationship is strong or strained (Silverstein et al. 2012). However, note how much stress Huiqing experienced during her father's last illness. The other interesting part of this was the apparent need to bring love into the motivation to care for her mother. This is discussed in Chap. 5.

Managing Tension and Conflict in the Discharge of Filial Obligation

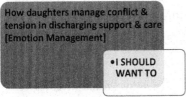

Image of managing conflict and tension (emotion work)

Emotion Work

Qingzhao was the oldest child in what she characterised as a 'not so traditional' matriarchal family with two working parents, a sister and three brothers. She described her mother as an angry, violent woman and her parents as always quarrelling. According to her, the children were verbally abused and beaten. Qingzhao was afraid of her mother and said she emerged from childhood with a strong sense of moral integrity and obedience, but nothing else.

At the time of her interview, Qingzhao's father had died and her mother lived alone. Qingzhao contributed financially to her mother and joined her family for lunch every Sunday. She related how 'wonderful' it was to spend time with her brothers and sisters. However, when her mother was mentioned she remarked, 'I really don't want to see her much. I don't enjoy'. When asked why she talked to her at all, Qingzhao responded: 'Because it's my duty'.

Although Qingzhao's duty did not extend beyond financial support and family meals she had difficulty even with that. However, because her interpretation of filial obligation [framing rule] required her to maintain contact with her mother, Qingzhao's assessment of what she *should* feel during this situation [feeling rule] prescribed that she find a way to do it with love. This was a 'moral imperative' she had given herself. Nonetheless, the gap between her feelings and her attempt at emotion work were evident when she said: 'My heart is so confused. That's why... I'm trying to make clear ... how she bring me up and... what happened between me and her'.

Qingzhao shared how she evoked positive feelings by reminding herself that her mother 'give birth of me and she really bring me up and educate me'. She reported how she tried to manipulate her feelings through exhortation: 'I have to do something as a return for what she has done to me'. However, this was not enough, so Qingzhao explained how she invoked a rule reminder:

> I just wonder what [will] happen if she just pass away. Would I feel regret much or [would] I feel happy? I just wonder. So every time I think what [might] happen...I have to [ask, should I give myself]...the chance to love her, to forgive her at [that] moment or not? Or after she died I regret, regret, regret. So that you know is a lot of troubles here inside my heart. (Qingzhao)

Qingzhao tried deep acting, attempting to evoke memories with warm feelings that were no longer present. She said:

> When I [am] in bed...sometimes I try to find out how my mother loves me; how she take care of me when I was a teenager...And, I find the memories, and she [was] really good sometimes. She give me money to study outside for the secondary education other than only in the school and she make me beautiful dresses and she sometimes bought me shoes and bought me rings to put on. And she's good. But I don't know, sometimes she's so bad tempered. (Qingzhao)

She noted how she drew on another rule reminder to examine the appropriateness of her feelings: sibling approval.

> My brothers and sister will see that I'm still a child of my mother and I have to do what they do to my mother. (Qingzhao)

Qingzhao claimed that as part of 'Chinese tradition' she instructed (exhorted) herself 'to play my role to love the family', including trying 'very hard to love my mother'. She said if she was unable to genuinely change her feelings, she *should* at least attempt to change her display to appear to feel what she did not. When she spoke about the recent encounters she had with her mother Qingzhao remarked: 'Whatever she say, I say ok, ok, ok...I just ask, [do] you want tea, [are] you hungry, [are] you cold? What do you want?' If her mother yelled at her in response, Qingzhao said she walked away; 'Or I just keep my mouth shut'. This is surface acting, what Hochschild (1983: 33) described as deceiving others about what we really feel, but not deceiving ourselves.

Qingzhao exclaimed that she could not envision a situation in which her mother would push her so far that she would terminate their relationship. However, her anger appeared very close to the surface, and never seemed to dissipate. Moreover, Qingzhao imposed limits on what she was willing to do for her mother. Projecting to a time when her mother might become disabled she said she would not be her mother's caregiver or invite her mother to live with her. She explained, 'I think maybe we [will] find a helper and stay at her place and I'll go visiting her' or 'maybe... put her in some elderly house.... But we have to talk first. Yeah. We brothers and sisters must talk. It must be a group decision'.

Declining to Provide Support and Care

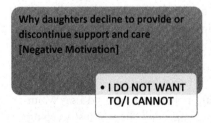

Image of negative model of motivation

Negative Relational Motivation

Sheu-Fuh's parents divorced when she was ten. She had not seen her father since. Her mother had recently died, however, prior to that, from the time she was a small child, Sheu-Fuh said her mother had abused her. She described the beatings she had received three to four times a week:

> It can be she could be using bamboo. She could be using [a] hangar. She could be using [a] belt. She could be using twelve canes tied together.... I remember this terrible incident...when I was in primary four, that's probably about 11 years old, when she would make me take off all my clothes and tie me to a chair and she would just cane me. (Sheu-Fuh)

The offences for which she was punished were minor, according to Sheu-Fuh. In her words, 'Maybe I cooked the wrong thing or I cooked it the wrong way or I just didn't clean a thing properly'. She remembered: 'Every day to me is like hell. Every day is like, is this going to be my last day?' She was afraid her mother was going to kill her, so when she was 14 she ran away and went to the police. She was 'back home by the very next day because nobody believed my story'. After a second unsuccessful attempt to flee some years later, when she was 20, Sheu-Fuh ran away for good. This time she had support from her school and eventually the authorities. She was legally emancipated.

Despite the beatings, Sheu-Fuh said she respected her mother as a filial child, but that she had only allowed herself to feel this after her mother's death. In her view, her mother had not fulfilled her obligations to her in any respect. After stating that she had been 'too scared to go near her' during her lifetime, she recounted the one and only time she had reached out to mother following her emancipation. She had learned that her mother was dying of cancer, and she called her. During that call Sheu-Fuh said:

> Mom...I know about your cancer...I am praying for you and I say Mom I'm sorry, you know. And, she started crying...and she was just weeping over the phone. ...She cried and she cried and she cried...I was just listening to her and after what seems like a long time I just say Mom, you know, trust God, you know. Just believe in God. And, I'm praying for you. (Sheu-Fuh)

Sheu-Fuh's mother asked for her forgiveness, an act that Sheu-Fuh said liberated her and caused her to 'embrace life'. However, she could not motivate herself to do more. Five months after this she again felt compelled to do something. However, she said: 'I just didn't want to because I was afraid that the moment I get in that house… something might happen to me… and I can't leave'.

Sheu-Fuh is an example of negative motivation. However, the analytical category described as '*I do not want to/I cannot*' has a broader meaning, which includes inability and unbalanced exchange. This is discussed in greater detail later.

Integrating the Typology of Support and Care™ and the Analytic Categories

Having established the typology of support and care and explained the analytic categories through the daughters interviewed for this book, it is now possible to show how the typology and the analytic categories are integrated to facilitate the investigation of the research questions.

As is apparent in Fig. 4.2, in the first three stages of the typology (support, temporary care, caregiving), all of the analytic categories are implicated in support and care. This is not true of the final stage (outsourced care), in which the daughters' motivation is no longer relevant beyond their reasons for discontinuing care and the post-care exchanges between the daughters, their parents and their domestic helpers.

In the following four chapters, the stages of support and care are investigated through the typology's framework as set forth in Fig. 4.2 above. At the end of this, the research questions are reviewed and answered.

Conclusion

The aim of this chapter was to explicate the structure through which the analysis of the interviews was conducted. To begin, context was provided to show the ways in which the daughters were in between traditional and contemporary norms. This was followed by an introduction to the typology of support and care.

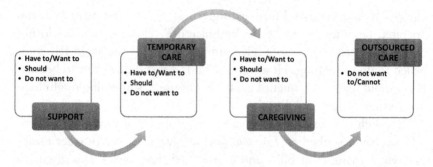

Fig. 4.2 Model showing the norms and mechanisms involved in the provision of support, caregiving, and outsourced care

The typology presented four types or stages: support (N = 64), temporary care (N = 24), caregiving (N = 8), and outsourced care (N = 7). Support required the least amount of time and effort from the daughters and consisted primarily of financial support and meals or telephone conversations with parents on a regular basis. Temporary care involved medical emergencies or circumstances in which a parent was briefly incapacitated and being cared for either at home or in the hospital for less than six months. Caregiving was interpreted as hands-on, long-term care in the home with or without assistance from a domestic helper. These first three stages of the typology focused on the daughters' motivations and how they discharged care. The fourth stage, outsourced care, expanded on the relevance of domestic helpers and explored nursing home care with or without assistance from a helper. At each stage of the typology examples were provided through reference to one or more of the daughters. As seen in Fig. 4.1, progressing through the typology, fewer daughters were engaged in support and care activities.

Once the typology was established, the conceptual and theoretical norms, previously organised into three broad analytical categories, were reintroduced. In Fig. 4.2, structural and relational norms of motivation showing why support and care were provided ['*I have to/I want to*']; coping strategies showing how tensions and conflict were managed in the discharge of care ['*I should want to*']; and negative motivation showing why some might have chosen not to provide care [*'I do not want to/I cannot'*] were integrated with each of the stages of support and care throughout the typology. In this way, a structure was created in which the research questions could be answered.

The actual accounts of the interviewed daughters were then presented to illustrate the key analytic categories. The first three narratives pertained to filial motivation: structural norms motivating support [*'I have to'*]; support motivated by relational norms of love and gratitude [*'I want to'*]; and structural and relational filial norms combined [*'I have to + I want to'*]. The fourth turned away from filial motivational norms to examine the tension and conflict involved in discharging filial obligation. One daughter's narrative illustrated how she used emotion work to bridge the gap between what she actually felt and what she believed she *should* feel to reduce tension and cope with her support situation [*'I should want to'*]. Finally, the fifth narrative returned to motivation, highlighting why negative motivation might result in the refusal of daughters to provide care [*'I do not want to/I cannot'*].

Each of the next four chapters is devoted to one stage of the typology. Chapter 5 considers support; Chap. 6 investigates temporary care; Chap. 7 probes caregiving; and Chap. 8 explores outsourced care. At every stage in the typology what has been learned from the literature is integrated with the conceptual and theoretical models, and the daughters' personal accounts, analysed in the context of contemporary norms and the changing roles and status of Chinese daughters.

Notes

1. The true names of the women in this book have been changed to protect their privacy. All of the names are fictitious.
2. Baby Boomers are generally characterized as those born between 1946 and 1964. Gen X generally refers to those born between 1965 and 1980.
3. In mainland China, some of the women said they lived with parents or in-laws during pregnancy or up to three years after a child was born so parents could provide child-care. When the child started kindergarten at age three, the daughters' nuclear family moved into their own home.

References

Hochschild, A. (1983, 2012). The managed heart: Commercialization of human feeling. Berkeley: University of California Press.

Lin, J.-P., & Yi, C.-C. (2011). Filial norms and intergenerational support to aging parents in China and Taiwan [special issue]. *International Journal of Social Welfare, 20*(Supp.s1), S109–S120.

Silverstein, M., Conroy, S. J., & Gans, D. (2012). Beyond solidarity, reciprocity and altruism: Moral capital as a unifying concept of intergenerational support for older people. *Ageing and Society, 32*(7), 1246–1262.

5

Support of Ageing Parents

Review of Support and Introduction to the Chapter

Support is the first stage of the typology, requiring the least investment of time, emotional resources, and instrumental help. Financial subsidies and companionship are the most common expressions of support, accompanied by the intermittent performance of commonplace tasks. All are undertaken for healthy parents and include meals, visits, phone calls, shopping, outings and vacations, supervision of domestic helpers and the occasional medical intervention (Table 4.1).

In this sample 64 daughters provided support to 156 support recipients. The comparison of parents and in-laws reveals a clear distinction in that 65% of support was provided to parents, 28% was provided to in-laws, and 7% to others.

The aim of this chapter is **to understand why daughters are willing or unwilling to offer support to parents who are able to take care of themselves, and to determine how they manage the difficulties encountered in doing so.** Relying on the interviews, the processes underlying motivation for support, limitations on the willingness to provide

© The Author(s) 2018
P. O'Neill, *Urban Chinese Daughters*, St Antony's Series,
https://doi.org/10.1007/978-981-10-8699-1_5

support and differences in the support provided are examined in the context of the changing roles and status of Chinese daughters and contemporary Chinese cultural norms.

The examples presented in the previous chapter, illustrate the three kinds of motivation emerging from the data and the literature: structural norms of filial obligation, ['*I have to*',] relational norms of affection, gratitude, and reciprocity ['*I want to*',] and combined structural and relational norms ['*I have to* + *I want to*']. These serve as departure points for discussing what is underpinning present day support motivation. In this chapter, narratives are further used as analytical tools to facilitate the identification and discussion of the research questions through a range of individuals and circumstances. Additionally, they allow us to highlight prominent themes emerging from the data.

How Structural and Relational Norms Are Motivating Filial Support Among Daughters

The breakdown of support motivation for parents and in-laws among the 156 support recipients is shown below in Table 5.1.

Among the 64 daughters providing support, the majority (43.5%) were motivated by structural norms of filial obligation followed by structural and relational norms of gratitude, affection and reciprocity combined (41.5%) and relational norms (15%) alone. Nine daughters cited religion as a reason for providing support, although always in conjunction with one of the three main analytical categories. Six daughters referred to lack of affection as a reason for not providing support.

Table 5.1 Motivation driving support for parents and in-laws

Motivation type	Mother	Father	Mother in law	Father in law	Other[a]	Total
Structural	12	14	26	14	2	68
Relational	14	8	0	0	1	23
Structural + relational	30	23	2	2	8	65
Total	56	45	28	16	11	156

[a]4 grandmothers, 4 aunts, 1 uncle, 2 adopted parents

Forces Underpinning Structural Filial Support Motivation

This section explores how structural norms are learned and internalised, how and why they have changed from the past, and why they are still driving support among these daughters.

Daughters Following Parental Role Modelling

Bo's outlook in the previous chapter was an example of structural obligation (duty) in which she was compelled to follow her father's example, learned through role modelling. As she explained, 'Because he does it like this and I follow his example' (Bo).

Role modelling has been portrayed in the literature and among these daughters as a powerful tool for the transmission of filial obligation norms within Chinese communities. As Ning, a Hong Kong Baby Boomer, elaborated, 'they are taking care of their parents and when I look at them I will be seeing that this is the way that we will do.... Whatever they do I will be doing the same thing'.

Statements similar to Ning's such as, 'My mother...will never tell me.... But, I learn from her behaviour, how she takes care of her mother' (Yet Kwai) and, 'What my parents do, I do', (Ah Kum), were heard frequently in the interviews. As seen with Huiqing in Chap. 4, childhood conversations between the daughters and their parents could be sparse. Learning moral values through observation under such circumstances would have been essential.

Today dual working parents, universal compulsory education, declining intergenerational households and ubiquitous Internet and telephonic communication could be driving further change in the transmission of traditional values. Because there is wider access to information and less time spent interacting with parents, some scholars have observed that the importance of the family, as the vehicle for the transmission of values, has been diminishing. The daughters also projected that it would be more difficult to educate children at home in the future.

Gender Specific Taught Responsibility

Unlike their male siblings, the daughters interviewed for this book were often taught to undertake gender specific tasks when they were barely toddlers. Because their mothers were busy and many families were still large, as youngsters these women learned to multitask. They helped with domestic chores, worked in the family business, ran errands, and supervised their siblings outside the home. Bo, for example, said she did housework and was required to watch over her sisters during school recess. Daughters, especially if they were the oldest, also tutored younger siblings because some parents were not sufficiently educated to do so. All the while, these girls imposed the obligation on themselves to do well in school.

The imposition of these multiple obligations on young female family members could effectively cultivate in them a predisposition to internalise duty, responsibility and gender specific behaviour, especially with respect to their parents and siblings. The young daughter became a substitute for or an assistant to her mother, understanding her subservient role in relationship to the male members of the household. Lihua, a Hong Kong Baby Boomer, was brought up in this manner and offered a glimpse into how it influenced her belief system:

> Girls...need to work hard and...do everything in the family.... I [will] give you an example. If...my father and the sons...go for [a] movie...the girls ...will stay home taking care of other things....and [when they come] home after the movie they [will] need to have some delicious food for entertainment [which] you need to prepare. (Lihua)

When asked how she felt about the gender division within her family, Lihua replied, 'If you find there is no...difference than the others next door... you feel it's alright'.

The Importance of Domestic Helpers to Sustaining Traditional Gender Roles

As Lihua's situation showed, just as it existed in childhood, gender stereotyping carried over into adulthood for many of the daughters. They were neither relieved of domestic responsibilities, nor expected to be relieved, even though many had become working professionals. Most of the daughters claimed their husbands declined to help with housework, cooking or caring for children.

Meeting the demands of these assorted commitments has produced important normative change in Singapore and Hong Kong, where the employment of foreign domestic helpers (FDHs) in the home has become the single most important factor keeping women in the workplace. Over half the Hong Kong and Singapore daughters interviewed for this book employed FDHs and those who did not expected to. This was slightly different in Kunming, where domestic helpers were neither commonplace nor foreign. As Yuet, a Kunming, Gen X explained, FDHs were more likely to be found in the tier one cities such as Shanghai and Beijing, especially among the wealthy. In the smaller cities, helpers who were not family members were mostly uneducated Chinese women from the rural areas (CDHs), and even then language could be a barrier to employment:

> Most of the people here locally, unless they are educated they don't speak English at all. They speak a local dialect. They don't even speak Mandarin. (Yuet)

Additionally, in Kunming there was resistance to hiring helpers. Many of the daughters there said their parents did not want a 'stranger' living in their home. Luli, a Kunming Gen X, explained:

> I don't think my parents would support this kind of idea. A lot of friends around me their parents don't like the so-called nursing worker. They think it's inconvenient as they're not familiar with each other. They may feel shy or timid when facing a stranger who takes care of you. (Luli)

Luli indicated, she would take care of her parents because that would make them feel more comfortable. Similar expressions were heard from most of the Kunming daughters. Otherwise, when a CDH was hired, there appeared to be a protocol. Wenling, a Gen X from Kunming, described how she understood the process:

If we need to look for a housekeeper, first we will choose the one we know something about this person's background. So, they will ask their friends or our not very remote relatives. Someone will recommend and it will be more safe for the family.... If we cannot find one we just go to the company. (Wenling)

In the future, dependence on domestic helpers is likely to grow if women continue to work. Especially in mainland China, recently coming out of 35 years of the One Child Policy, working women sandwiched between children and elderly parents may be unable to fulfil their obligations to both their family and employer without them.

Oral Transmission of Traditional Family Obligations

For centuries devotion to the family has been part of Chinese cultural ideology, tied to traditional notions of filial piety and Confucian values. Although the hierarchal system that gave rise to it might no longer exist, the importance of the family has remained intact. Regardless of the extent to which attitudes have been reframed to reflect the exigencies of contemporary life, in this group of Chinese women, traditional normative expectations regarding one's family obligations continued to be subtly transmitted through what might appear to be casual remarks, but which had deeper meanings. Lihwa, a Hong Kong Baby Boomer, provided an example of how this happened:

> You will listen to my grandmother saying…who is good to his grandmother, who is not good to his mother... his mother is so and so. And the son is so and so. You know this is [a] casual remark, [but] then you will know what she is expecting. (Lihwa)

Whether it was subtle or direct, the transmission of traditional Chinese values to these daughters from their parents was ubiquitous, regardless of where they lived or how old they were. Those who were the recipients of these messages often verbalised sentiments similar to Ai's, a Singaporean

Baby Boomer reflecting on how the importance of the family was transmitted to her:

> Essentially, when I was young we were always taught that family was the most important thing. And, I have always felt that basically…So, whatever we do, at least for me, they will always come first. (Ai)

The primacy of the family and how it has underpinned support motivation is illustrated by Huiliang, who said the obligation to put family first was 'ingrained in us when young'. She remarked, 'We just knew that we have people that we have to take care of' because this was 'passed down through the ages as an obligation…. It's something you have to do it, like it or not'.

As a young adult, Huiliang studied and then worked in Europe for several years. Her mother had died, and Huiliang was residing in France when she decided to go home to look after her father and grandmother. She said this decision 'was a big struggle' because 'obviously, I wanted to get on with my life', adding that 'I still look at it sometimes as a sacrifice… I gave up something because of this obligation'.

When Huiliang returned home and moved in with her grandmother and father, both were healthy and mobile, requiring no care. She indicated she could have sent money to fulfil the obligation to support them. She felt more was owed. Huiliang, however, was not immune from the influence of contemporary filial norms. Upon returning to Singapore, she hired an FDH to look after her family, went back to work and immediately began construction of her own home. Within three years she had moved out of her father's house, leaving the two older people with the FDH. When asked why, Huiliang responded that the nagging she received from the old folks upset her and she wanted to remove herself from a potential situation where she would raise her voice and later feel guilty.

Although Huiliang's 'ingrained' traditional duty to her family generated an expectation in her as to what her behaviour should be, the nature and extent of her duty was no longer automatically accepted. Rather, it was weighed against her own needs to achieve an acceptable balance. This is discussed in greater detail below.

Family Obligation Distinguished from Filial Piety

Although parental support has historically been linked to Confucianism and filial piety (Cook and Dong 2011) there is evidence to suggest that in the minds of some of the daughters, commitment to family might have been distinct from these ideologies. Ai explained:

> I don't think I do all this because I'm filial, to be very honest. That's why I don't put much weight in the word because to me it's worth nothing.... Some people just provide financial needs to their parents and nothing else. And, it is very often these days in Singapore we do that... So, to me what is it really to be filial? But, it's more important that they are my family and that's why I am doing what I'm doing. (Ai)

Huiliang's reasoning for returning to Singapore could be interpreted as familism rather than filial piety. Further support for this view can be seen in the comments of Weici, a Singaporean Gen X:

> So, maybe it's not a filial piety anymore, it's more like, where [are] all [the] responsibilities now that...they don't have this Confucianist thing?... We are all cremated anyway, so nowadays there is no need to clean [the] gravestone so the filial piety part is not even physically possible anymore. (Weici)

Finally, several Hong Kong and some mainland daughters, like Chunhua, did not know the terms filial piety or *xiao*.[1]

Structural Obligation Mediated by Contemporary Norms

Perhaps the perseverance of family obligation and traditional gender norms has been surprising, given the modern lifestyles of the women interviewed for this book. However, even though their beliefs had a foot in the past, these women also regarded themselves as being different from their mothers in both attitude and lifestyle:

I didn't want to live like my parents, you know, I wanted to be financially independent, I wanted to be sure that I can take care of myself. I didn't want to be dependent on anybody. (Huiliang)

We are also taught the old values because you know it is from my Mom's side and all that, and yet on the other hand, you get to also learn to think for yourself because of education. (Ai)

In the past, one of the historical justifications for son favouritism was that the son was expected to support the family financially when the parents became old. A daughter's value was derived from carrying out her husband's filial obligation, or if unmarried, caring for her natal family at home. In contemporary Asia, however, many Chinese daughters contribute financially to the family, the same as sons, and in some cases seen among these women, instead of sons:

[My parents] told me, I don't have [a] son, so you as my daughter and your sister, both of you have to take care of me when I'm old. (Ah Kum, Singapore Baby Boomer)

My brother [is] not taking care of my parents, so [it was] left to me.... So, I look at myself more like a man now. (Jaihui, Hong Kong, Gen X)

Yes, if I have two daughters, I must make a daughter to be a son. (Yan, Kunming Gen X)

In this critical way, the roles and status of daughters have changed, and their families have derived substantial economic benefits from it. Parents have acquired a potentially greater reservoir of long-term financial security and more resources to invest in their other children. The potential burden of supporting an unmarried adult daughter has also virtually disappeared. Yet even though they are generating stable incomes to be enjoyed by their parents rather than being financial liabilities, daughters are still obliged to be the providers of emotional and instrumental support to their parents. This is a net increase in their filial obligation. The only appreciable difference is that the obligation has shifted. All of the daughters in this book who were providing financial support, whether married or not, did so for their own parents, not their in-laws. Thus, the seminal question remains, why do daughters agree to take on so much responsibility?

Are the learned behaviours and inherited family obligations so strong among these women that filial beliefs are preserved despite conflicting evidence that the structural elements of filial piety are waning? Is commitment to the family so resolute that it supersedes competing demands on contemporary Chinese women's time and resources? Among these daughters, opinions varied, but most tried to find a balance. Consider the following comments by two Singaporeans, the first one a Baby Boomer and the second from Gen X:

> From my parents' generation, especially my mom, she live[s] for the family, whereas for me, yeah, I do care about the family but I also live for myself. (Huian)

> Family is important, but I think first and foremost it's self. Because, like I said, if you can't look after yourself, you can't look after anybody else. (Nuo)

Self-sufficiency has given modern Chinese daughters greater bargaining power, which has affected several aspects of family life, particularly marriage. The following statements are expository, made by a Hong Kong Baby Boomer, Hong Kong Gen X, and a Kunming Gen X daughter respectively:

> It's like we're going to hold out. If we don't get what we want then forget it. We don't care. (Tao)

> Maybe [you] cannot find the Mr Right.... You know [he is] very difficult to find and you know now you can earn the money. No need to get the money from other people. Like my mother. They need to stay at home as a housewife. For the financial supporting [it] need[s] to come from my father or from my brother or my sister. [For me] up to now [there is] no need to [get married] because I'm ok. The financial? For me [it] all is from me.... Yeah just take care of [it] by yourself. Also, if I have Mr Right it's a burden. (Sying)

The first thing is financial independence. So, if he disagrees I will do it with my own money. That means the economic is the baseline for the decision-making power. (Yuet)

This state of mind has appeared to carry over into the decision to live with one's in-laws. Granting that housing size in Asian cities today has not inspired intergenerational living, daughters-in-law have also been declining to co-reside, as this Gen X Singaporean explained:

My Mother-in-law articulated that she expects him [her son] to look after them...And so, we lived under the same roof for half a year. Yeah, I couldn't manage that.... I was horrified.... I had a very bad experience so [we] moved out... (Zhenzhen)

Like Zhenzhen, after their marriage, Qingzhao (Chap. 4) and her husband also lived with his family, which lasted only six months. When the newlyweds moved out and contacts with his parents dwindled, Qingzhao's husband attempted to initiate more. Qingzhao helped him understand why they should not do this:

And then I calmly talk to him that you must understand that the marriage is between two people: you and me. I just marry you...And I have nothing to do with [your] family because they don't like me and not because I don't like them. So, [from] this moment maybe we just live together...and [have no] concern about the other persons. (Qingzhao)

In mainland China, young married couples have very often continued to live with the husband's parents after childbirth, remaining together until the child begins kindergarten at age three. I asked one Kunming daughter living with her in-laws if she would rather live with them or not, to which she replied, 'not with them, of course'. I then asked if she was looking forward to moving out, to which she responded, 'Yes! I am very much looking forward to that day' (Xiaoli). Other Kunming daughters replied similarly. Even when they were fond of their in-laws, they said living apart was viewed as a way to avoid conflict. Older women, who were already in-laws, expressed the same sentiment.

As mentioned previously, duty has been the primary motivation driving the daughters in this book to support their in-laws. However, among most of the married daughters, the husband-sons were motivated by the same duty as their wives. Some, like Qingzhao's husband, did not especially like their mothers and supported their wives against them. Other husbands intervened between the daughter and the in-laws. Yuet, for example, remarked that, 'that's the tricky part about the Chinese husband. They always stay in the middle. They prefer the role of mediator … for both women. The war is always between women.' For still others, their husbands were apathetic, as Lihwa articulated:

> He really does not care. His road to his mother is quite similar to my road to my family. That means he is supportive financially and then he [is] also the brain to them. (Lihwa)

In a reinterpretation of filial obligation, the interviewed daughters were not only choosing to live apart from their in-laws, they were seeing them less. Although many of them were visiting their own parents at least once a week, others saw their in-laws once or twice a month or only during festivals or holidays. Some of the daughters said they had agreements with in-laws to see their grandchildren, but might not spend time with them themselves. It was far more common among these women to see financial arrangements made for in-laws rather than commitments of time.

One can speculate that being relieved of the duty to contribute all but financial support to in-laws (which their husbands provided) has allowed adult daughters to focus on their families of origin, which is a more natural relationship. For example:

> Many girls, that is married girls, try to hide some money, some things for their parents' family, behind their husband….So, nowadays, we would rather give birth to a girl instead of a boy. (Wen, Kunming Baby Boomer)

> You talk to these mothers nowadays they'll say they prefer to have daughters rather than sons, you know? Things have changed a lot… daughters tend to be closer to their mothers than the sons are. (Huiliang)

This is a major shift away from traditional filial piety and Chinese values. Additionally, although the duty to provide support has not vanished, there appears to have been notable change. Whereas the ideological belief in filial obligation has remained deeply internalised, executing it has achieved an element of voluntariness. For example:

My parents, the way that they are brought up is whatever the parents say, that's the final decision and no arguments also. But, I'm kind of caught in between, because for me it's always about reasoning. It's about logic. It's about convincing. (Te')

As seen with Huiliang, Chinese daughters might now be considering their personal desires more, deciding what they are willing and unwilling to do in light of how they have interpreted filial obligation.

Daughters Desire Independence But Not Necessarily Individualism

Most of the daughters' parents had encouraged them to be independent. Luli recalled how she grew up in Kunming:

Maybe because my father was a college graduate 40 years ago, he may [have] received some of new opinion or value different from the traditional Chinese. He just told me you can do what you want. You can go where you want and just do as you like. From when I was a very little child, my father just told me this. (Luli)

There are several considerations underpinning this. Ning explained one of the most important factors:

The life has changed...I have many relatives. But come to my level now, they [daughters] don't have that many close relatives. Even [if] they have them...they are far away...So, they can't depend on us...they have to be trained to be independent, on their own. (Ning)

Independence, however, has come with a caveat that conveys the paradoxical situation of modern Chinese women. Although they desire independence, most of the daughters distinguished it from Western style individualism. For example:

I feel that being independent means I can do things on my own. I don't have to rely on a person or don't have to be dependent on a person.... But... I equate [being] individualistic more to self-centeredness. Yes, but I don't think being independent is being self-centered.... They are different. (Huizhong)

Jai, a Gen X Singaporean, explained how these seemingly conflicting norms may be accommodated:

How do I reconcile? I think maybe it's a very Asian thing or Chinese thing; you tend to be a little bit more self-sacrificial than others... (Jai)

Jun, a Singaporean Baby Boomer added, 'that you are not alone. You need to... consider others in things that you do'.

These comments are representative of how the women in this book thought. Even though they said they wanted independence, traditional Chinese collectivism appears to have remained an integral part of their internalised values.

Proceeding Cautiously in a Time of Changing Norms

Understanding that they were charting new territory, and given their traditional childhoods, perhaps these daughters were simply proceeding cautiously. Comments such as the following suggest this might have been the case:

We will also want our own way, maybe not so much as the Gen Y because maybe during our time it's like we are slowly *testing the waters*.... Ok, maybe I want to do this. [I'm] not sure what it's like, [or] would society accept [it] or whatever. (Meifeng, Singapore Gen X; *Emphasis added*)

I don't think my generation is the sort to complain because we realise *we can't have our cake and eat it*. We will want to continue to work but at the same time we will have to raise the family. So, we take it in our own stride. (Shu, Singapore Baby Boomer; *Emphasis added*)

By balancing their own needs with those of their parents, daughters showed traditional respect, even though in most cases they said respect must be earned:

> I respect my parents' generation for what they have done, but respect is not an automatic thing, at least for me. It must be earned, regardless of whether you are older than me or not.... Filial piety cannot be like default. (Nuo)

Face was also preserved, and for both parents and daughters it has continued to silently traverse the entire ensemble of Chinese cultural norms:

> My Mom, she just explained...to me...about Face, losing Face and this traditional thing that we have to do because we have to maintain our connection with the extended family. And we do not want others to look down on us. (Rou, Hong Kong Baby Boomer)

Daughters Declining to Transmit Filial Obligation to Their Children

Nearly all the daughters reported that they neither expected nor wanted their children to take care of them in old age. They were aware they would likely live longer than their parents, and that their families were smaller, so there would be fewer children to 'share the load' (Weici). However, more than anything else, it was the perceived burden, which almost none of the daughters wished to see imposed on their children. Weici explained:

> Because firstly, it's a burden on them. I feel sometimes the burden not so much financially, the feeling is...ok yes your parents have raised you and you owe them something, but is it right to feel that you have to repay? I don't want the repay part, you do it out of love. So that's why I [would] rather you not do it to me unless you are doing it because you really want to. So, don't repay me for what I did for you... that's not measurable in the first sense and it's [a] mother's duty anyway. (Weici)

Similar remarks were made by most of the daughters, evincing the growing momentum away from structural to combined motivations, and especially to relational norms, as the impetus and rationale for providing care to older parents. In the following statement one can also see how this shift in motivations to provide care has driven movement away from the unconditional care previously required for in-laws:

> So that duty thing that I had to suffer because I married into that family [is] something that I don't want to force on someone else…I did it because I had to…I'm married to the family. What else can I do?… You see that was the thinking then, 30 years ago, 40 years ago… And even [though] I was educated enough to find my own job and I was working, I mean there's still that lingering [thought]…you always have to wear two hats. You are working with the [one] hat [and then when] you are at home with…the [other] hat… She [mother-in-law] never fails to remind you that … 'you are liable to me, never run away'. That's why I don't want to put that poster on my daughter-in-law's head…I felt chained or locked in and I don't want to give that feeling to someone else. (Weici)

The influence of education and employment were also seen. Contemporary Chinese women, accustomed to having power and authority in the work environment, might be reluctant to forfeit such status at home:

> These women, when they are at work, they make decisions for millions of dollars. They manage people and when they are back [home] they have to listen to this mom in-law who has barely any education and she has to do things the [mother-in-law's] way…And she comes back [home] stressed and she still want to, you know, to agree to all these [things], so I think it makes it, very difficult for the women. (Jun)

Many of the daughters' mothers had no choice but to accept traditional norms of filial obligation. Although the daughters interviewed for this book had greater choice than their mothers, most were still unwilling to completely sever themselves from the traditional Chinese values transmitted to them in childhood. Nonetheless, they intended for caregiving to end with them. As Weici observed: 'That [is] my duty. [It] is my life, ok, but it's not one I want to pass on to my children. So, I've cut the line'.

Forces Underpinning Relational Models of Support Motivation (Affection, Reciprocity and Gratitude)

Chunhua's story (Chap. 4) exemplified how relationships are featured in motivating support. She and her mother had always been close. Chunhua's parents earned her respect by keeping the family together and supporting their children's dreams.

Respect was often pivotal to the relationships with parents among these daughters and a condition precedent to affection and gratitude. If one parent was an abuser, respect for that individual could be lost. Alternatively, the recipient of abuse might gain respect by not abandoning the children. Likewise, hardships suffered by one or both parents could earn respect, especially if it was perceived as being a sacrifice for the sake of the children. Huizhong expanded on her parents' sacrifice:

> I feel that, yes, they sacrificed a lot of time for the family. And... I find that they are really, very fantastic...They give a lot of support to us as kids.... (Huizhong)

There were many different scenarios found in the interviews in which respect was implicated in the quality of a daughter-parent relationship. It is hard to imagine a situation in which affection and gratitude could drive support motivation without it.

Gratitude for Education

The vast majority of the daughters interviewed for this book expressed prodigious gratitude for the ability to attend school. For example:

> Because of her then I can have good life for myself. Because she give me [a] good education. Because on her theory she said the children if they want to study she will pay for them and never reject unless they don't want to study. (Changying, Hong Kong Baby Boomer)

When I was a child, I hope that my parents would support, really my education. They've done it well. They support all of my education, my sisters and my brothers. They are really great. In China, you know about 20 years ago it's not easy for parents to support all of their children to get higher education. But my parents they did it. So, I'm really grateful for them. (Luli)

Most of the daughters recalled how their mothers had been denied access to education. Statements similar to the following were repeatedly heard in the interviews:

We looked at my parents' generation. Then the daughters never went to school, only the sons; Whereas, for my generation, my parents sent all of us to school. Whether you are a daughter or son, it doesn't matter. So...I think it boils down to the fact that because of the education level... we are able to achieve quite a lot. (Xiurong, Singapore Baby Boomer)

Among the women in this book, the desire to learn was instilled in most of them by their parents at a very early age.

I think they maybe keep on saying that you must receive [a] good education. You must be capable to manage yourself, your own life. And if you have no good education you have no future. (Lihwa)

Some daughters hoped to fulfil their parents' 'unfinished business' because the parents regretted not having the opportunity to study. Bo, for example, noted how her family valued education, saying 'the only thing that no-one can take away from you is your knowledge. So, if you want to be respected, if you want to be someone good, you have to study hard'.

Education was also the pathway to a good job, which could equate with copious personal benefits. Niu from Singapore and Wen from Kunming reflected on this:

In China, there is a saying that knowledge can change your fortune. Many people from the poor family in the countryside, if they study very hard and they enter the university, after graduation they become white collar, or they become leaders or they have a chance to do business, they become rich. They can support their family. (Wen)

Without an education, I would not be able to work. I would not be able to
be financially independent. I would not be able to be what I am today.
(Niu)

More than any other factor, the importance of education to the daughters in this book should not be minimised. Parents who supported their
daughter's education almost always created an irredeemable obligation on
the part of their female offspring (Berman 1987).

Gratitude for One's Upbringing

In addition to education, gratitude for the care, encouragement and support received in childhood drove feelings of reciprocity among these
daughters, and this was linked with both duty and affection. The daughters were grateful to their mothers for giving up their jobs and staying
home with the children, for remaining in bad marriages and for supporting the family without any help from their husbands. They were grateful
to their parents for the gift of life, for their hard work and sacrifice, for
allowing them to pursue their goals and for shaping them into who they
were. Expressions of gratitude such as, 'they allowed me to become what
I am today' and 'it is the least I can do' were frequently heard from these
daughters. Jai explained how gratitude factored into her motivation to
support her parents, saying, 'Yes, I think it's time for me to take care of
them given that they did their part when I was younger and fully dependent on them'.

Jai's words were not new. Probably women of her mother's generation
had made similar statements. The difference was context. Parents' obligations and children's expectations have changed. It might be that it is no
longer enough for parents just to provide food and shelter.

Gratitude for Help as an Adult

Mutual obligations and exchanges between parents and children carrying
over into adulthood can form a special type of reciprocity (Croll 1995;
Ng et al. 2002). Parents perform services for adult children such as baby-
sitting, cooking meals and helping with housework. Whether intended

or not, the effect is to strengthen the incentive motive of adult children to care for their parents, either as payback or when parents are in need.

Among these women, one daughter each from Singapore and Hong Kong, and three daughters from the mainland received help with their children from their own parents. In each case, it was part of an overall pattern of reciprocity extending from childhood. However, for the women in this book in general, the decline in intergenerational households and greater geographic distance between the households of the adult children and their parents contributed to a dearth of on-going exchanges of this kind. Further, as previously mentioned, in some instances the introduction of domestic helpers deprived parents of opportunities to perform services for their children.

Although traditional models of adult reciprocity have diminished, new forms of adult exchange have been forthcoming. Yuet related a story that exemplifies this:

> I travel a lot. [In] one month I travel to northern China, and then down to Guangzhou, the southern part, then I travel back to Xinjiang and then I travel to India then Bangkok…. My dad accompany me to the airport every time. Sometimes we have early birds flight… But because he worry that I'm a girl and security and safety matter, he accompany me every time to the airport and pick [me] up…every time. I really appreciate that. Even I tell my husband, I expect you to love my daughter as much as my dad love me. (Yuet)

The Need to Feel Loved and Give Love to Parents

The giving and receiving of love was strongly implicated in support motivation among these daughters. Arguably, it was only natural that they wanted to feel loved by their parents, even as adults. For those, like Chunhua, who felt genuine affection from their parents, the desire to reciprocate that affection could be one possible outcome.

However, among the daughters who did not feel loved *by* a parent, as the story of Qingzhao demonstrated, a strong compulsion could also exist to feel love *for* a parent even in the face of conflicting evidence that it was not merited. Both Bo and Huiqing mitigated negative feelings for their mothers when the latter exhibited signs of vulnerability. In each case, there was no prior history of affection, closeness or interdependence to justify such a change in feeling. Similarly, Sheu-Fuh generated feelings of love for her father even though he had abandoned her.

Love has been recognised in the literature as having an historical linkage with filial piety (Wong and Chau 2006). However, without trying to further explain why the need for reciprocal parental love was so prevalent among the women interviewed, we can look at how affection can be generated to bolster support arising out of filial obligation.

Forces Underpinning Combined Structural and Relational Motivation to Provide Support

Creating Love to Support Duty

As a female, Yet Kwai said she had no status within her family. Although she was a highly accomplished professional woman, all of her achievements could not elevate her position:

> You know, my father told me that it's too bad you are not a son. He likes the kind of social status that I've got. He always carries my name card with him, but it's too bad I'm not a son. (Yet Kwai, Hong Kong Baby Boomer)

During her interview, Yet Kwai related a series of incidents over the course of her life in which she felt rejected by her father. These hurt her deeply, however, her attempts to make her grievances known over these and other affronts had been ignored. Proclamations of love for her father had similarly been met with impassivity and lack of emotion.

Despite her self-perceived status as a 'second class citizen', Yet Kwai proclaimed her unconditional love for her family and a strong sense of filial obligation, especially toward her father. To generate a belief that her father was worthy of the love and attention she bestowed on him, she excused her long and unsuccessful history of trying to be good enough, and disregarded the perceived injustice, mistreatment and rejection he had inflicted on her and other members of the family. Comments such as, 'I don't think he meant it', and 'even though so much he also love us', were repeatedly made. Yet Kwai also reminded herself of the good things her father had done for her, reining in her expectations:

I'm grateful...I don't know if I always [felt] bad about myself in my earliest years but I still... have a father. But, different fathers will have different relationships with their children. It's not like...I'm from...a broken family... My father is always there ...Of course I know my limits. I will not ask for more than I...am allowed. (Yet Kwai)

Yet Kwai claimed she felt appreciated by her father. However, it was not her father but her mother telling her that he appreciated the things she did for him. In truth, Yet Kwai was closest to her mother and felt protective of her because 'I think she will be hurt by my father emotionally'. She also appeared to have modelled her own feelings and behaviour on her mother's:

Emotionally, whatever I can do for my parents' family, I will try my best to do so because I'm the oldest. Like my mother, she's the oldest in her family; she's taking care of her family and I have to take care of my mother's family. And, I have to be good and work so I have the ability to take care of them. (Yet Kwai)

After commenting that obedience and respect were expected from and given to her father, 'even though you don't get respect in return', Yet Kwai explained how her belief in God had helped her to compensate for what was lacking in her life. In her words, '[when] I [was] growing up, I have a father, but I don't receive the love... But, I have a father, God in heaven'.

Equally important to her were three men she referred to as 'mentors'. As a young adult, they gave her attention, acceptance and encouragement, allowing her to see 'what is missing in my family'. Supported and empowered, Yet Kwai generalised the positive feelings she had for these men and gave herself permission to love her father.

Yet Kwai's reasons for supporting her elderly father appeared to be rooted in an Asian cultural model of filial responsibility. She seemed to have internalised what was considered right and what ought to be done (Holroyd 2001). However, Yet Kwai also showed how obligation could be linked with affection and how affection could be used to justify support that might not be deserved.

Yet Kwai's relationship with her father was not a loving one in the classic sense. However, even among the daughters in this book who said they felt loved, demonstrations of affection from their parents were extremely uncommon. That said, norms have been changing. All the daughters who were asked said they hugged and kissed their children and told them they loved them. Perhaps this change in behaviour reflected something that had been lacking in these women's childhoods, which they were attempting to compensate for; or perhaps love was tied to something entirely different, for example gratitude.

Why Love, Gratitude and Duty Were Inseparable Among This Group of Chinese Women

In conducting the interviews, every daughter was asked to explain why she was willing or unwilling to provide support or care for her parents, whether she was actually doing it, had done it in the past, or had not done it at all. Probing beyond this, the daughters were asked if they could distinguish between love, gratitude and duty as a reason for providing support or care for their parents. Many could articulate which of these motivating concepts underpinning filial obligation was the most important or the least important. However, there was a general disinclination to eliminate any of them, and most of the daughters were hesitant to separate them at all. Luli's response illustrates the prevailing point of view:

As a child, yes it's my obligation to take care of the parents. I must do this for them.... And, I think, even though, if this is not my obligation, my responsibility, I should take care of them as I love them, they love me. Yes? And another grateful, yes, too. My parents, they raised me up and they taught me to be a person of this kind. Yes, I think I'm really grateful for them. Sure, I need to take care of them. Actually, I don't think I need to divide the three separately. I think they are just some kind of combination. We cannot say I take care of my parents because of grateful, because of my obligation, because of love. I think they are the same. They are together. (Luli)

To understand this, it is important to remember that in the Chinese culture, feelings of love, gratitude and family obligation have historically been interrelated in a way that has been different from contemporary relational norms in the West. As discussed earlier, overt expressions or demonstrations of affection were not prevalent among these women and their parents. Inquiries into this were repeatedly met with responses such as: 'No. Not the Chinese culture' (Juan, Hong Kong Baby Boomer). Rather, it was the repeated small acts of kindness that the daughters remembered. Zhaohui, a Gen X woman from Hong Kong, told a story from her childhood that illustrates this.

One time, when Zhaohui was overseas at a retreat, her father sent her a letter. The letter contained a drawing of a heart with hands and feet. To her this meant: 'love is action'. She said this had remained with her ever since, and added, 'It also means that you don't have to say it all the time but you need to do it. You have to show it'.

The daughters interviewed for this book recited many tender and unselfish gestures gifted to them by their parents, like preparing their favourite foods when they were sick, talking to them and sharing their feelings, buying them special things, showing concern for them, sacrificing for them and guiding them to become good human beings. They cited practical reasons such as providing shelter and clothing, and allowing them to become educated. Not all the women felt loved, but most did. As Sying remarked, 'Chinese people never say love. But, maybe they do something'. Qiaohui, a Singaporean Baby Boomer added, 'I think in my generation particularly in the Asian culture, you know, we don't speak of love. When my parents care for me...I know they love me'.

The performance of good deeds for the daughters in this book generated both love and gratitude that were inextricably intertwined with traditional Chinese cultural norms such as duty. These were generally indistinguishable except when negative feelings for a parent were found. In these instances, limitations or conditions on parent support could apply. This is discussed later in this chapter.

Christianity as Combined Structural and Relational Motivation to Provide Support

Traditional Chinese religious beliefs are an inchoate composite of Buddhism, Taoism, indigenous practices and superstition (Goh 2009; Liu 2003). Temple visitations and family shrines focused on ancestor worship are tied to filial piety, which instructs the living to revere their elders in life and their ancestors after death. As can be seen from the following statement, ancestor worship particularly operates as a structural norm of filial obligation, grounded in obedience and devotion to parents:

> The traditional Chinese will worship their ancestors because they believe that they will be blessed in their life if their ancestors are happy people… So that is why, this filial piety came into [being]…it's a belief that if you are a bad son or a bad daughter…your parents are going to…make your life very difficult…when they die. So, it's kind of like, a belief that they have that if you don't look after your parents, if you don't worship them or if you don't pray to them after they are gone then you are going to be in a lot of deep trouble, your life is going to be a big mess, you are going to be very unlucky and stuff like that. (Huiliang)

However, it can also be viewed as a very enjoyable practice, as Xiaoli explained:

> Every year twice, the winter and the summer we will [go] to the graves and clean them up and take some food and take some flowers and say something to them. It's the culture. It is a part of my culture, not a duty. We are very glad to do that. And at that time, we can see our other families. Another kind of celebration. (Xiaoli)

In either case, the strength of these beliefs among the 64 Baby Boom and Gen X daughters appeared to be waning. Only three subscribed to any form of traditional 'religious' practices; 28 claimed to have no religious belief; one identified as a Muslim and 32 called themselves Christian. Among the Christians, few came from Christian families. For one thing, in mainland China 'religion' had been officially banned for many years after 1949, and so few of these women had participated in any religious practices until recently. In Hong Kong and Singapore many of the daughters had been required to observe traditional Chinese rituals during childhood. However, the deeper meaning of these activities had not necessarily been internalised:

> When my grandfather passed on, we had to lug our stuff… to his grave-stone and do all that gravestone stuff, which I could never figure out what they were doing … It was something we had to do and so we just went along with it even though we didn't see any point in it …because father said, 'go' so we go. Father said, 'do', we do. (Weici)

It could be that for these daughters, Christianity answered some of the questions unexplained by traditional Chinese religious practices or the absence of value transmission by parents. Meirong, a Hong Kong Baby Boomer, articulated a sentiment heard elsewhere:

> I think I know how to live my life and the values and the order, all the things that I have learned. [But,] …my own life is from the Bible, not from my parents. (Meirong)

There was also an element of accountability to Christianity that was consistent with the upbringing of these Chinese daughters. The similarities can be seen in the following remarks:

> I still believe there is a God. So, whenever I do anything I trust someone is watching. So, doing something good, righteous [like] be fair, be true to others and yourself, these are the core messages, I believe, because I do believe one day, if you've done something wrong, you will pay in a different way. (Bo, who attended Catholic school but did not convert to Christianity out of respect for her parents)

> In Chinese…we also believe every person has god watching you. Some god, maybe you don't know who it is, just watching you and you do everything. That's the Chinese way. (Xiaoli, who observed traditional Chinese practices)

Christianity was also compatible with many of these women's Chinese values, as Zhenzhen's statement reflected:

> There are some…religious teachings [that go] hand in hand with the traditional values I've been brought up with as well; things like respecting your parents, you know, that sort of thing, loving your neighbours. …. I think what is the most difficult was like, for example, perhaps we should put God first before anything else. (Zhenzhen)

As seen with Yet Kwai, the 'love of God' could also have drawn some of these Chinese daughters to Christianity if they had been born into families where they felt unloved or treated unfairly. Together, Christian love and obligation might have constituted a reason to offer support to parents that otherwise might not have existed if the parent-child relationship lacked warmth or was distant.

For some of the Christian daughters, their relationship with God motivated support for a parent. For others, religious beliefs did not factor into their support decisions, or Christianity was combined with traditional Chinese values. However, for these Chinese women and perhaps for Chinese women generally, parent care motivated by Christian values could represent a new normative trend.

Conditions, Qualifications, and Limitations on Support Motivations for Older Parents

Regardless of whether support was motivated by structural norms of filial obligation or relational norms or both, qualifications and limitations on providing support to older parents appeared in several ways among this group of Chinese women. First, only conditional or reduced support was offered to parents who did not fulfil what their daughters perceived their parental obligations to be in childhood. Second, some adult daughters who professed a willingness or an expectancy to support their parents made themselves unavailable to do so. Third, some daughters were willing to provide only the most basic, minimal support for their in-laws. Fourth, structural impediments such as the distance between households could limit parent support. Finally, in one instance a husband would not allow his wife to see her own mother.

Conditional or Reduced Support

The first limitation on support motivation was seen with Qingzhao, who forced herself to dine with her mother, but would do no more. In these cases, the relationship between the parent and the daughter was strained from abuse or rejection. A more common scenario was where a father had abandoned the family or the parents had divorced. Ah Cy, a Singapore Gen X, explained the difficulty she had deciding what, if anything, to do for her father, who had remarried:

> It's my mom's wish that…we should be wary of what…the motive [was] behind him [father] wanting to contact us …So out of respect of her wishes, I don't contact him…But I'm wondering, if she's not around … I sometimes struggle… (Ah Cy)

The second limitation on support motivation, often referred to as the gap between filial belief and filial behaviour, is seen in the story of Qiaohui.

Unavailability

Qiaohui was the eldest child in a traditional family with one son and four daughters. Her father had died and her mother had lived alone ever since. Fortunately, Qiaohui's mother was in good health and able to take care of herself. Qiaohui supported her financially. She also loved her mother and wanted what was best for her. However, she was conflicted. On one hand, she believed in 'looking after our parents' and said, 'sometimes I feel that if I'm not…caring for her [mom]… I'm not a filial child'. She added that she depended on her 'mother's approval'. On the other hand, Qiaohui was a modern, unmarried working woman who enjoyed her lifestyle, and had spent many years working abroad. When contemplating the discharge of filial obligation, she wondered whether she could be a caregiver if called upon:

> It's a very scary thought. Would I be prepared to do it? Yes, I would, although I don't think I'm going to be very good at that. I don't think she's going to be an easy patient. (Qiaohui)

Qiaohui tried to explain why she felt this tension and conflict:

> I ask myself, am I trying to get a job overseas so I can get away from her? So that's where I think the conflict and the feeling comes in, that on the one hand I think it is good for me to go and good for us to have that space. On the other hand, I feel so guilty for leaving her alone, you know, 83-year-old-mom is alone at home. (Qiaohui)

The problem was that when Qiaohui returned home, after three days, 'it goes downhill'. She related how her mother monitored her activities so that if she went out she felt guilty. She said she did not understand why she had such a sense of obligation: Was it expected of her or did she expect it of herself? Was it love or duty that motivated her?

Qiaohui claimed she was 'in [a] dilemma' and felt 'a bit lost'. If she remained at home she would have to live with her mother. The family owned a large flat and Qiaohui said people would wonder if she, a single daughter, did not live there when there was so much space. Besides, she said, she did not 'want her [mother] to be miserable'. However, Qiaohui's mother got on her nerves:

> Every time I come back, I go off feeling so angry…because she will be upset with what I said… And she'll say, 'yeah you guys don't care about me. All you care about is your father'…. I'll go back [overseas] and tell myself, why do I want to live that way because it's so unpleasant …although of course, you know, Sunday comes, I call her and still [it is] like nothing has happened. (Qiaohui)

Ultimately Qiaohui concluded that she would look after her mom if she had to, 'but that's probably not my strength …I think my capabilities [are] to go and earn the money to be able to afford to do that'.

Shortly after her interview, Qiaohui took another job overseas. With that in mind, some points should be made. Because her mother was still healthy, Qiaohui was only required to provide support, not care, to be 'filial'. She met this obligation by paying her mother's bills, making occasional visits home and calling her mother every Sunday night. This was the compromise she had reached with herself to balance her traditional values and personal needs. Nonetheless, Qiaohui felt guilty. She wanted her mother's approval; however, making her mother happy required Qiaohui to sacrifice much of what she enjoyed in her own life. This was a very common dilemma among the women interviewed for this book. The same expressions of conflict and feelings of guilt were repeatedly conveyed to me. Moreover, the same could be said for the myriad Chinese women I have met and known over the years.

When Qiaohui is finally faced with the decision of whether to move home to undertake the hands-on caregiving of her mother, it is likely to be challenging, given that in the past her mother has rejected the services of an FDH. Meanwhile, perhaps it can be said that there is safety in removing herself from the source of her conflict and postponing the decision.

Minimal In-Law Support

The third limitation on support motivation pertained to the Chinese daughters' provision of support to their in-laws. As noted previously, in-laws received less commitment of time from the daughters than did their parents. If relations became strained contact could even be severed altogether or limited to infrequent polite exchanges. The daughters were also generally unwilling to take time off work or to leave employment for their in-laws, particularly at the support stage. Some deliberately moved great distances from in-laws to minimise contacts. One daughter made sure the FDH she hired did not speak Chinese so that her mother-in-law could not give her instructions.

Structural Impediments

Some of the daughters also lived far from their own parents due to work and other commitments that could not be avoided. This was particularly so in mainland China. Although this could be a barrier to daily physical contact, the daughters compensated through regular telephone calls and attendance at meals, birthdays or holidays like the spring and autumn festivals and Chinese New Year. It should also be noted that distance had no negative effect on the financial support the daughters provided to their parents.

Husband's Objection

The final limitation on support motivation was unique among this group of women. During ten years of marriage Ah Cy was only permitted by her husband to see her own mother on birthdays and holidays because he did not like her.

Except for geographic distance, all of the qualifications and limitations discussed above had a single source: the quality of the relationship. In assessing the point at which the quality of a relationship intersected with support, the daughters' expectations of themselves were higher for parents than for in-laws.

Managing Tension and Conflict in the Discharge of Filial Support

The daughters have shown that the motivation to support their parents was not clear- cut, but rather, was often entangled with emotion. One's emotional state might be even more vulnerable in the actual discharge of filial support.

This section explores the relevance of 'appropriate' feelings related to the quality and quantity of support provided by the daughters to their ageing parents. As Hochschild (1983) suggested, 'appropriate' feelings are prescribed by framing rules that define and give meaning to situations. In the context of this book, the framing rules of these daughters can be viewed as being synonymous with Chinese cultural norms, and their interpretations of them. As discussed earlier, the literature suggests that in traditional Chinese culture there has been a gender driven role that women have been expected to fulfil. This ideological mandate could be deeply embedded in a daughter's mind from an early age, defining or 'framing' her obligations. Feeling rules would have then prescribed how she *should* feel about these obligations. However, if there was a discrepancy between what she actually felt and what she believed she *should* feel, emotion work might have been necessary to reconcile the contradictions and create a culturally acceptable display, or even to change a daughter's feelings to align with her normative values. The story of Jaihui below illustrates how emotion work can be implicated in parental support.

Emotion Work to Generate a Willingness to Support Parents

Jaihui was the eldest child in a traditional family that also included three sons. When she was one year old she was given away to a family friend. Rejoining her family at age five, she quickly learned of her low status in the family hierarchy. As she described it:

> They don't care about [the] daughter. When I was young I was brought up in this situation. They pamper the son so well. Everything they gave my eldest brother. (Jaihui)

Jaihui explained that during childhood she only saw her father once a week and seldom saw her mother. She related how her mother never looked at her homework, and the only value transmitted to her was the difference between right and wrong. According to Jaihui, she and her parents rarely conversed. When they did, she said she 'never answered back' even if she knew they were wrong.

Jaihui recalled several instances of her parents' injustice. For example, at age 13 she developed a fungus and needed to go to the hospital. Her mother sent her there in a taxi, telling her to look for her uncle who was a doctor. After being examined, Jaihui was told she had a very serious condition requiring surgery and she would need signed parental permission for anaesthesia. When neither of her parents could be located, she underwent the operation without it. This hurt Jaihui deeply because just before it happened her brother had undergone a tooth extraction and the entire family had been in attendance for support.

Years later, after completing high school, Jaihui expressed her desire to study abroad, to which her father responded, 'Why [do] you want to study so much? Just go find a husband and get married'. Persevering, Jaihui applied for and was accepted to college in New Zealand, where all three brothers soon followed. Upon graduating, each child was asked to come home. Only Jaihui agreed, observing that, 'they can't force my brothers to come back, and they don't care about him [dad]'. However, as soon as Jaihui returned to Hong Kong her parents sold the family home and moved to New Zealand to be with their sons. Jaihui was forced to live with a friend.

A year after they left, Jaihui's parents migrated back to Hong Kong, but having sold their home had no place to live. Jaihui rented and paid for a separate flat for them, with neither her parents nor her brothers contributing to the rent. Ultimately, burdened by the expense, she bought her own flat, and her parents moved in with her.

At the time of her interview, Jaihui was divorced and living with her father. Her mother lived in mainland China, but returned to Hong Kong for two days each month. According to Jaihui, her mother suffered from chronic depression caused by separation from her sons. Whenever she saw her, Jaihui's mother tearfully recounted how much she loved and missed them. However, it was Jaihui, not the sons, who was the sole support of both parents.

Jaihui's Coping Strategies Although she did not know it, Jaihui used emotion work to cope with supporting her family. Her framing rules were heavily influenced by traditional Chinese values:

> I will accept the fact this is life…. [The way] I [was] brought up; like my godmother might tell me yeah, yeah, they like boys. You're a girl, too bad, you're a girl. You have to look after them. I mean… I've been educated [in such a way that] …. I just think this is a life traditional…Now I'm ok. (Jaihui)

If Jaihui's framing rules instilled in her a need to support her parents, her feeling rules created an expectation in her to love them. Jaihui insisted she did love her parents, however, as seen in the following statement, she was conflicted:

> I'm not saying that I don't have love with my parents. Of course, ...I love them. I'm not the person who speaks out, but I love them ... Even though they didn't treat me very well when I was young. (Jaihui)

As she continued to speak, it was clear that a discrepancy existed between what Jaihui really felt and what she believed she *should* feel:

> I don't feel anything. I guess it's like because of this kind of environment growing up... maybe I lost the love or passion thing from people. I mean that is like I don't get my passion or love from my family. (Jaihui)

To change the quality of her feelings, Jaihui attempted to suppress her unwanted memories by replacing them with pity:

> I know I have a very bad feeling. But when I look at them I [feel] pity. I'm sorry [for] them. They're getting old. My mom is...alone, by herself. And then my brothers [are] not taking care of her. *So, all this feeling cover all my memories.* [Jaihui; *Emphasis added.*]

Jaihui said she tried to keep herself busy to avoid having to think. She admonished herself. But neither action could change what she felt:

> Not much feeling. It's like I need to look after them, take care of them. That's it. Spend some time with them. But when I sometimes look at them, getting old, then I will go and scold myself, why don't you spend more time. You [would] rather stay outside with your friend[s]... don't go back home...It's like...I don't really have much feeling on them honestly...But every time when I see them, then I will feel... pity about them getting old [and think] I should have done better on that. (Jaihui)

Jaihui reminded herself she was the 'glue' that held the family together. The message, heard from so many of the daughters, was that if she did not attend to her parents' needs, who would? She reinforced this emotion work with a rule reminder from her mother: approval and praise. Jaihui recalled:

> But my mom...did mention once to me... nowadays you are the only person who supports my life. She told me this.... Then she says how 'I wish I have four daughters or three daughters and one son rather [than] one daughter three sons'. (Jaihui)

Jaihui moved back to Hong Kong at her parents' request, lived with her father, and supported both parents financially. However, she was unable to generate a desire to spend more time with them. Jaihui was also unwilling to care for her parents if they became disabled, a position she legitimised on the ground that she had to work. She stated she would hire a nurse and if things got too bad she would send her parents to a nursing home. According to Jaihui, it would be a 'family decision', made by Jaihui and her brothers.

Through Jaihui's story we can see how important feelings are in providing support for parents, and how potentially important emotion work can be when there are seemingly irreconcilable tensions. As will become evident moving through the typology, there appears to be a direct correlation between feelings and the quality and quantity of support and care. Successful emotion work can positively alter feelings and display between daughters and their parents. However, emotion work is not always successful.

Refusal to Provide Support: Poor Relational Quality

The literature suggests that parents' misconduct, emotional remoteness, and other adverse behaviour when their children are young can have negative consequences for parental support and care when the children reach adulthood. As seen with Qingzhao, adult children may lack genuine feeling for parents' well-being, or experience relationship strain, as witnessed in the narrative of Huiqing.

Among the daughters in this book, declining to provide *any* support for a parent was rare. Four refused to support their fathers, even financially, because the parents divorced or the father deserted the family. In each of these cases there was little or no contact between the daughter and father over the life course. Furthermore, the fathers were blamed for the mothers' suffering and hard lives, caused by raising the family on their own. The other two instances in which support was refused involved abuse of daughters by mothers. The beatings Sheu-Fuh received from her mother were discussed in Chap. 4. The other was the emotional abuse of Bik, a Hong Kong Baby Boomer.

Bik's mother was a concubine, whose status in the family was tied to her ability to bear sons. Bik was an unwanted daughter, given away when she was three years old to family friends. At age 12, she was returned to her birth mother following the death of her natural father; however, her mother was a stranger to her, and she was cruel. She informed Bik that if she did not help with the housework she would not be fed, and she refused to pay Bik's school fees. Bik was not permitted to study at home or even to bathe. After passing her O level exams at age 17, Bik left school, and went to work. She walked out of her mother's house and never saw or spoke to her again.

Conclusion

Support is the first stage of the typology and there was very little interference with the daughters' daily lives. Possibly for this reason, all of the women provided some form of support to their parents or in-laws. Support can assume different forms, as shown in Table 4.1. However, the standard among these daughters was financial aid and visiting or having meals with family members.

Structural norms of filial obligation, individually and in combination with relational norms of affection and gratitude, motivated support among these women. For parents, combined support motivation was more prevalent than the individual motivational models, whereas structural norms motivated most of the support for in-laws.

Teasing out the processes underlying support and the elements driving it, role modelling of parents during childhood was found to still be a common method for teaching children how to provide support for others. Role modelling has long been associated with the transmission of Chinese cultural norms and intergenerational transmission processes more generally. Among the women in this book, it was especially important when parents had little time to spend with their children. By observing their parents, the daughters learned respect and what they should do when their own parents became elderly.

As young Chinese girls, the women in this book were particularly receptive to supporting others, because they were indoctrinated into traditional gender roles at an early age. Being assigned childhood responsibility for the household and siblings often translated into an irredeemable sense of obligation and accountability to the family in adulthood. This could result in excessive burden being placed on these contemporary daughters who were working and taking care of the home. Some changes in traditional filial norms, however, were revealed and more women were employing domestic helpers to manage their household chores. Nonetheless, stress and exhaustion were implicated.

Feelings of obligation were also reinforced through family members' subtler modelling and transmission of family obligation or beliefs about the centrality of the family. The subjugation of self to the family was seen in the story of Huiliang, a woman who sacrificed a promising career abroad to return home to support her father and grandmother. Huiliang's story also raised the question of whether family obligation originated with filial piety or familism.

These daughters, however, were different from their mothers because education and employment had made them more self-sufficient. They were providing financial support for their parents equal to that of their brothers, and in some cases, instead of their brothers. This engendered further normative change within the family, and the daughters gained greater bargaining power and control over their own decisions. Notably, this manifested in marriage negotiations, the refusal to reside with in-laws, and increased exchanges with their own parents. The daughters had become more independent, although they distinguished this from individualism, which was not always viewed positively.

Structural obligations were mediated by contemporary filial norms; however, these daughters were proceeding cautiously. Although filial obligation could be a matter of individual interpretation, many of the daughters retained the internalised values transmitted by their parents. As a result, they were likely to balance their own needs with those of their parents, and in the process, show respect and maintain Face for the family. They were, nonetheless, declining to transmit traditional filial obligation norms to their own children.

Respect that was earned was the core of relational motivation, whether it was based on gratitude or affection. Gratitude was expressed for one's birth, upbringing and later life exchanges, although the latter could be affected by geographic distance or domestic helpers. However, by far, the greatest effect on gratitude was education. Nothing meant more to these Chinese women than the education they received and the independence, status and financial security they had derived from it. They were universally and deeply grateful to their parents for the education they had been allowed to undertake.

In addition to gratitude, the relevance of love and affection to relational motivation was immeasurable. The giving and receiving of love with one's parents was widely desired among these daughters, and it also combined with both gratitude and duty. To highlight the importance of love to filial obligation the narrative of Yet Kwai was presented. Yet Kwai was a woman of great achievement with strongly internalised familistic values. Her story demonstrated the lengths to which a daughter would go to gain her father's love and generate love for him in return. It further emphasised how love and duty drive support for one's parents. However, Yet Kwai's account also epitomised the conflict between contemporary norms and traditional values and how one may need to go outside the family to fulfil one's needs as a precondition to offering support. Further, it raised the question of a daughter's traditional place within the family, when demonstrations of love have historically been denied to her, and what that meant.

The paucity of overt expressions of love in Chinese families led to an examination of the relationship between love, gratitude and duty as motivators for parental support. Unlike in the West, perceived parent love resulted from the parents' actions, particularly acts of kindness and generosity, for which their children were grateful. Feelings of love and gratitude were often inseparable given that both originated from the same source. Feelings of love and gratitude could also generate a sense of duty, because loving and grateful children might believe they 'owed' their parents for what they had been given. Where feelings of love in the parent-child relationship were absent, Christianity could provide an alternative source for generating positive feelings for parents.

Several limitations, qualifications and conditions on support were found among these women. Conditional, reduced or minimal support might be all that was offered to parents who had not provided for a daughter in childhood; or to parents-in-law who were either disliked or not cared about. Geographical barriers resulting from family members living far apart could hinder instrumental, but not necessarily emotional or financial support. One daughter was prohibited from seeing her mother because her husband disallowed it. Occasionally, there were also gaps between filial belief and filial behaviour. The latter was depicted in the story of Qiaohui who professed to love her mother and wanted to support her, but continued to seek overseas employment. Qiaohui's story also allowed us to see the tension and conflict some daughters experienced between internalised norms of filial obligation and contemporary norms of self-fulfilment.

Conflict and tension between traditional and contemporary norms was common among these daughters, who could be torn between what they felt and what they believed they *should* feel. The story of Jaihui, showed how one daughter attempted to bridge this gap and reconcile her feelings through emotion work. Jaihui grew up the sole daughter in a household where son favouritism prevailed. After a childhood characterised by emotional abuse and neglect, she was obliged to support her parents when her three brothers refused to. Even though she provided a home and paid her parents' expenses, Jaihui struggled to convince herself she should spend more time with them, when she really did not want to. She tried to generate feelings for her parents by pitying them. Her emotion work, however, was unsuccessful, and her story illustrated how important positive feelings are, even at the support stage.

In extreme cases, support could be refused due to negative motivation. Divorced fathers could especially be excluded from it, but so could mothers. Sheu-Fuh, who was beaten by her mother, and Bik, who was emotionally abused by hers, could not generate a willingness to support them.

The next chapter moves the discussion from support, the first stage in the typology, to the second stage, where some actual hands-on caregiving was required and where the demands on the daughters were greater.

Notes

1. In Mainland China, filial piety is referred to as xiàoshùn (孝 順).

References

Berman, H. J. (1987). Adult children and their parents: Irredeemable obligation and irreparable loss. *Journal of Gerontological Social Work, 10*(1-2), 21–34.

Cook, S., & Dong, X.-y. (2011). Harsh choices: Chinese women paid work and unpaid care responsibilities under economic reform. *Development and Change, 42*(4), 947–965.

Croll, E. J. (1995). *Changing identities of Chinese women; rhetoric, experience and self-perception in twentieth-century China.* Hong Kong: Hong Kong University Press.

Goh, D. P. S. (2009). Chinese religion and the challenge of modernity in Malaysia and Singapore: Syncretism, hybridisation and transfiguration. *Asian Journal of Social Science, 37*(1), 107–137.

Hochschild, A. (1983, 2012). The managed heart: Commercialization of human feeling. Berkeley: University of California Press.

Holroyd, E. (2001). Hong Kong Chinese daughters' intergenerational caregiving obligations: A cultural model approach. *Social Science & Medicine, 53*(9), 1125–1134.

Liu, t.-s. (2003). A nameless but active religion: An anthropologist's view of local religion in Hong Kong and Macau. *The China Quarterly, 174*, 373–394.

Ng, A. C. Y., Phillips, D. R., & Lee, W. K.-m. (2002). Persistence and challenges to filial piety and informal support of older persons in a modern Chinese society: A case study in Tuen Mun, Hong Kong. *Journal of Aging Studies, 16*(2), 135–153.

Wong, O. M. H., & Chau, B. H. P. (2006). The evolving role of filial piety in eldercare in Hong Kong. *Asian Journal of Social Science, 34*(4), 600–617.

6

Temporary Care of Ageing Parents

Review of Temporary Care and Introduction to the Chapter

Temporary care represents the second stage of the typology of support and care. Although the duration is not long, less than six months, it is characterised by emergencies, injuries or the acute illness of a parent, which are stressful events. Temporary care is more than support. The daughter providing such care must generally invest more than a nominal amount of time. Moreover, temporary care *can* interfere with the caregiver's personal life and may involve sacrifice.

As shown in Table 4.2, for a situation to qualify as temporary care within the typology, the parent must be hospitalised or cared for by the daughter in either the parents' or the daughter's home for six months or less. Most hospitalised parents received visits, and sometimes homemade food from the daughters in this book, who also interfaced with medical staff and monitored their parents' medications. Home care consisted of hands-on care, supervision of a domestic helper, driving parents to appointments and overseeing medications. Both current and past temporary caregiving experiences have been included in this chapter.

© The Author(s) 2018
P. O'Neill, *Urban Chinese Daughters*, St Antony's Series,
https://doi.org/10.1007/978-981-10-8699-1_6

The first thing that stands out is how much less temporary care was provided by these daughters than support. One hundred and fifty-six parents received support from 64 daughters, whereas only 24 daughters provided temporary care to 32 parents. This might be attributed to the youth and good health of most of the parents. However, another explanation, supported by the data, is that parents were generally cared for by their spouses as they grew frail, until their condition reached a crisis level.

Among the 32 care recipients, 24 were parents and five were in-laws. Additionally, there were two aunts and an uncle, all cared for by one daughter. Among the 24 daughters providing temporary care, 62.5% were Baby Boomers. The prevalence of Boomers might be linked to the older age of their parents.

This chapter moves beyond the previous one, examining why the daughters were willing or unwilling to provide temporary care, how they resolved the tension and conflict incurred in discharging this type of care, and why care was terminated. The differences in stress between home care and hospital care are explored, as is the distinction between the Hong Kong, Singapore and Kunming daughters in the provision of temporary care, and the intersection of care with employment. Disparities between the temporary care of parents and in-laws are considered, and the limitations, qualifications and conditions of temporary care are probed. Finally, just as the daughters' own voices were heard in the previous chapters, so are they here.

How Structural Norms of Filial Obligation and Relational Norms of Affection, Gratitude and Reciprocity Motivate Daughters to Undertake Temporary Care for Parents

As will be recalled, motivations for support and care have been grouped into three key analytical categories: structural norms of filial obligation, ['*I have to*'] relational norms of gratitude, love and reciprocity, ['*I want to*'] and combined structural and relational norms ['*I have to* + *I want to*']. Among the 24 temporary caregivers, two thirds were motivated by combined structural and relational norms, and religion alone drove

Table 6.1 Motivation driving temporary care for parents and in-laws

Motivation type	Mother	Father	Mother-in-law	Father-in-law	Other[a]	Total
Structural	0	2	2	2	0	6
Relational	4	4	0	0	0	8
Structural + relational	5	9	1	0	3	18
Total	9	15	3	2	3	32

[a]2 aunts, 1 uncle

temporary caregiving in one situation. There were no instances related by the daughters in which temporary care was refused altogether due to negative motivation, other than as discussed in Chap. 4. Table 6.1 shows how structural and relational norms motivating temporary care were distributed among the 32 care recipients.

The reader is reminded that each *daughter* in this book is tied to the same motivation or set of motivations throughout the typology. However, the motivational profile of each *stage* in the typology shifts as the number of daughters and type of care change (e.g. from 64 to 24; support to temporary care).

Forces Driving Structural and Relational Motivation for Temporary Care

In Chap. 5, many of the forces underpinning the daughters' motivation for support were discussed in the context of traditional values and normative change. In this and the ensuing chapters these themes are expanded upon, probed more deeply and enhanced by exploring related paradigm shifts. In furtherance of these objectives, this chapter takes a slightly different approach than Chap. 5. Here, all the key analytical categories are examined through a single daughter. Weici's experience shows how one daughter was motivated by structural norms of filial obligation and relational norms of affection, gratitude and reciprocity in the context of temporary care for each of her parents and her mother-in-law. Her story also illustrates how emotion work could be involved in providing temporary care in the face of stress or conflict. Finally, it demonstrates how and why care might be terminated.

Structural and Relational Motivation and Emotion Work in Providing Temporary Care; Differences Between Parents and In-Laws

Weici, a college educated, married Baby Boomer, had three sisters and two brothers. Her parents and mother-in-law were still living. Weici's parents were divorced and neither they nor her mother-in-law lived with her at the time of her interview.

Weici and Her Parents

> My father was a very abusive man and my grandfather was an abusive man too. So…our youth…was spent being constantly in fear of my father blowing up and throwing things and smashing things, destroying furniture, and beating up my mother. And, we would…accompany her to the hospital, sit with her when they stitched her up… At that time, it was quite traumatic. (Weici)

According to Weici, besides being violent, her father was an unfaithful husband, although, he provided financially for his family and he could also be kind. Weici remembered one Christmas when he bought the children a Christmas tree. In her view, her father had fulfilled his obligations to the family. It was Weici's mother, however, whose strength and love sustained her children:

> My mother was the one that gave us emotional support…even though… she was abused. She…kind of put us on the footing that…we are not emotionally unstable…. She didn't blame my father for anything and she didn't turn us against him… We could come to her… when we needed something or we had some problems. She would always listen. She didn't have a lot of advice but she was very [good at] listening… And…up until now she still does that. (Weici)

Weici related a story about her mother that defined their relationship. After Weici and her sister were in college, their mother learned to drive and got a job as a van driver for an airline. One winter, Weici sent her mother a photograph of herself in the snow at her college in America. Her mother said, 'ohhh, it's so cold'! The rest of the story is told by Weici:

So, she would go to these auctions that [the airline] would have for people who left stuff on the plane… She would go there and look, keep on looking … [She] said, 'I want to get you a coat'. So, she finally found this coat…. [It was a] brown coat with a hood and it was really warm and she bid for it and she told all her friends, 'you cannot bid for it ok? I want it for my daughter' …and she got it and I think she only gave $20 for it. It was a down coat and I still have it until today. (Weici)

Weici said she was proud of her mother and she respected her too. This woman, who was orphaned as a child and uneducated, took control over her life and then divorced her husband. At the time of her interview, Weici's mother lived with an FDH in a senior citizen community and her father lived with a friend.

Weici explained the difference between how she felt about support and care for her two parents. Regarding her father, there appeared to be limitations on what she was willing to do. She said:

He provided for us. So up to today, I guess if he ever needed help or anything, we won't hesitate, but there won't be any great love going on, it would just be a duty we had to do, as a duty [for what] he did to us…It will be more of a financial thing. I won't hold his hand or hug him or anything. (Weici)

For her mother, it was completely different:

For me, [it] would be because I care for her, and…because she also put up with so many things that we did because we were children [and] all that, so, for her it would be a real mother-daughter bonding. I mean, I love her for what she did for us, that she stayed to put up with my father so that we could…have a whole family even though it wasn't wholesome; and…. [in] that sense, I don't have any problem if she needs me. I would go to her and help her out willingly. (Weici)

Up until the time of her interview, Weici's father had not required any care. However, Weici did provide temporary care for her mother, and readily so. A couple of years before the interview, Weici's mother fell and injured her shoulder. For two months, Weici moved into her mother's house and took care of her. She described it:

> I went to my mother's house and I stayed with her. So, I would rush back from my mother's house [to my house] to make sure everything was ok in the house. I rushed back to my mother's house to [spend] the night because in case she has any problem... I would sleep through the night with her on a hard floor, on a plank...on a thin foam mattress, small little pillow... [and] tolerate that for two months. (Weici)

Weici explained how difficult this was, because her mother was used to doing things her own way. They she added:

> ...but I was more forgiving in the sense because she is my mother. Sometimes I would get irritated with her ...but...I could be myself with her. I could vent, I didn't have to hold it in...and she also knew that I was giving up so much just to stay with her on the floor... (Weici)

Weici's care for her mother was motivated by love and gratitude. What follows is temporary care motivated by duty.

Weici and Her Mother-in-Law

After Weici married she and her husband moved in with his parents and lived with them for two years. This was a time Weici did not remember fondly. She portrayed her mother-in-law as 'a real naggy, demanding' woman who abused Weici's father-in-law for not being 'good enough' and she recalled how she too had difficulties with the woman. After explaining how she would 'do the things that keep the house clean', even though her sister-in-law 'would come back and do it all over again', Weici chronicled some of her other issues. For example:

> I would do her laundry and it was like, no, you didn't iron it this way... or....no, daddy likes the shirt the other way or something like that, so it

was pick, pick, pick, you know, you don't do anything right…Finally…the week before I moved out, I think I finally said, 'oh, I know how daddy wants his shirt ironed now'. (Weici)

Weici managed her negative emotions through avoidance:

I was at work most of the time and then I just go back to bed. The moment I came home, I would just eat what she cooked, I would do all the dishes, clean up everything and just go to sleep. (Weici)

At the time of the interview, Weici's mother-in-law lived alone in her family home. However, a few years earlier she had fallen and fractured her hip, and she had come to live with Weici and her husband. Weici described how she oversaw her mother-in-law's convalescence by telling her domestic helper: 'whatever she does, you just let her do it'. For six months the mother-in-law disrupted the household. Weici recalled:

Well…at that time, she couldn't really move very far but she was calling the maid, every single [minute].… So, one time I said, why is the laundry not done? [The helper responded,] 'Madam, Ah-Mah [referring to Weici's mother-in-law] keeps calling me all the time, I've got to make her tea, then I've got to clear her tea, then I've got to make her bed…'. (Weici)

The mother-in-law's irritating behaviour did not improve over time:

Because she would say, 'this is not right, that's not right,' you know, [and then] when [my husband] Elliot is at home, [she would say] … 'how come you are not buying [Elliot's favourite foods]'? So…I said 'mommy, just give me a list of things I should get for Elliot and I'll go and buy [them] and you go and cook it'. Ok, so she'll stand next to the stove…she'll tell my helper how to cook…and she'll tell [me]…you forgot this, you forgot [that]… then after that, I'll tell her, 'It's not that I forgot, you never tell me'. But fine, ok I forgot… I didn't want to cause ripples because I knew my husband was stressed in the sense that his brothers and sisters were not helping. And he didn't have the courage…[to] say, 'excuse me, can you all each take mother for a little while?' (Weici)

Elliot was unconcerned with what his mother was doing to his wife. Weici recounted:

> He never cared because she treats him like the lord, everything she is serving to him, you know. 'Elliot, you want tea? Elliot, you want coffee? Elliot, get him a cake'....So, he didn't have any problem, he was the duke on high, the master of the house and he was treated like that. (Weici)

Weici was also actively involved in her mother-in-law's care. She recalled: 'I'm chauffeuring, I'm driving, I'm taking her to the doctors, I'm carrying her back and forth for her check-ups'.

Weici's Emotion Work When she was not providing care, or coping through avoidance, Weici practiced emotion work (although she did not know this). When she was called upon to manage her emotions, she resorted to exhortation [deep acting]. Below Weici talks about her emotion work:

> I don't want to get angry with her. I don't want to feel bitter towards her. I don't want to hate her so much that I can't stand to see the sight of her. So, somehow or other, I managed to put up [with her]. I'm always given, always felt this traction, this no, no, no, don't do this, no, don't get angry. Even though sometimes she said some of the stupidest things, I said, swallow it, put up with it and then it [wasn't] that bad anymore. Yeah, I don't feel like stabbing myself or stabbing her, whatever. (Weici)

When she became angry ('I just want to choke her...') she suppressed her emotions by excusing her mother-in-law's behaviour:

> She's elderly, she probably cannot be changed...and she always wants to be right. She's human and if she wants to be right, I'm not going to change it by correcting her. So, there's no point me forcing my correct view or logic or whatever on her. (Weici)

Weici reverted to avoidance before her emotions escalated, and again practiced exhortation:

She was driving me nuts so what I did was, 'ok fine mommy...I can't talk to you anymore.... When I find out the answer I'll come back to you'. And basically, I just walked away. It was easier just to walk away then to slam my fist or to shout at her... Better to bite your tongue than create trouble then for the rest of the how many years of your life, she's going to hate you for it...It was more of shut up, shut up, shut up, you are not going to win, give up, give up, give up. (Weici)

Gift Exchange The time finally came when Weici felt that what she owed her mother-in-law (or her husband) was outweighed by the emotional burden of caring for in her own home:

So, I put up with it and after a while, it finally got to a point where I really couldn't stand it anymore, and I said ok, honestly, if I don't say something soon I'm going to live with her for the rest of my life. (Weici)

She went to her husband for permission to ask her mother-in-law to leave:

So, I said... 'When is she going home?...I know you are getting all the favourite food that you want to eat which I don't cook. But the helper is not doing her work...I'm doing it. And I cannot do it anymore because I have to fetch the children from school, tutorials, and classes and all the rest of it'. So, I sat down and said to him, 'Try not to be angry.... I'm really suffering here. Please, you [have] got to help out'. (Weici)

Negotiations were held with Elliot's brothers and it was decided that a domestic helper would be hired to live with the mother-in-law in her own home. Weici took charge of this project and her mother-in-law left. She recalled:

So that was all done and... I very nicely [said] to her, 'Mommy, I don't mind you staying with us but I'm sure you want to go back to your own place'. 'Oh yah, yah, yah, I want to! I want to! Yah you just set it up for me then I'll go back'. So, on that ...[we] put her in a nice car and took her back and said 'Mommy your house [is] all cleaned up already'. I said, 'The helper is coming next week and I'll come by every evening and bring you some food'. (Weici)

After this, Weici said one of sons commented: 'If you want to give an academy award, give it to mommy, she's an academy winning actress when it comes to her mother-in-law'. Note the emotion work evidenced in her son's statement and hers. Thanking him, Weici commented:

> At least you realised that I do not show my true colours in front of people, that's what my mother always said. '[If] you are angry with the person, [you] don't have to let them know you are angry...' (Weici)

She added that at times, when she returned home after seeing her mother-in-law, she walked through the door into her own home and yelled. Hearing this and seeing her expression, she recalled her sons would say, 'Went to see Ah-Mah [grandma] today, right'?

Why Relationships Matter in Temporary Care

Weici's story very clearly illustrates the extent to which relationships begin to matter at the temporary care stage of the typology. She was motivated by both structural and relational norms to provide parent care, which for her mother was affection. Although it was not easy, Weici exercised patience and understanding, and communicated with her mother directly and honestly. The two enjoyed a seemingly healthy emotional relationship that enabled Weici to provide temporary care for two months in uncomfortable and sometimes stressful conditions.

Weici had not been required to care for her father, but her feelings were unambiguous. She said he would be taken care of because he provided financially for his family. Although she did not explicitly say what she would be willing to do, she suggested help would likely be financial, indicating that she would not support him emotionally. Presumably, this was because of the abuse he had inflicted on Weici's mother. However, the emotional distance from her father that she experienced in childhood might also have been implicated.

Finally, there is Weici's mother-in-law, whom it is fair to say, Weici did not like or respect. Weici tolerated her out of duty and courtesy to her husband, but one can see the strain this put on her, even with the help of an FDH. Eventually, when she could no longer endure the situation, she confronted her husband and negotiated a face saving move everyone could accept.

Underpinning Motivations Driving Temporary Care

In Weici's story, some of the elements underpinning motivation, as discussed in the previous chapter, are observed. Weici had traditional values, evidenced by her definition of filial obligation:

> For me it would be, making sure that your parents are not in want of anything. And that they had someone to look after them when they could no longer look after themselves.... like you look after your own children except that they are old people and they'll be more fussy. (Weici)

Weici had a role model in her mother, who held the family together at her own expense. Moreover, she observed both of her parents taking care of their parents:

> He [father] even still gave money or he looked after my grandparents...needs and...my mother... even though she would never get any help from [her] mother-in-law, she looked after my grandmother for a while when my grandmother was ill. And she was the only daughter-in-law who did that. (Weici)

Weici was willing to subjugate her personal interests to the family, when necessary. She lived for two years with her in-laws and cared for her mother and mother-in-law when they were in need. These acts appeared to have been undertaken out of respect for her husband, or norms of obligation for her mother-in-law and both love and gratitude for her mother.

The influence of contemporary norms could also be seen. Weici made time for herself and escaped unpleasantness with the in-laws. Further, she placed limitations on what she would do for both her father and her mother-in-law. Weici additionally relied on religion, saying that 'God is always asked...[to] help me, and he has [helped] me with my mother-in-law'.

Managing Tension and Stress When Temporary Care Conflicts with Work

Weici did not work, and although her situations were stressful, she was able to manage the disruptions and still have time to pursue her personal activities, at least with respect to her mother-in-law. The following narrative addresses the conflict between home life and work during temporary care. In this case, Rou's father was cared for in his own home with the help of an FDH, and then he was hospitalised.

Temporary Care by a Working Daughter

Family was important to Rou, who shared that most of her values came from her parents. Even though the relationship between the parents was 'all the time very bad', Rou claimed she was very close to them both.

In the last few months of his life, Rou's father was incapacitated, and although the family tried to keep him in his home and her parents had a domestic helper, it was difficult for everyone. Rou recalled having to go to her parents' home many nights when her mother could no longer tolerate the demands of caregiving. She explained how '…because my mother will feel very uncomfortable and she will cry and then she will phone to me and then I have to comfort her. And then I will go back home and comfort my father… So, I will try to mediate [between] the both of them'. Rou also described how her relationship with her father changed during this time when he fell in the bath. She said: 'I think that something shifted at that moment…because I have to pick him up together with my maid…and he knows that he has to depend on somebody even in bathing'.

Then her father was hospitalised and her own life spun out of control:

> I would view the life as very hard for me…. I will take quite a lot of the caring role [upon myself]. I buy him some food and go to the hospital daily or two times daily to feed him because the nurse is so busy and he cannot get the food that he would like to have. (Rou)

During this time, Rou was working full time and trying to complete her PhD. She described her situation:

I work here day and night and I remember at that moment I will cry to myself. They said that I have...some anxiety symptoms because the PhD is so harsh for me...I remember I would sit in that chair, I would cry every morning because every time I feel that I cannot control myself, and also [it was] so hard to engage in this kind of study...because I should spend my time with my parents. (Rou)

Rou recalled that working a demanding job while studying for the PhD and caring for her father made her feel 'torn between all these parts'; but she maintained she had 'to endure because I'm the eldest daughter in the family [and] the decision maker'. She observed, 'If I collapse my mother will also collapse'. Rou expressed gratitude for having 'a very good husband and also a very good family, including my brother' who helped her get through this challenging time. However, she remembered how her own health had suffered:

After my father's death, I have been sick for about three to four months. I know that the burden is so hard, the burden is so great, that it makes you sick.... Even though I go to [the] doctor, a number of doctors, I cannot be helped. I cannot retain my health ...I understand I have to endure this period because my body has already suffered a lot. I cannot get enough sleep and sometimes my father will bring out his temper because I think he suffers a lot. I have to pacify him as if he's a child. (Rou)

One thing all the temporary caregivers had in common was that when a parent was hospitalised, in a final illness or there was a family emergency, the parent became prioritised by the family. As Hwei-Ru, a Gen X Singaporean noted: 'It is sometimes quite difficult to strike a balance, and you just have to set your priorities'. Nonetheless, of the 23 temporary caregivers in this book who were working at the time of the crisis, only two took leave: one, until an FDH could be hired, and the other until the parent could be stabilised. That raises the issue of *Work-Life-Balance*.

Work-Life-Balance

Work-Life-Balance is a contemporary concept promoting harmony between the home and the workplace. Flexible working hours, fewer working hours, part time work, and the granting of employee leave, when needed, are central to its core objective of spending more time with the family. Rou did not attempt to invoke *Work-Life-Balance* during her father's final illness. She was unwilling to take leave from her job, like most of the daughters who said they had to work or wanted to work. Wenling, a Gen X daughter from Kunming, explained why, after taking time off when her child was younger, she would never do it again:

> I tried for half year then I just realised, this is not...work needs me but I need work. Because staying at home makes me feel like I am far away, isolated from the society. ...my world will become smaller- smaller and smaller. I just put all my focus on my husband and my daughter. I lost myself. So, I think I'm still young. I still have my dreams.... I will always work, no matter what. If it's both my husband and I am too busy, you know, to take care of her [daughter], I'll find someone to share the burden, but I will never stay at home. (Wenling)

As an interesting aside, Wenling added that working also promoted a sense of value, not only from job satisfaction but from how others perceived her. She related a story she had read in the paper about a boy who called his mother worthless because she stayed at home. Wenling remarked that mothers had to set an example for their children. Referring to the article again, she emphasised, 'for me I can never accept that in my daughter's eyes if I am such a person'.

Whether they were from Singapore, Hong Kong or mainland China, most of the daughters said they could manage both home and work with the help of their parents, siblings or domestic helpers, even though it was stressful. Very few expressed conflict between work and family, although some said they felt guilty for not spending enough time with their children. Chunhua elaborated on the challenge:

As a woman in a country like China, at a certain level [it is] still quite traditional, although it is developing so fast. Of course, for example, if you have, if a child [who has] a problem then people always blame the mother. They think the father's responsibility is just the breadmaker… And then for women you really have to take a lot of jobs in your daily life… and this is why I said we really need a kind of wisdom to really develop your perspective towards your life and to balance the life. (Chunhua)

In mainland China, and to a lesser extent in Hong Kong, an additional factor was in play. If a woman left the workforce too long she could become unemployable. Yun, a Gen X from Kunming explained:

It depends on how many years you stay at home as a full-time mother or housewife…. It only one year I think it's ok, you can go back. But, more than two or three years maybe it's a little bit difficult. You have to kind of catch up on everything and get training and maybe some employers don't want it. (Yun)

The most frequently cited strategy used in a family emergency involved appraising the situation, deciding whether family or work required more attention, committing to whichever that was, then if work was affected, seeking approval from the employer to accommodate the situation. In times of crisis nearly all the daughters said they could make arrangements with their employers by working fewer hours, taking a few hours off during the day, having flexible hours, or taking work home. In situations of longer duration, like the final illness of a parent, leave might be requested, as long as it was reasonably short. Praise for understanding employers was widespread among the daughters and jobs were sometimes selected based on how supportive the employer was of family obligation. The statement below is a good example of what many of the daughters said.

I feel that family is more important…my job is important, but…let's say suddenly… somebody at home needs my attention. I would apply for leave and go and attend to that person…I don't think there will be a situation where I have to resign because of family. Definitely we can work out something. I can still keep my job but at the same time, I can attend to my family's need. (Huizhong)

Indeed, most of the daughters reported that family was more important than work. The daughter making the statement below changed jobs five times to accommodate her family:

> You can move jobs, you can move company but we have…responsibilities to our kids, to our husband and family…I can lose a job but I do not want to lose any relationship with my loved ones, so they are definitely more important. (Jun)

Paradoxically however, most of the daughters also admitted that work consumed the majority of their time. As one daughter reported, 'at this time, my family doesn't really need my time. So, I spend more time working' (Shu). For those who tried to balance work and home, although they tried, most indicated they could not always give 100% to both. Juan, a Hong Kong Boomer explained that, 'both [work and family] are important but for the work…you have to…put your 100% effort in it. If you put 100% effort in it then to the family it will become less'.

Differences Between Hong Kong, Singapore and Mainland China

Some comparisons between the daughters can be drawn. The commitment to family and work and the prioritising of family were virtually identical among all the daughters interviewed, regardless of where they were from. However, in practice it differed slightly. The only two daughters who took leave to provide temporary care, Te' and Ah Kum, were both Singaporeans. Jai, a Gen X Singaporean, also sacrificed her career aspirations when her mother developed Parkinson's disease. She explained why:

> So, I would have to sacrifice my own career and aspirations for the family. But, that's fine… because I know that if that desire comes again, I can always do it. I'm much younger than my mom. I think she needs me more than me fulfilling my own career aspirations. (Jai)

Five Singaporean and three mainland daughters brought parents or in-laws into their own homes to provide temporary care, whereas only one in Hong Kong did. The provision of temporary care by daughters in their parents' home was also more prevalent in Singapore, where seven care-recipients remained in their own homes. All the temporary care recipients in Hong Kong, with one exception, were hospitalised.

In Singapore, the concept of '*Work-Life-Balance*' was popular among the daughters. For example:

> I think one of my top priorities right now is to…work less… to achieve a *Work-Life-Balance*. What I really want…is to focus on finding…my life partner and…having my own kid. (Jai)

> I'm glad that working here allows us to have *Work-Life Balance*. That's why I chose here as my career…after I gave birth, because it's not as demanding as my previous work in terms of hours, in terms of expectation and all that. So…. I'm able to manage better now. (Hwei-Ru)

The mainland women were also aware of the concept, but practiced it more informally. As discussed above, both mainland and Hong Kong women were more likely to remain in the workplace regardless of the circumstances. The following statements of two Hong Kong Baby Boomers were indicative of this perspective:

> Conflict between work and family life? Not much…. While I am working I am… fully committed to my job. (Juan)

> I'm really a career woman. And you can imagine as a woman you have a full-time job, you have a full time role as a wife. You have a full-time job as a mother. Sometimes there's really certain conflicts of time and energy. And… I am… always too serious with my work. And maybe for some time I've been a little bit negligent onto my other roles. (Lihwa)

As seen with Rou, Hong Kong and mainland daughters were also very likely to push themselves to the edge of exhaustion, trying to manage both family and work. Yow, a Hong Kong Boomer gave an account of her internal struggle to justify working:

> So, when you have too many cases…you have to take [them] home… And I could …work until 4:00. And, sometimes I really pity myself…. I don't

need the money to support myself. Why do I…have to work like this and stay up the whole night when people…are sleeping soundly in bed with the quilt. Especially during winter time. I pity myself so much. (Yow)

But she did not stop working.

Like Yow and Rou, many mainland and Hong Kong daughters reported being 'stressed all the time' from trying to balance work and family life (Chang-Chang). However, the availability of a job-threatening workforce in mainland China and the Hong Kong government's lack of enthusiasm for promoting *Work-Life-Balance* suggested it was unlikely that mainland and Hong Kong women would follow the family friendly Singapore model.

Limitations, Conditions and Qualifications Related to the Provision of Temporary Care

Differences Between in Home and Out of Home Care

Weici and Rou illustrate the difference between providing care in one's own home as opposed to the parents' home or hospital. Care in one's home appeared to create emotional strain arising from the disruption of the household from the omnipresent parent. Care in the parents' home or hospital seemed to engender more physical strain resulting from the constant travel between venues.

In this sub-sample of 24 temporary caregivers, all but two daughters continued working and those who brought parents into their home hired domestic helpers to provide care. Two of the daughters provided temporary care for cognitively impaired in-laws. Shuang, a Hong Kong Baby Boomer, cared for a stroke victim, and Lian, a Singapore Gen X, cared for a dementia patient. Although their involvement was limited, it did not completely alleviate the stress. Lian described taking care of her father-in-law:

So, I get stressed because my helper get stressed. They brought their own helper but my father-in-law will take advantage of [the] helpers in the sense that he will yell and shout at them. And my helper told me that, you know, sometimes after she cooked and served my father-in-law food, if he didn't like it he will just throw it back at her. (Lian)

Lian's father-in-law disrupted the household to such an extent that she developed migraines and could not sleep. She said her performance at work suffered. The experience was so unpleasant that her father-in-law wore out his welcome. Lian and Shuang, like Weici, discontinued care and sent their in-laws back to their homes when they could no longer tolerate the caregiving situation. Shuang explained how her husband eventually made the decision to send his mother home:

> [It was] very tough…There was the time when he feels that she should not stay here because she's affecting…the well-being of…our life here…. This outburst of the temper often comes with a cry that she wanted to go back to her own home. So, maybe after discussing with the brothers he feels that maybe… this is what she wants. So, when her condition improved [so] that she could walk they feel that she should really go back to her own home and feel peaceful and at ease then. (Shuang)

Three in-home caregivers went to their parents' home to care for them. All three of these daughters lived in mainland China where the distance between their own home and their parents' home was far. The other in-home caregivers invited their own mothers to stay with them. Jun and Jai's mothers were brought home to die. The time was short and care was discontinued by death. Zhenzhen cared for her own mother twice following surgeries. The first time she kept her mother for a month, the second time she kept her for two weeks. Even though Zhenzhen said she loved her mother, she recalled that having her at home could be challenging:

> It's not the physical part. But, I would think that the emotional and psychological part, it is a little more stressful, honestly speaking, because she gets bored and she expects us to be home, and she basically needs somebody to talk to. And, we're so busy unfortunately, so that becomes the stress…that you have work commitments and yet there's a mom waiting for you at home. So…you try to rush home so that she gets somebody to talk to…At one stage…I was saying that she was marking mental attendance. (Zhenzhen)

The daughters' chief complaint about hospital or out of home 'care' was the amount of time it took, particularly for temporary caregivers who continued working. Below, Huizhong describes the hospital visitations she made for three weeks after work every day, arriving home about 9:00 p.m. every night. All the stories regarding hospitalised care were very similar to this one:

> When my father-in-law was hospitalised…I…had to visit him every day at the hospital and at the same time, I had to have time at home, house work, my office work and so on, so actually I find that it's the demand on the time…. It's not the amount of time spent with him, it's actually the travelling…. From work, you travel to the hospital because it will take some time, and then at the hospital, you stay for half an hour, one hour, and you travel all the way home…. [This took] between…about three and a half to four hours every night [after work]. (Huizhong)

Among these women there was scant evidence of a correspondence between the number, length and duration of visitations to the hospital or to a parent's home and the quality of the relationship the daughter had with the parent. Perhaps that was because most of the hospitalised parents were fathers, and caring for a father also supported the mother. Face within the family was also implicated. Family members expected the daughters to provide care, and failure to live up to such expectations might have resulted in disapproval. Further, hospital care or care in the parents' home could involve all the siblings, even if the daughter was the primary caregiver. This provided some respite for caregiving daughters, for example by alternating visits with sisters and brothers. The limitations that did exist were more likely to result from the daughter's unwillingness or inability to stop working, thereby restricting the amount of time she had to spend with the disabled parent.

Home care was slightly different. The duty to take a parent or in-law into one's home was not generally dependent on the quality of the relationship. However, once a parent and particularly an in-law was in the home, the relationship became important. What this suggests is that the willingness to *provide* care was more related to structural norms of obligation and the disposition of the wife to support her husband than it was to the relationship between the daughter and her husband's parents. For example, Shuang explained that she brought her mother-in-law home, 'because my husband feels that she…was in a critical situation and she need…[us] to…watch her closely so that she doesn't get into a worse condition and if it comes to that stage…we can give immediate attention to her'.

However, the willingness to *continue* care might have been dependent on the relationship between the caregiver and care recipient. Perhaps that is why the majority of temporary care was provided to parents rather than to in-laws. The relationship was easier to sustain. Many of the interviewed women said they preferred daughters to daughters-in-law, and they also preferred to take care of their own parents. Discussions with the married daughters were similar to the following:

Q   Do you feel closer to your own mother or to your mother in law?
A   To my mother.
Q   Given the choice, who would you rather take care of?
A   My mother (Shuang)

Hwei-Ru explained why:

I think because the parents…bring up the children and they would appreciate that the child is the one who is taking care of them. And it's really their own children.…Daughter-in-law or son-in-law is actually…not 100% their own, so I think…it's just naturally that I care more for my mom [than] my parents-in-law. (Hwei-Ru)

There was also a difference between mothers and fathers. No fathers were cared for in a daughter's home unless they already lived together. As mentioned previously, this might be explained by the fact that among these daughters, mothers took care of their husbands in their own homes if the mother's health allowed it.

Other Qualifications, Conditions and Limitations

Conditionality, structural impediments such as distance, and gaps between filial attitudes and behaviour were not seen in the provision of temporary care among these 24 daughters. Moreover, only three women said they would refuse to provide temporary care, although none of them had been asked to do so, and their position was specific to their mothers. Lian said she would not provide *any* care again in the future but would contribute only money. Given that both of her parents were dead, she was speaking of her in-laws. Two of the daughters providing hospital care reported their unwillingness to provide emotional support.

Among those not actually providing temporary care, most in Hong Kong and Singapore maintained that they would hire an FDH to perform the hands-on caregiving. Several daughters indicated the type of care provided and where it was provided would depend on whom the care was for. Very few expressed a willingness to take extended leave from work, consistent with what has already been discussed. However, until these women are actually faced with the decision, it is impossible to know what they will do.

Differences Between Support and Temporary Care

> If parents are healthy, then there's no issue, but when somebody falls sick, then you find that …your time is very stretched. (Huizhong)

With temporary care, the balance between parental and personal needs appeared to tip slightly in favour of parents. Although most daughters continued to work, they *did* allow parents' care and well-being to interrupt their lives. However, limitations applied, and by definition, care was temporary. If it was expected to have an end date and if it did not occur within a reasonable time, the daughters could terminate it in consultation with family members.

As stated at the beginning of this chapter, the principal difference between support and temporary care was the level of commitment required. However, there were subtle distinctions within this. For one thing, although daughters like Jaihui accept responsibility for parent *support* because nobody else would do it, at the stage of temporary care, the daughters were stepping forward and taking charge. Te' and Rou were good examples of this. These women not only directed their parent's care, they were the emotional backbone of the family, holding it together.

Although with home care, decisions regarding where care was to be implemented and by whom appeared to be made collectively by the siblings, some daughters volunteered for this duty. For example, below is how Jai explained her decision:

> I don't think I was expected to, but it was just a natural... thing that I be the one to take care of her, because I'm technically the most educated in the family and I don't have other financial commitments... All I had was work commitment...so I volunteered for it. (Jai)

The assertiveness seen at the temporary care stage, but not in evidence at the support stage, has two possible explanations. The first is that it was role modelling by the daughters' mothers, as seen from the following statement:

> Actually, my mother is a very submissive, very gentle lady. [But,] at the time of crisis she will stand up very firm, very courageous and [be a] very decisive lady. (Rou)

Additionally, some of these women were accustomed to taking responsibility. Te', for example, was preparing for marriage and running a multi-million-dollar project at the time of her father's crisis.

This leads to another difference from support, and an important one. Stress increased substantially at the temporary care stage. When Te', for example, was asked to indicate on a scale of one to ten, with ten being the most, what her stress level was, she replied: 'Ten.... I'm trying to recall. I think my fuse was very short'.

Huiqing, discussed in Chap. 4, told her dying father to 'let go'. Other daughters did the same. It was not only that these women were trying to manage the balance between work and home; it was the emotional element as well. Daughters could be called upon to perform unpleasant tasks regardless of whether their parent was cared for at home or hospitalised. They related stories of diaper changing, bathing, and feeding parents through a tube, assisting with dialysis and dealing with behavioural problems. This had two further ramifications. Some temporary caregivers, like Rou and Te', experienced a shift in the nature of the relationship with their parents when they perceived them as vulnerable. The other was that there appeared to be a link between stress and *emotion work* at this stage that was not found with support.

Looking back on the *support* emotion work done by Jaihui, Qingzhao, and even Yet Kwai, suggests that the objective was to maintain the relationship, and to ensure that it continued to exist. It was protracted and seemed to involve a desire on the part of the daughters to be accepted and valued by their parents, and reciprocally, to care about them. If stress existed, it appeared to be self-imposed by personally interpreted framing rules and feeling rules, not by the circumstances.

In contrast, the emotion work done during temporary care was immediate and related to managing stress. As seen with Weici, there was pressure to maintain one's equilibrium, control one's emotions, and not exhibit anger. Conditions were more intense, especially if the parent remained in the caregiver's home. Although framing rules and feeling rules might have necessitated emotion work to provide support, with temporary care the breadth of the work was greater and more integrated with societal expectations in addition to personal ones.

The entirety of the in home temporary caregiving daughters experienced this pressure. They all expressed how difficult the situation was. If they did not do emotion work they practiced avoidance, and some did both. There *did* appear to be a relationship between the necessity of doing emotion work, the frequency and intensity of contacts between the caregiver and the care recipient, and the nature of the care being provided. Emotion work was really not seen among the daughters caring for their parents in the hospital where care appeared to be more related to exhaustion and concern rather than tolerating the disruptions and demands of a parent living in one's home. Moreover, in hospital care, the daughters could remove themselves from the care environment and the care recipient. Similarly, supporting a parent by dining or visiting with them, *in itself,* was less likely to become a stressful activity, especially if other siblings were present.

All of this suggests that when providing support and nothing more, emotion work may be based on the relationship alone. With temporary care, emotion work appears to be based on the relationship plus the care-giving activity and the ease with which one can remove oneself from the situation when it becomes too stressful.

Conclusion

Temporary care is the second stage in the typology of support and care. Among these daughters, it took place in their home, the parent's home, or the hospital and lasted six months or less. In this sample, 24 daughters cared for 32 care recipients. Three quarters of the temporary care recipients were parents. Baby Boomers provided most of the temporary care. Even more than with support, temporary care was largely motivated by combined structural and relational norms.

The focus of this chapter was Weici, who had provided temporary care at different times for both her mother and her mother-in-law. Weici grew up in a dysfunctional family in which her father beat her mother. Her mother held the family together, but once the children were grown she found a job and became self-sufficient, divorcing her husband and earning Weici's respect. More than that, her mother's willingness to listen to her children and the repeated acts of loving kindness made Weici love and feel gratitude for her mother, motivating Weici to care for her with patience and understanding, even sleeping on the floor to do so. Weici was grateful to her father for supporting the family and supporting her education, however, she felt no affection for him. Thus, although her father had not yet required care, she was willing to provide financially for him out of duty, but not to provide for him emotionally.

The story of Weici's mother-in-law was in stark contrast to her own mother. Weici had developed a dislike for the woman when they had lived together and had implemented a management style consisting largely of avoidance. After her father-in-law died, Weici and her husband declined to live with the mother-in-law. Nonetheless, when the mother-in-law broke her hip, duty obligated Weici to take her in. She related how her mother-in-law disrupted the household and abused Weici's FDH. Weici practiced emotion work to change how she felt and acted. After six months, her mother-in-law was sent home.

From Weici it was possible to see how relationships affected the temporary caregiving experience. Caring for her mother was done out of love and gratitude, whereas caring for her mother-in-law was her duty. Although both experiences were difficult, it was Weici's attitude and how she felt about each party that defined the situation and the amount of stress accompanying it.

Weici was a traditional woman from a traditional family. Her mother was a strong role model. Through her, Weici learned to subjugate her own interests to the family. However, contemporary norms were also seen in her need to set limitations by taking time for herself and ultimately instigating the removal of her mother-in-law from the home. Further, Weici relied on her Christian faith to help her through the difficult times.

Religion, in this instance, was part of the emotion work undertaken in providing temporary care for her mother-in-law, not the force driving care. Weici prayed to God to control her temper and to mitigate the negative feelings she had for her mother-in-law. However, she also exhorted herself to change her display and continued her practice of avoidance. Conversely, Weici appeared to have done no emotion work with her own mother.

If Weici showed us why relationships matter, Rou's story illustrated the difficulties encountered when one's responsibilities exceed one's ability to manage. During her father's final illness, Rou worked a full-time job, wrote her PhD thesis and cared for her father, first at home then in the hospital, while supporting the rest of the family emotionally. She was exhausted and overwhelmed but said she never considered altering her circumstances. After her father's death, it took Rou several months to recover her own health.

Rou's situation raised the question of *Work-Life-Balance.* In this regard, Hong Kong, Singapore and mainland China were different. Most mainland and Hong Kong daughters, like Rou, were likely to remain in work and drive themselves to the edge of their ability to cope. Hong Kong's proximity to and interaction with mainland China and the mainland's work ethic were likely to be implicated. Conversely, the Singaporean daughters were more likely to take leave or change jobs to accommodate the needs of their families. Social engineering and family friendly policies initiated by the Singapore government might account for this difference.

The dissimilarity of Weici and Rou's experience highlighted the reason why there is no 'one size fits all' formula for understanding the limitations of temporary care. Home care was accompanied by emotional strain resulting from close and constant proximity to the care recipient. Although it might not have affected the initial decision to bring a parent into the home, once care began, the relationship *did* matter: It was associated with the amount of stress and emotion work required to withstand the situation, the decision over when to discontinue care, and whether to renew the invitation should care be needed again. This could be why more daughters said they would rather care for their own parents instead of their in-laws, and daughters who were parents said they preferred to be cared for by their own children.

In contrast, caring for a parent in hospital or the parents' home appeared to cause more physical exhaustion and stress resulting primarily from worry over the parent's condition and its effect on the remaining family members. Relationships were not as important, and the decision to terminate care was beyond the daughter's ability to control. The greatest limitations to hospital care or care in the parents' home were the daughter's employment and physical stamina.

Conditionality, gaps between filial belief and behaviour and structural impediments, such as distance, did not appear to limit temporary care. However, distance could affect a daughter's exhaustion level if she was visiting a parent after work and getting home late at night.

The essential differences between support and temporary care were the disruptions to one's life and the commitment needed to get through it. However, other dynamics were at work as well. Principally, most of the daughters appeared to become more authoritative and assertive during times of crisis. This could have been attributed to the role modelling of strong mothers or the nature of the daughters' employment responsibilities.

Temporary care additionally involved a level of stress not seen at the support stage of the typology. Daughters could be required to undertake hands-on care that was not only unpleasant but that could result in a role reversal with vulnerable parents.

The forces driving emotion work were also different. Emotion work conducted in furtherance of parental support was directed at preserving the relationship and motivating daughters to spend time and be cordial. Any stress was likely to be self-imposed due to the daughter's interpretation of framing rules and feeling rules telling her this was what she *should* want. In contrast, emotion work undertaken in the performance of temporary care was more related to controlling one's emotions in the face of intense pressure. The daughter *should* maintain a pleasant outward display, exhibit no anger, and attempt to *feel* no anger. Arguably, the work was greater and more constant because the daughter could not walk away indefinitely, especially if the parent was in her home.

One of the primary questions addressed in the next chapter is whether the importance of relational norms and the intensity of emotion work increase as caregiving moves from temporary to more permanent conditions requiring more effort and causing greater stress.

7

Caregiving of Ageing Parents

Review of Caregiving and Introduction to the Chapter

The third stage in the typology of support and care is caregiving, or long-term care. It is distinguishable from temporary care in two principal ways. First, it is of unlimited duration. Additionally, it takes place <u>only</u> in the caregiver's home.

The activities of caregiving, shown in Table 4.3, describe the kinds of endeavours associated with long-term care in the domestic setting, characterised by hands-on care, with or without assistance from a domestic helper (FDH/CDH). Among the 64 daughters in this book, eight were providing or had provided caregiving for 10 parents, with 70% of the care recipients being mothers. Additionally, three in-laws formerly received care from one daughter. As discussed, the preponderance of mothers as care recipients (as opposed to fathers) may be explained by a tendency seen in temporary care. Most of the fathers were taken care of in their own homes by their wives, with possible assistance from a domestic helper until hospitalisation was required.

© The Author(s) 2018
P. O'Neill, *Urban Chinese Daughters*, St Antony's Series,
https://doi.org/10.1007/978-981-10-8699-1_7

Even more than it was with temporary care, 88% of caregiving among this group of women was provided by Baby Boomers, with two of the daughters providing both temporary care and long-term care at different times. In both instances, temporary care was undertaken for the father and long-term care for the mother. Among the full-time caregivers, two quit their jobs. Another daughter took time off while seeking re-employment, but later resumed working. The others continued in employment. Three daughters had support from siblings, and all but two hired a domestic helper. Finally, all eight caregivers identified themselves as Christian and six of the eight relied on their religion to help them endure the burden of caregiving.

Like the previous one, this chapter examines why the daughters were willing or unwilling to provide caregiving, how they resolved the tension and conflict incurred in discharging this type of care, and why care might have been terminated. The limitations, qualifications and conditions involved with caregiving by these daughters are also probed, however, the emphasis and approach in Chap. 6 shifts slightly to explore the discharge of care more deeply.

All the daughters in this book provided some form of support. Because the demands on their time, energy and emotions were nominal, it allowed us to focus on the forces underpinning their support and care motivations. Progressing to temporary care, with fewer daughters and greater demands on them, the relationship between the daughters and their parents and the daughters' employment became relevant to understanding each of the elements in the axis of analysis. At this third stage of the typology the length and intensity of the caregiving experience, and the commitment to it, suggests a need to investigate more thoroughly the daughters' coping strategies, especially for accommodating tension. Again, the daughters' narratives are used to tease out the epistemology of caregiving.

How Structural Norms of Filial Obligation and Relational Norms of Affection, Gratitude and Reciprocity Motivated These Chinese Daughters to Undertake Caregiving of Their Parents

Among the eight caregivers, 37.5% were motivated by combined structural norms of filial obligation and relational norms [*'I have to + I want to'*], 25% by structural norms [*'I have to'*], and 37.5% by relational norms of affection, gratitude and reciprocity [*'I want to'*]. There were no instances, related by the daughters, in which care was refused altogether [*'I do not want to/I cannot'*] due to negative motivation, other than as discussed in Chap. 4. Among the 10 care recipients, combined structural and relational norms motivated *half* the total care and all of this was for mothers. Combined norms were associated more with fathers in temporary care. The distribution of structural norms of filial obligation and relational norms of affection, gratitude and reciprocity among the care recipients is shown below in Table 7.1.

This chapter begins with two case studies. The first, Huan, is an exploration of care motivated by structural norms of filial obligation. The other, Ai, examines care motivated by relational norms of affection, gratitude and reciprocity. Huan and Ai approached the caregiving experience from opposite perspectives. Ai, a single woman, provided care for her own mother out of love and gratitude, without any help. She said she did not believe it would be possible to do this without feeling close to her parent. Huan, a married woman, cared for her husband's parents and grandmother out of duty, with three domestic helpers. Based on her

Table 7.1 Motivation driving caregiving of parents and in-laws

Motivational type	Mother	Father	Mother-in-law	Father-in-law	Other	Total
Structural	1	0	1	1	1[a]	4
Relational	1	0	0	0	0	1
Structural + relational	5	0	0	0	0	5
Total	7	0	1	1	1	10

[a]Grandmother-in-law

childhood experiences she defined herself by traditional Chinese values. For example, she said, 'from my upbringing I have to respect the old people'. Ai lived alone with her mother. Huan lived with her husband's extended family. The two women's lives and their motivations for caregiving were different. But, did this matter?

Structural Norms Driving Caregiving

Huan grew up in a poor and traditional Chinese family where she was the oldest child of five. As a child, she helped her mother (a housewife) with chores, tutored her four younger brothers and supplemented the family's income by sewing and making plastic flowers. According to Huan, education and elevated status were important to her parents and she became a nurse at her father's suggestion. Reciting her system of values, Huan said, 'you must be a loyal servant'; you must be 'obedient' and have a 'good manner'; you must give money to your parents and 'to the old people in China'.

As a traditional Chinese woman, once married, Huan's life became centred on her husband's family. Although she gave money to her parents after she began working, she never expected to care for them. At the time she was interviewed, Huan's father had died and her mother, who had dementia, lived alone with a domestic helper. Huan said she met her mother every few weeks for dinner. She and her youngest brother shared her mother's expenses, but her other brothers did not contribute any form of support. In fact, Huan supported two of them.

At the time of her interview, Huan had lived with her husband's family for 37 years. She described their relationship as good and said that maintaining family harmony was important. For this reason, sensitive communications with her in-laws were channelled through her husband and if she had a difference of opinion from them, she said she would 'bear it down'. According to Huan, she learned this from watching traditional Chinese films, which she asserted, 'are always teaching you, anything if you don't like [it], you just bear it. Women have to bear it, bear the suffering'. Expanding on this, Huan said:

Yeah, this is the ethics, the society expects [from the] woman; you must be tender, gentle, loving and kind. And you have to accept the things that are not happy or you have to protect your family members. You have to make a harmonious family. Make everything happy. (Huan)

Huan reflected, 'it's already deep rooted in our mind that you have to be a good daughter, a good wife, and a good mother and a good friend'. She acknowledged that this put pressure on her, but added 'when you do it on your own will…it's happy…' She disclosed the most important thing to her was her husband's support; however, she also said she relied on her Christian religion as part of her problem-solving strategy.

Over the course of several years, often at the same time, Huan provided care for her father-in-law, mother-in-law and her husband's grandmother, all of whom lived with her. For nearly 20 years, until his death, Huan helped her chronically ill father-in-law through a succession of illnesses, including asthma, ulcers, hernia, cataracts, hypertension, heart disease, and later Parkinson's disease and liver cancer. Overlapping ten years of this she also cared for her husband's grandmother who was blind, had heart disease and later a stroke. The grandmother could neither bathe nor feed herself, and Huan recalled the grandmother's care consumed much of her time. However, Huan's most difficult experience as a caregiver was with her mother-in-law.

Huan's Mother-in-Law Huan knew her mother-in-law was depressed after her husband's death. However, it was not until she refused to bathe, take her medications or change her clothes that Huan said she began to suspect something else was wrong. In attempting to find an answer, Huan's sister-in-law took her mother to the hospital for an evaluation, but according to Huan, when the doctor's diagnosis was related to her, no cognitive irregularities were reported.

Despite the diagnosis, over the next four years Huan noticed a decline in her mother-in-law's temperament, and said she was puzzled when the older woman would not cooperate with instructions for her health care. When the elderly lady began to regularly exhibit signs of impairment, becoming angry, beating her chest, hitting the walls and threatening to commit suicide, Huan said she found herself 'shocked and astonished' over her 'very, very queer behaviour'. Her lack of knowledge of her mother-in-law's condition, combined with the old woman's erratic demeanour, drove Huan into a state of confusion and despair. She recalled:

> And before, I was in a dark place, in a dark hole. I don't know what to do.... I do not know what is happening to her. Is it just due to depression?... But why is it so long, the depression period? So, nobody is going to help me. (Huan)

Huan said she could not remember how she got through this difficult time. However, wanting information, she wrote to the doctor her mother-in-law had seen four years before. When he wrote back, he informed Huan that her mother-in-law had been diagnosed with dementia at the time of her prior visit. Huan said she was stunned.

After reassessing her mother-in-law, the doctor told Huan:

> This lady [has] got dementia, you have to learn how to take care of her, and you have to organise the family members and [you] have to make a decision how to take care of her because the disease will get worse and worse. (Huan)

Huan said, 'that aroused me...oh!! Big trouble'. She knew she had to educate herself on how to take care of her mother-in-law. This previously 'nice lady', who had been 'very gentle [and] very kind', had become 'another person' who was 'very agitated and easily angry and cannot cooperate with you, and always have no sense of safety'. Fortunately, soon after the second diagnosis, Huan received a promotional leaflet from the Alzheimer's disease Association. She recalled how, with new awareness, she contacted them. To cope, Huan said she also spoke with friends, but neither her friends nor her husband offered solutions. She explained how she was conflicted, depressed and frustrated, and how she tried to change her feelings to survive:

> Very depressed. I am very frustrated. Nobody can help me. And, I want to die. But I just said oh, every day is a new day. Try every possible means to

[do it] …because I have to respect my mother- in-law. She helped me a lot when my children are young, alright? That's a conflict. I have to respect this …lady but still she does something [that] makes me unhappy. I have to accept that. (Huan)

Huan's statement reflects her attempt to bridge the gap between what she actually felt and what she believed she should feel. Unbeknownst to her, this was emotion work. She finally enrolled in a course to learn how to care for and communicate with Alzheimer's patients. She joined a carer support group and placed her mother-in-law into day care. Huan described her state of mind, looking back on what she had learned:

I know the way, how to tackle all the problems. Of course, you can't solve [it in] one day. You just bit by bit [try] to learn how to cope with her, all right, because dementia is [a] very, very strange disease. Every case is differ-ent…. You have to learn and you have to talk with the carers, and join the association and listen to the professional's advice. And, you…must have a kind heart behind [it]. Love, …patience and acceptance …is the drive that makes you accept this people, this patient. (Huan)

In Huan's case, emotion work could be viewed not only as an attempt to create an appropriate display or to bridge the gap between what she felt and what she believed she should feel, but also as a coping mechanism to help her endure the caregiving experience. In her words:

I remember the professor saying every day is a new day. Use humour to ease the negative emotion. That's very useful for me…. Every day I have nega-tive emotion, when I'm taking care [of her]. But, later I learned the com-munication skill. We must accept the patient, not argue with her. [I] have to respect her, to encourage her and say, her drawing is very beautiful, you are a very nice lady and so, all kinds of praise words. She will be happy. If she [is] happy, I'm happy. I want to be a happy carer, all right? I don't want to die so early. If I am sick nobody will take care of the family. I always think of a broad view. The family is a whole. I can't collapse. If I collapse nobody will take care of the family members. (Huan)

After ten years, Huan's mother-in-law became incontinent, had diffi-culty swallowing, and developed pneumonia. When she required an IV drip, a nasal gastric tube to feed her, and a stretcher to lie on for bathing, the decision was made to place her into a nursing home. She remained there the last three years of her life.

Huan's story demonstrates how useful professional support and emotion work can be. Although her underlying motivation to care for her in-laws consisted primarily of structural obligation ['*I have to*'], she was able to effectively change her feelings and adapt to her circumstances.

Relational Norms Driving Caregiving

> To me the value is always there- that you're supposed to look after your parents. But, it has to come with feelings. If you don't feel that closeness and that you want to look after them, it's no point.... If [children] don't have that ...bonding with the parent, I don't think it's possible at all to do it. (Ai)

Ai was one of two daughters, and as she related it, had always been close to her parents. Now 50, she recalled how, during her twenties, she had struggled between commitment to her family and a desire to live independently. She chose to remain with the family, and since her father's death Ai had been the sole caregiver of her 80-year-old mother, who suffered from dementia.

Unexpectedly, I interviewed Ai twice, six months apart, allowing me to explore the effect of caregiving over time. During the first interview Ai elaborated on her motivation to care for her mother:

> My main motivation is that she looked after me when I'm young, and a lot of my young memories flash through my mind these days... So I feel that right now in the sorry state that she is [in], I feel moved, sorry, that I should have to look after her. (Ai)

Ai expressed that taking care of her mother was '*the least I can do*'. In her words, gratitude compelled her to feel 'responsible and obligated'. She added that, 'to be honest, I think religion is [also] a big part of my life'. Ai said it helped to remind her there was more to life than what she was doing.

The First Interview Following her mother's dementia diagnosis, Ai's father took over her care. However, two years into it he died from a heart attack. Ai recalled, 'Then I feel everything falls on me'. At the time, Ai was still working, however, her job required her to travel and her mother could not be left alone. Her mother was also in denial over her disability. Thus, every time Ai attempted to leave for a trip, stressful altercations erupted in which Ai insisted her mother must stay with Ai's sister and her mother alternatively argued that she could take care of herself at home or that Ai 'should find a job that's local' (Ai).

When Ai eventually began to absorb the full extent of her mother's condition, she quit her job and became a full-time caregiver. Describing the dull routine of her life, she explained how her mother had to be bathed, fed and entertained every day. Ai said she had difficulty finding enough activities to engage her. Three days a week her mother attended day-care where she was reasonably coherent. However, at night she became agitated and hallucinated. Ai recalled how she had to curtail her evening activities to stay at home, and how her circle of friends had diminished. She described how lonely and isolated she felt and how she had become bored, admitting that, 'it's starting to get to me to be very honest'. To help her cope, on Sundays she went to church where, she said, she prayed and complained to God.

Despite her complaints, Ai asserted that she had 'grown to love her [mother] a lot more as a person' and had 'some enjoyable moments with her'. She claimed she was 'able now to see her...like a childlike person rather than as a dementia person needing care'. Ai maintained she had 'gradually changed...from feeling sorry for her [mother]' to feeling that she 'has her adorable moments'. She commented that they had grown closer because of that, and the 'love part' was 'stronger than the day to day burden'. Otherwise, she said, she 'would not have been able to carry on'. Ai explained how she focused on the positive, adding that on the days when it became 'pretty bad', she tried to keep herself in equilibrium. When she was out of balance or depressed she said she 'handled it very badly', losing her temper, raising her voice, scolding, or even yelling at her mother. However, if her mother started to cry she said she stopped and apologised, then retreated until she had 'cooled down'. Ai related some of the difficulties associated with caregiving:

> When it first started, especially when I quit my job, it's like there's no hope in the tunnel. You know, it's like, is this going to be what I'm going to do every day? And it's the repetition. You know, you just have to keep repeating and repeating and the daily chores, you know, and then you get very angry, you get very resentful, you get very short tempered, and, you're wondering why are you doing this? (Ai)

Ai explained how she worried about losing control: 'Yes, I was afraid that I'm going to go out of control. So generally, I don't because I think if I ever smack her I think it would get worse and worse' (Ai). To illustrate her frustration, Ai described an incident in which her mother lost her dentures:

> Her teeth, gone. Where? Don't know? Oh, I tell you, I searched high and low and in all the unlikely places because you don't know where she's going to put it. We just couldn't find it. And, I called the day-care centre and said, 'did she leave it there?' And, no she didn't. And, I am asking her, 'Where did you put it?' And she is saying 'No I didn't do anything', you know, and… 'did you throw it away?' 'No, I didn't. Why would I?'…She's always doing…the right thing. But, it's not right to us, it's right to her, ok, so she lost it. And, I blew my top. (Ai)

Another set of teeth had to be made, which took two months to fit and involved repeated visits to the dentist plus a substantial cost. Once they were done, Ai told her mother not to take her teeth out unless she was instructed to. However, returning from church shortly after receiving the new pair of dentures, Ai recalled how her mother had lost them again. Describing how angry and frustrated she was, Ai said was screaming and yelling at her mother, asking, 'Where did you put it? Did you throw it down the drain? Throw it down the chute again?'

Ai finally found the new dentures in her sewing box, but never did find the first set. She said she resolved to work on her attitude: 'otherwise, I'll kill myself'. She noted how she had started reading self-help books to give her a better perspective, adding that, 'if I myself change, the situation is actually not as bad, I suppose'. In addition, Ai pointed out that religion gave her strength and hope to 'pull through' and to reaffirm that she was doing the right thing.

Six months after this interview, I saw Ai and asked if I could interview her again. I wanted to find out what, if anything, had changed, how it was affecting her and what she was doing to get through it. She agreed to talk with me.

The Second Interview:

> She's getting worse in doing simple tasks and then recently it's gotten even worse because she doesn't even know when she has poo...And, I have to check and I figured that from now onwards I have to probably...clean her as well. So that in itself ... seems like it's going to be like more regular and that worries me.

As her mother's condition worsened, Ai worried that 'if I have to do daily caregiving now in everything, I don't think I can'. Her mother had started wearing diapers when 'she has a bad stomach', and could no longer manage simple tasks such as folding laundry. Ai described how sometimes her mother's vocabulary was 'all wrong'. She was not as lucid as in the past and some mornings she was unable to recognise Ai. Ai remarked that she had begun calling her mother by her first name so that 'when she goes to day-care [and] people say who are you at least she is able to tell people her name'. She then recalled a recent incident that had pushed her over the edge:

> She was soiling herself and she kept telling me no, and I'm saying like 'are you having a stomach ache?' 'No, I'm OK'. So, I say fine. So, every time she soils I have to bathe her. She just finished bathing and then she soiled. So, I say, 'OK, we bathe again' because, you know, what else am I going to do? So, I put her then on diapers and it's again.... And, I'm going like 'are you really not having diarrhoea? How come you can't tell me when you are about to soil?' And, she's going 'I know there's nothing wrong with me'. So, that really, really ticks me off. (Ai)

Ai remembered that she was 'really, really angry that day'. She said she shouted so loud 'I think probably the whole block can hear my voice'.

Then she added, 'I am not surprised because I think some days I really get it up'. Ai recalled how after this event she hit her mother on the hand, and how much this concerned her. She also said she had become anxious about her own health: 'Yes, I am worried, to be very, very honest. And, I know I can't afford to. So, that's why I told myself to cool down. The consequences, yes, I'm afraid of a stroke'. If that happened, 'then, we are going to be two persons needing help…and, it's going to be terrible then because who is going to help me, I ask myself? Yeah, that's the scary point'.

Contemplating her situation, Ai explained that she had begun to consider hiring professional help:

> Thinking ahead, it's going to get worse, it's not going to get better. And, I'm asking myself, what am I going to do about it? I was actually very much against having a maid, partly because my mom can't communicate, partly because of what I hear from people… and… I've got no experience handling a maid. (Ai)

After reasoning this thorough, she ultimately concluded, 'that I already have one person who is causing me stress and if I have to be responsible for another one I think I am going to go crazy'. With that idea dismissed she turned to the nursing home option. She acknowledged that, 'I'm actually telling my sister, not asking, that we have to start thinking about putting her in a nursing home'. However, in the end, Ai admitted that she did not think she had the heart to do it.

With no support or hope for support, Ai asserted that her stress level had 'increased quite a fair bit' since we last spoke and that she was 'asking myself, can I do this like forever?' She said, 'I dread to go home because I don't know what I'm going to find'. Further, she reported, her mother was getting on her nerves more:

> It's like every little thing bothers me. It really, really bothers me and I know for a fact that my mom is actually quite a good patient, really…. But, I suspect it's also me…. As it adds up, you know, your fuse gets shorter and shorter. (Ai)

Ai explained that her anger was closer to the surface and that she was more often unable to tolerate the circumstances of her life. She pointed out that she had become resentful of her sister's unwillingness to help, relating that, 'every time we talk we quarrel'. To overcome her negative feelings, Ai said she performed 'a lot of psycho' on herself. However, it appeared that this was not enough. In addition to being frustrated and angry, Ai's feelings of loneliness and isolation had grown. Falling back on what to her was an untenable position, she nonetheless reflected that some days, 'I don't want to do this anymore.... I just want to send her to a nursing home and be done with it'.

The Third Meeting with Ai A year later I saw Ai again. During a long conversation 'off the record', she offered no information about her mother's condition or whereabouts, her own mental state, or whether she had hired an FDH.

How Much Does the Type of Motivation Matter?

Some scholars have investigated the importance of affection to caregiving. They have argued that it is 'positively correlated to the level of commitment' and the amount of care provided, and negatively correlated to the degree of stress and ability to manage the burden (Horowitz and Shindelman 1983: 18; Lyonette and Yardley 2003). They have also suggested that strained relationships might cause affection and concern to recede and caregiver burden to rise as the demands of caregiving become more difficult (Horowitz and Shindelman 1983; Whitbeck et al. 1991, 1994).

Ai had a strong loving connection to her mother plus a sense of duty owed to her family. Conversely, Huan appeared to be more motivated by duty and less emotionally attached to her in-laws. Clearly, both women suffered from caregiver burden. Huan said she was in 'a dark place, a dark hole'. She felt nobody could help her. She wanted to die. Ai stated she felt like 'there's no hope in the tunnel'. She claimed she was getting angrier and thinking about giving up or killing herself. Paradoxically, both daughters worried about their own health. However, instead of giving up, both searched for new ways to motivate themselves to continue caregiving. Why? Did the type of motivation matter?

Motivation as a Framing Rule

Hochschild (1979: 566) told us that framing rules are the 'rules according to which we ascribe definitions and meanings to situations'. In the broad context, this has very often been synonymous with culturally prescribed norms and practices. The caregiving literature has separated the norms and practices underpinning and motivating the support and care of parents by their children into structural norms of filial obligation and relational norms of affection, gratitude and reciprocity. Within the Chinese context, both structural and relational norms have historical ties to Confucianism and filial piety. However, because Hong Kong, Singapore and mainland China are transitioning societies, they have additionally been influenced by the contemporary attitudes and values that have accompanied urbanisation. Together, these have formed the basis of the framing rules the daughters in this book subscribed to.

The importance of motivation is therefore dyadic. First, it provides a tool with which to investigate why Chinese daughters provide care. Second, and perhaps more important, is that as a framing rule it establishes the *standard of care* owed to the care recipient (in this case, the parent). For Huan and Ai, how they interpreted their filial norms, or framing rules, how they felt about them and the actions they took in furtherance of them, would have consequences for their care recipients, but even more for themselves.

The Relationship Between Framing Rules and Self-image

Holroyd (2001) posited that internalised cultural norms compel Chinese women to do what they consider right to preserve their personhood. Mac Rae (1998: 145) asserted that, 'According to symbolic interactionists, human beings have self-consciousness and are motivated toward achieving and sustaining a positive self-image'. Aronson (1990) argued that failing to live up to culturally shared assumptions and obligations related to caregiving could end in self-criticism, shame and guilt. These forces are clearly seen in both Ai and Huan, even though in their interviews it could be discerned how structural norms were primarily driving Huan and relational norms were driving Ai. Although different, these were the individual framing rules each had imposed on herself to preserve her positive self-image, sustain her personhood and be free of guilt.

Huan's background was grounded in traditional Chinese norms. She looked at the family 'as a whole' and understood her place within the collective hierarchy. Her core belief was that, 'you must be tender, gentle, loving and kind, and you have to accept…the things that are not happy or you have to protect your family members'. She had a lifetime of learning how to 'bear the suffering', and in her own words, she had always expected the life she had. Unlike Ai, Huan's duty as a traditional Chinese wife was to care for her in-laws, not her own parents. She understood that she would not be released from her duty as long as she wished to live by the framing rules she had adopted, and she accepted this because 'this is the ethics'. Society expected it and she expected it. If successful, Huan would preserve her self-image as 'a happy carer' and a dutiful daughter-in-law and wife, assuring her status in her husband's family.

Like Huan, Ai grew up with traditional values. However, she was also influenced by contemporary norms. Although she was taught to put family first she noted, 'you…learn to think for yourself because of education'. Ai articulated how cognisant she was of living in a time of normative transition and the effect it had on her:

> I like freedom. I like independence. I am a very independent person. So, it does irritate me then, when…I'm in my 20s, my 30s and I just want to get out of my house and go and live alone and yet the traditional side of me is that…[if] I moved out then they [parents] are on their own. And, they are dependent on me financially. So, that stopped me also from moving out. That's why they have always lived with me. (Ai)

Tonkens (2012: 197) wrote, 'the process of managing feelings becomes more difficult during times of rapid social change'. Transitioning cultural norms made Ai aware that she had a choice, which created conflict. On the one hand Ai loved her mother and was grateful to her. However, these relational norms also made her feel 'responsible and obligated' because she had been taught to put family first. On the other hand, as a dynamic, self-sufficient woman, Ai wanted freedom and independence.

The tension between Ai's framing rules and her self-image had already emerged earlier in her life. Ai wanted to work overseas, but did not go. Reflecting on this, she said: 'Could I have just dumped it and gone? I probably could, but I would probably feel very guilty'. However, placing her own needs above her family would have violated Ai's framing rules, thereby damaging her positive self-image and personhood, or selfhood as Aronson (1990) described it.

How Framing Rules and Self-image Are Implicated in the Discharge of Care

Due to the differences in their framing rules, Huan and Ai began the caregiving experience with disparate expectations of themselves. Huan treated caregiving as a hard job, referring to her mother-in-law as a 'patient'. She took appropriate, well considered and informed action in caring for her patient. Her reward came not from her patient who had dementia, but from her 'boss', her husband. If she carried out her duties professionally and the patient was happy, she would receive her husband's approval and retain her positive self-image. For Huan, that approval was what kept the exchange in balance.

During all the years she provided care, the only time Huan remembered being on the edge of tolerance was when her husband accused her of making his mother angry. She interpreted this as an insult to the very core of her personhood. Not only was her sacrifice unappreciated, the trust and respect she had earned were ignored. Huan said she was so shocked and hurt she 'that [the] incident stay inside my heart for several years'. She recalled:

As long as my husband can understand what I'm doing, [that] I'm not hurting my mother-in-law, that's Okay. Nobody should query what I'm doing. It hurt because other people suspect what I'm doing. You understand? (Huan)

Ai, in contrast to Huan, was more emotionally invested in her mother, the care recipient. She started from relational framing rules of love, irredeemable obligation, and placing family above self. However, the potential for conflict already existed even before she commenced caregiving.

Whitbeck et al. (1994) reminded us that adult parent child relationships are complicated. They argued that helping parents could have a negative effect on the quality of the relationship if feelings of obligation grew and the exchange was thrown out of balance. Cicirelli (1993) further suggested that the greater a mother's dependency and the more assistance provided by the daughter, the greater the caregiver burden and the lower the quality of the parent-child relationship.

As her mother's disease progressed, caregiving became more difficult for Ai. Her positive self-image, earned from putting family first, struggled under the weight of caregiver burden and the relationship began to become unbalanced. During the second interview Ai spoke frequently of hiring an FDH and even putting her mother into a nursing home, although the latter she did not think she could do.

Based on her framing rules, it was likely that anything Ai did to terminate or significantly diminish her own role in the caregiving relationship with her mother would result in guilt and self-deprecation. Conversely, the cost to Ai for maintaining the status quo might have been her own health and well-being. Ai was in a double bind and we will probably never know what choice she made.

Asking the question again, **does the type of motivation matter**? As we have seen with Huan and Ai, if motivation is viewed as a framing rule, becoming the standard by which female Chinese caregivers measure their performance and judge themselves, perhaps it does not matter. It can be argued that the type of motivation (structural, relational) is not as important as the caregiver's commitment to it. If the caregiver believes she has fulfilled her commitment to the standard she has defined for herself, whatever that is, she is likely to preserve her self-image and be free from shame and guilt.

How Feeling Rules Are Implicated in the Discharge of Care

O.M.H. Wong and Chau (2006) wrote of carers suffering cognitive dissonance caused by the overwhelming nature of caregiving. Hochschild (1983: 90) called this 'emotive dissonance' derived from the conflict between what one feels and what one believes one *should* feel. Wong and Chau (2006: 612) gave the example of a caregiver who believed in traditional norms [framing rules] prescribing that parents should be cared for 'stoically and without hesitation' [feeling rules]. Yet anger and resentment still surfaced, leading to conflict between what she felt and what she believed she *should* feel. Ngan and Cheng (1992) called this caring dilemma, describing it as a love-hate relationship between a caregiver and care recipient in which the carer loves the patient but may also want them to die. Aronson (1990) emphasised the role of guilt and shame, which serve as *rule reminders* to tell us whether we are in compliance with culturally prescribed normative expectations of what a caregiver should be, a *framing rule*. Because framing rules are implicated in one's positive self-image, caregivers are highly motivated to feel emotions that are culturally appropriate and acceptable to them (Mac Rae 1998). *Feeling rules* tell us what we should feel in the context of our framing rules and the situations we are in.

Huan's framing rules had always obligated her to maintain a display that was 'tender, gentle, loving and kind' and to 'accept the things' she was not happy with. Her feeling rules required her to 'have a kind heart' and develop the 'love and patience' to become a 'happy carer'. Ai's framing rules required her to place her family's needs above her own. Her feeling rules mandated the strengthening of the loving parent-child bond as essential to discharging her filial obligation.

However, in the process of caregiving, both Huan and Ai experienced a *gap* between what they actually felt (despair, hopelessness, anger, caregiver burden) and their individual feeling rules. As a result, both Huan and Ai attempted to bridge the *gap* between the negative emotions they felt and what they believed they *should* feel through emotion work.

The Importance of Emotion Work to Caregiving

Emotion work is the 'act of trying to change the degree or quality of an emotion or feeling' (Hochschild 1979: 561). In addition to being a useful tool for preserving a person's positive self-image, it is a helpful and important schema for coping with stress (Hochschild 1983). This is especially true for those who are required to endure and continue caregiving. Both Huan and Ai did extensive emotion work.

To become a 'happy carer', and 'make a harmonious family', Huan said, 'I have to educate myself first before I can give the love or give care to [my mother-in-law]'. With knowledge of what her feelings should be, Huan prayed and talked to friends so that she could 'bear it happily'. She exhorted herself to change her unhappy mood by invoking the phrase 'every day is a new day'. She used humour to adjust her display and ease her negative emotions. She exhorted herself to provide care with a 'kind heart' and to develop love, patience and acceptance of her mother-in-law. She relied on her training as a nurse, viewing herself as a professional and her mother-in-law as a 'patient'. This is deep acting. By Huan's account, her emotion work was successful. She was not only able to change her display, but her feelings.

Hochschild (1983: 68) argued that the deeper the bond the greater the emotion work required. That was certainly true in Ai's case. She performed deep acting by invoking loving memories of her mother's care for her, and she *visualised* her mother as a 'childlike person' with 'adorable moments' to avoid viewing her as a dementia patient, and to love her more. She relied on religion to give her perspective and hope, and she prayed and complained to God to change her emotions. She walked in the park to calm herself and 'open up' her perspective. She looked at the positive side of caregiving to get through its dull repetition. Ai distracted herself with activities to 'cool down' when she was upset, and she suppressed her emotions when she was angry. She deliberately attempted to change her attitude to survive the caregiving experience, or to make 'the situation…not as bad'. She read self-help books to try and find more meaning in life because she could not alter her circumstances. Without feeling a parent-child bond (her feeling rule) she was not sure she could carry out her filial obligation. Accordingly, she worked hard to ensure it was there.

As caregiving became more burdensome and her 'fuse' got 'shorter and shorter' Ai tried to invoke feelings of gratitude for 'little things' like not having the financial problems some did. She told herself if she did not calm down she would get a stroke. Ai might have been partially successful at the emotion work she performed. However, she was unable to completely change her feelings. This might have been due to her inability to resolve the conflict and tension between her desire for freedom and filial obligation.

Both Ai and Huan were adamant that they could 'not collapse', and they performed the emotion work necessary to keep their feelings and emotions, and thus caregiving, in balance. Besides Huan and Ai, five of the remaining six caregivers did emotion work. They invoked memories from their childhood; like Huan, they reverted to their professional training; they prayed for patience and strength; and they practiced avoidance to calm down.

One of the seminal themes emerging from the conversations with the women in this book was emotion control. Nearly every daughter spoke of the importance of family harmony and early childhood training to avoid conflict. One could even argue that Chinese daughters are culturally predisposed to emotion work.

Emotion work has many benefits for caregiving situations in which controlling one's emotions is both difficult and essential. As seen, it is a mechanism that can be called into use at will and relied on to diffuse anger, relieve stress, and create desired feelings. If successful, there can be a protective affect for the caregiver's own health. Arguably, it can also protect care recipients from potential abuse by their caregivers. Conversely, if emotion work is unsuccessful it may damage one's positive self-image and result in feelings of shame and guilt (Aronson 1990; Mac Rae 1998). Further, as Hochschild (1983: 90) pointed out, surface acting (as opposed to deep acting) can lead to strain if carried out excessively or over an extended period of time, causing the caregiver to become emotionally detached, numb or devoid of feeling altogether (Hochschild 1983: 21). Finally, if the interpersonal, or 'gift' exchange becomes unbalanced, the caregiving arrangement may shift.

The Importance of Support in Dealing with Conflict and Tension

Perhaps because of her nursing training, when her mother-in-law's deterioration became intolerable, Huan sought and followed professional advice. She wrote to the doctor, enrolled in a class to learn about dementia and joined a carer support group, integrating everything she learned into a new support strategy. In addition, Huan employed three domestic helpers and relied on religion. She surrounded herself with knowledge and reinforcement.

Like Huan, Ai relied on religion, but Ai tried to manage caregiving almost entirely on her own. Instead of joining a class or support group she walked in the park. She worked on crafts and read self-help books. Ai had no relief from her caregiving burden other than day-care and she was reluctant to hire a domestic helper, even though she knew she needed one.

A significant difference was found in Ai's ability to manage caregiving between the first and second interviews. As her mother's dementia grew worse Ai began to wonder if she could continue. She mentioned that her stress level had increased. Every little thing bothered her and she dreaded going home because she did not know what she would find. Ai asserted that the stress was cumulative, her anger was closer to the surface, and her mother was getting on her nerves more. She was shouting at her and even hit her, something she thought she would never do. Ai felt increasingly lonely and isolated and was resentful of her sister. She worried about her own health. She even contemplated placing her mother in a nursing home, a thought she could not bear.

Ai's negative feelings might have been driven in part by tension between her traditional and contemporary values. However, she also lacked social support. The relevance of support has been noted in the caregiving literature. For example, in a study of 60 elderly Singaporeans and their 50 caregivers, Kua (1989) found that carers who lacked social support were more inclined to depression and anxiety, particularly if they lived alone with the care recipient and were otherwise socially isolated. In a study from mainland China, L.-Q. Wang, Chien and Lee (2012) tested the efficacy of a mutual support group among family caregivers of dementia patients. The participating family members said that sharing their feelings and exchanging information empowered them and reduced their negative feelings and stress. A Hong Kong study of 30 caregivers of schizophrenia patients, similarly found that participation in a six-month support group allowed the carers to acquire new skills and problem solving strategies, facilitated exchanges of information and generally empowered them (Chien et al. 2006). In a separate Hong Kong study of elder abuse among the family caregivers of 122 dementia patients, Yan and Kwok (2011: 533) found that having an FDH helped to lower verbal abuse by the primary carer. They suggested this might have been due to less caregiver burden through relief from domestic chores, but also that the presence of a third party might 'increase the caregiver's sense of self-awareness'.

Part of what differentiated Huan and Ai was the amount and type of support they availed themselves of. This was also true of the other six daughter-caregivers in this book. All but one had help from either sisters or support groups, or they received professional training. The one daughter, who like Ai tried to manage alone, also experienced a high degree of stress, and like Ai her support came primarily from religion.

Limitations, Conditions and Qualifications to Caregiving

Interpersonal Exchange

When the burdens of caregiving outweigh the rewards, the exchange becomes imbalanced and a change in behaviour or the situation is likely to occur.

Among the five daughters caring for parents with dementia at home, two eventually institutionalised them. In Huan's case the parent's physical disabilities required it. In the other, the daughter and her domestic helper could no longer control the mother's erratic behaviour and emotional outbursts. The three remaining dementia patients were still living with their daughters at home at the time of their interviews. In two of these cases, domestic helpers were the primary caregivers and there was sibling support. Both of these daughters indicated that if caregiving became too difficult, placement in a nursing home was an option. The other case was Ai.

For the three caregivers of acutely ill mothers, two of the care recipients remained at home until they died. The daughters supervised and assisted, but care was primarily provided by a domestic helper. These women also had sibling support. Li, who had no support, placed her mother in a nursing home only when it became impossible to care for her at home.

The Quality of Care and Length of Caregiving

Among these women, the quality and length of long-term in-home care appeared to depend to a great extent on the daughter's ability to tolerate the stress according to her framing rules and feeling rules, and further, how these intersected with both her relationship to the care-recipient parent and her self-image. Firmly embedded in this was the strength of the daughter's framing rules and whether she experienced conflict between traditional and contemporary norms. In addition to this, the daughter's willingness to undertake the emotion work needed to cultivate attitudes that were appropriate and acceptable to her, and her ability to garner enough support from a domestic helper, siblings or professionals, were all implicated in maintaining a reasonably balanced relationship. In the case of the acutely ill, the length of care could depend on how long it took the disease to progress to its conclusion or to a point where hospitalisation or institutionalisation was inescapable.

Limitations Based on Who Care Was Provided For

Among the women in this book, care recipients who had closer relationships with their daughters were more likely to receive caregiving from them. Parents, for example, received more care than in-laws. This was also true of the extended family. Family members who were farther removed, both emotionally and geographically, were less likely to receive care, and were generally not considered in caregiving decisions.

Health Concerns of the Caregiver

Half of the caregivers expressed unease over what caregiving was doing to their health and what would happen if they became incapacitated. The implication seemed to be that if this issue could not be addressed then caregiving might have to be terminated or modified by, for example, employing a domestic helper or institutionalising the parent. The concern seemed to be who would be left to take care of the parent, and more important, who would take care of the caregiver herself if she became unwell.

Conclusion

This chapter concerns the third stage of the typology of support and care: caregiving. Among these women, caregiving was unlimited in duration and took place in the caregiver's home. There were eight daughters providing long-term care for 10 parents: seven mothers and three in-laws. Baby Boomers provided most of the caregiving. Two of the daughters terminated their employment to provide caregiving, six employed domestic helpers and three had sibling support. All eight were Christian and six relied on religion as a form of support. Half of the caregiving support was motivated by combined structural norms of filial obligation and relational norms of affection, gratitude and reciprocity.

Two narratives were presented to illustrate motivation for caregiving. In the first, structural norms of filial obligation were explored through the story of Huan, a woman from a very traditional background. She accepted Chinese cultural norms unconditionally and had learned from childhood to serve others and 'bear the suffering'. Huan cared for her husband's father, grandmother and mother. However, it was the latter, suffering from dementia, who drove Huan to despair.

As Huan came to understand the severity and irreversible nature of her mother-in-law's disease, she set about to educate herself. She sought professional help, joined a support group and relied on her experience as a nurse. She placed her mother-in-law into day-care and performed emotion work to change her own attitude and outlook to accept her situation.

In the second narrative, motivation driven by relational norms of affection, gratitude and reciprocity was examined through the story of Ai. Ai was interviewed twice, six months apart. She loved, and was grateful to her mother, and had also been taught that, 'family is the most important thing'. However, in contrast to Huan, Ai embraced the contemporary norms of freedom and independence. As the caregiver of her mother, who had dementia, Ai experienced tension and conflict between her own and her mother's needs.

Like Huan, Ai placed her mother into day-care; however, she had no other support besides self-help books and religion. Over the course of caregiving her burden became worse. Ai experienced severe stress and became short tempered. She did extensive emotion work, and worried about losing control. Between the first and second interviews there was a distinct difference between Ai's ability to manage. She had also become lonelier and more isolated.

In the process of discharging care both Huan and Ai adjusted their motivation for caregiving. Huan used emotion work to move away from structural obligation and develop greater feelings of affection for her mother-in-law. Ai attempted to increase her feelings of love for her mother, but also increasingly relied on structural norms of obligation to overcome the conflict she experienced over caregiving. Their stories thus led us to ask how much the type of motivation mattered. The literature has suggested that caregiving motivated by relational norms has a more positive outcome than caregiving motivated by structural norms. However, these two narratives appeared to show that other factors may have been in play. In trying to understand this unexpected outcome, motivation was viewed as a framing rule.

Hochschild (1979: 566) defined framing rules as how 'we ascribe definitions and meanings to situations'. These situations can be as narrow as a single event or as broad as cultural norms and practices. In the context of caregiving research, present day Chinese ideology and coping behaviour can both be viewed as framing rules, bifurcated into traditional norms based on Confucian notions of filial obligation, and contemporary norms influenced by both traditional Chinese culture and urbanisation. Hong Kong, mainland China and Singapore are all transitioning societies where structural and relational norms are often combined. As a framing rule, motivation establishes both the standard of care and the ideal by which caregivers measure their own performance.

According to symbolic interactionists, people are motivated to take actions that protect their positive self-image (Mac Rae 1998). Likewise, in the Chinese context, Holroyd's (2001) cultural model suggests that the desire to maintain personhood is what drives daughters' in discharging filial obligation. Huan's approach to caregiving was underpinned by traditional Chinese norms, so if she lived up to them, her self-image would be preserved. Ai, conversely, was torn between traditional and contemporary norms, arguably undermining the commitment to her framing rules of loving her mother and putting family above self. Although her needs were in competition with her mother's, if Ai abandoned her framing rules she would forfeit her positive self-image.

Huan's framing rules provided a precise roadmap for her to follow that enabled her to set specific goals to sustain her sense of personhood. She approached caregiving as if it was a job. If her performance met the approval of her 'boss', her husband, her expectations would be satisfied and her positive self-image would be sustained. In contrast, Ai entered the caregiving journey with an irredeemable obligation and framing rules that were in conflict. Lacking direction, as her mother's dementia grew worse, Ai's caregiver burden increased. However, she continued her caregiving activities at her own expense, conceivably to avoid guilt and self-deprecation, as Aronson (1990) suggested.

Feeling rules prescribe what feelings are appropriate in the context of one's framing rules. In the process of caregiving, both Huan and Ai adjusted their feeling rules. Huan said she should respect and accept her mother-in-law and have a kind and loving heart. Ai said she should increase her love for her mother. To bridge the gap between what they felt and wanted to feel, both women did extensive emotion work.

According to Hochschild (1979: 561) emotion work is 'the act of trying to change the degree or quality of an emotion or feeling'. Huan relied on the advice she was given by the professionals and the carer support group. She integrated humour to alter negative emotions and exhorted herself to develop an attitude she deemed acceptable. She performed deep acting by relying on her experience as a nurse and visualising her mother-in-law as a patient, rather than a family member. She relied on friends and religion, and if all else failed, she retreated to her longstanding belief to bear the suffering. Huan was successful in changing her feelings to conform to her self-image as a 'happy carer'.

It appeared that Ai did more emotion work than Huan. She performed extensive deep acting to invoke happy memories and visualised her mother as an adorable child. She read self-help books to develop a more positive outlook. She suppressed her anger and frustration, and relied on religion. All of this enabled her to continue her caregiving work. However, it did not resolve the conflict between her own and her mother's needs or the tension between her traditional and contemporary norms. Ai could neither completely embrace modern values toward parent care nor abandon traditional norms of filial obligation. In this context, the ability to choose was a double-edged sword and Ai's indecisiveness was seemingly the cause of psychological distress. During the second interview, she spoke increasingly about hiring a domestic helper or putting her mother into a nursing home.

The other six daughters caring for their parents were not unlike Huan and Ai. Five did emotion work, including deep acting, to help them get through caregiving, and they developed strategies to control their display. In fact, control over emotions was a prominent theme among the daughters in this book, most of whom were trained from childhood to avoid conflict and preserve harmony.

Emotion work has many salient features. If successful, it can help to diminish anger and stress and promote appropriate feelings. It may also have a protective effect for both the caregiver and care recipient. If unsuccessful, however, it may damage one's self-esteem and instigate feelings of guilt and shame. Moreover, protracted surface acting may lead to strain and overuse of emotion work may lead to feelings of detachment and lack of emotion. If the exchange becomes unbalanced, change is likely to occur.

One thing that helps maintain balance in the caregiving relationship is support. One can see the difference it made in Huan, who availed herself of professional and peer support and Ai, who did not. Like Huan, five of the remaining six caregivers sought support from family, professionals and peers, and four relied on religion as well. The importance of support has been noted in the caregiving literature.

The limitations on caregiving among these daughters included social, or 'gift' exchange when caregiving became too burdensome. The quality and length of care could depend on one's framing rules and feeling rules, the willingness to do emotion work, and the desire to maintain a positive self-image. Who care was provided for could also be contingent on the closeness of the relationship. Finally, the health concerns of the caregiver could influence whether care continued.

The next chapter looks at the relationship between daughters, care recipients and foreign domestic helpers, in the context of what happens when a domestic helper becomes the primary caregiver, or when caregiving at home is terminated.

References

Aronson, J. (1990). Women's perspectives on informal care of the elderly: Public ideology and personal experience of giving and receiving care. *Ageing and Society, 10*(1), 61–84.

Chien, W.-T., Norman, I., & Thompson, D. R. (2006). Perceived benefits and difficulties experienced in a mutual support group for family carers of people with schizophrenia. *Qualitative Health Research, 16*(7), 962–981.

Cicirelli, V. G. (1993). Attachment and obligation as daughters' motives for caregiving behavior and subsequent effect on subjective burden. *Psychology and Aging, 8*(2), 144–155.

Hochschild, A. R. (1979). Emotion work, feeling rules and social structure. *American Journal of Sociology, 85*(3), 551–575.

Hochschild, A. (1983, 2012). The managed heart: Commercialization of human feeling. Berkeley: University of California Press.

Holroyd, E. (2001). Hong Kong Chinese daughters' intergenerational caregiving obligations: A cultural model approach. *Social Science & Medicine, 53*(9), 1125–1134.

Horowitz, A., & Shindelman, L. W. (1983). Reciprocity and affection. *Journal of Gerontological Social Work, 5*(3), 5–20.

Kua, E. H. (1989). Psychological distress of families caring for the frail elderly. *Singapore Medical Journal, 30*(1), 42–44.

Lyonette, C., & Yardley, L. (2003). The influence on carer wellbeing of motivations to care for older people and the relationship with the care recipient. *Ageing and Society, 23*(4), 487–506.

Mac Rae, H. (1998). Managing feelings: Caregiving as emotion work. *Research on Aging, 20*(1), 137–160.

Ngan, R., & Cheng, I. C. K. (1992). The caring dilemma, stress and needs of carers for the Chinese frail elderly. *Hong Kong Journal of Gerontology, 6*(2), 34–41.

Tonkens, E. (2012). Working with Arlie Hochschild: Connecting feelings to social change. *Social Politics, 19*(2), 194–218.

Wang, L.-Q., Chien, W.-T., & Lee, I. Y. M. (2012). An experimental study on the effectiveness of a mutual support group for family caregivers of a relative with dementia in mainland China. *Contemporary Nurse, 30*(2), 210–224. https://doi.org/10.5172/conu.2012.40.2.210.

Whitbeck, L. B., Simons, R. L., & Conger, R. D. (1991). The effects of early family relationships on contemporary relationships and assistance patterns between adult children and their parents. *Journals of Gerontology, Social Sciences, 46*(6(Supp. 6)), S330–S337.

Whitbeck, L., Hoyt, D. R., & Huck, S. M. (1994). Early family relationships, intergenerational solidarity, and support provided to parents by their adult children. *Journal of Gerontology, Social Sciences, 49*(4(Supp. 2)), S85–S94.

Wong, O. M. H., & Chau, B. H. P. (2006). The evolving role of filial piety in eldercare in Hong Kong. *Asian Journal of Social Science, 34*(4), 600–617.

Yan, E., & Kwok, T. (2011). Abuse of older Chinese with dementia by family caregivers: An inquiry into the role of caregiver burden. *International Journal of Geriatric Psychiatry, 26*(5), 527–535.

8

Outsourced Care

Review of Outsourced Care and Introduction to the Chapter

The final stage in the typology is outsourced care. In the first three stages the three key analytical categories of conceptual and theoretical norms were explored to explain *why* the daughters were willing or unwilling to provide support and care and *how* they navigated the conflict and tension involved with caregiving when their parents moved from good health to poor health. This fourth stage of support and care initially focuses on the dilemma the daughters faced in outsourcing parent care and then why they discontinued their own care activities or declined to accept them in the first place [*'I do not want to/I cannot'*]. The remainder of the chapter highlights domestic helpers (FDHs/CDHs): why they were hired; the issues involved with their employment; how they affected the daughter-parent relationship; and finally, the *emotion work* they were required to do to manage caregiving. The role of domestic helpers is examined in the context of both home and institutionalised care and the transition between them. The elements of outsourced care appear in Table 4.4.

© The Author(s) 2018
P. O'Neill, *Urban Chinese Daughters*, St Antony's Series,
https://doi.org/10.1007/978-981-10-8699-1_8

Seven daughters either previously or at the time of their interview, institutionalised a family member. A total of eight family members were placed into nursing homes or hospitals: Three mothers, two fathers, two mothers-in-law and an uncle. Among these, three family members received supplemental care in the institution from a domestic helper hired by the daughter. Three of the daughters previously provided in-home caregiving (two with domestic helpers) before institutionalising their family member, and were included in Chap. 7. Five daughters remained in employment while their family member was institutionalised.

As with the previous chapters, the actual accounts of the daughters illustrate the subjects under discussion. However, this time the domestic helpers are heard from to achieve a different perspective, especially about the daughter-parent relationship.

The Dilemma Over Outsourcing Care

Transitioning norms were particularly visible when it came to outsourced care. Both the daughters and their elderly parents, according to them, held diverse views on domestic helpers and nursing homes. This was especially the case in mainland China, where there was a general reluctance to embrace either one. For this reason, all of the women quoted in this section lived in Kunming.

Daughters Reluctant to Hire Domestic Helpers

When asked how they felt about hiring a domestic helper for their parents, there were a variety of responses from the mainland daughters. However, love was a major factor:

> If I take care of my parents myself, it's better than a housekeeper…the housekeeper does not have the love as us, love as deep as us. And she just take it as a kind of job. It's a job. (Chenguang)

Concern was also shown for the parents' safety and well-being:

It's common, [hiring a domestic helper] but we do not choose that way because our parents are healthy and are more safe [with their children] than with the strange person, I think. (Xiaoli)

There's also one concern, and even worries about helper because most of the helpers they don't really get much trained. They might be like some salesman in the market today and tomorrow they will be the helper. So, secondly, we don't think they will put their whole heart for the patient because they don't have any touching and they [are] completely a stranger. So, that's one thing we really worry about because it has been ... reported by the newspaper and also television, talk about helper they actually abused the patient. (Yuet)

According to their daughters, the parents did not want strangers in their homes.

I don't think my parents would support this kind of idea. A lot of friends around me, their parents don't like the so-called nursing worker. They think it's inconvenient as they're not familiar with each other. They may feel shy or timid when facing a stranger who takes care of you. (Luli)

Parents also wanted to remain independent:

She [Mother-in-law] is still healthy and wants to live in her own way. She said that as long as I can take care of myself I want to stay alone. She refused to have a helper. (Chunhua)

In mainland China, unlike Singapore and Hong Kong, care was neither subsidised nor regulated by the government. Thus, the expense could also be an issue. Contemplating the hiring of a CDH, who would ordinarily have been a woman from the rural area, Chunhua remarked:

I think now it is becoming more and more difficult, unlike before. The labour cost has also become more expensive in China. And I think even the farmers have more choices than before. They don't always have to do the labour work... now the young generation of farmers...also got a very good education.... So, this is why the labour cost is also more and more expensive. (Chunhua)

The vastness and cultural diversity of the mainland could also be problematic:

Another issue is also the language and culture difference....for example get someone from the Philippines, then the whole family has to be English speaking. Otherwise it's hard....and also have some culture difference... even the way of cooking... I mean probably some of the well educated people with better income, affordability as you say, with better affordability, I think you know, some already have. But ...it's not many. (Chunhua)

Finally, it should be noted that, although these daughters all lived in the city, some of their parents remained in their home towns in the countryside, where domestic helpers of any kind were rare.

Daughters' Reluctance to Institutionalise a Parent

We should also respect their idea. But, you know, our concern is, like my parents' generation, not all of them can accept to be in the institute, the care centre and especially they have five children [who] have the capacity to take care of them. So, also we don't want to put them into the institute if we have the capacity to take care of them. (Chunhua)

Institutionalising a parent in a nursing home was less accepted in Kunming than it was in Hong Kong or Singapore. Some daughters characterised it as 'cruel'. Others said they had never thought about it for their parents. Many expressed their parents' desire to remain in their own homes. There could also be an issue of Face. Yan referred to this in the context of nursing home placement, saying, 'ah yes, loss of face.... a lot of people think my children is no good, trick me. My family is not good.

I fail to teach my children'. I asked Yan if this meant the parent would be perceived as being a 'bad parent' who was institutionalised because the children would not take care of him or her, to which Yan responded: 'Oh yes!! You know, you know'!

For those who were opposed to institutionalising their parents, a common practice was to move them closer but to allow them to remain independent as long as possible. Chunhua's remarks below elaborate a very common plan found among these daughters and the feelings underpinning it:

> My brother and my sister, we have already started to plan for my parents because they have really spent their life for us. So, now they are approaching 70 years old and although they always said they can take care of themselves, we know there will be time coming [when] they will not be able to take care of themselves. So, now we are thinking of moving them close to anyone of us… we … brothers and sisters will do whatever we can to support them…. So, one day if one of them cannot manage their daily live then they have to stay with us. (Chunhua)

This type of solution was largely made possible because some of the daughters, born before the One Child Policy, had siblings to share the responsibility. Large families also afforded another solution, proposed by Yan, who said she preferred to give money and have her brother take care of their parents, who did not want to go to a nursing home:

> I like my job. I like studying in particular. And I don't like to take care of [my parents] ….I can cook delicious. I can sweep a floor. Everything I can do….But if I choose to take care of my parents, I need to give money. If we take care of them…. I become a nurse, doctor, housekeeper. It's very tiring I think. …I think if they want to [go to the] old place. I send them to there. But, they don't! (Yan)

Yan's comment reflects the influence of contemporary norms, and although tradition was still strong among the Kunming women, the transition to new models of filial obligation could be seen, as discussed below.

Why Daughter Caregiving Was Outsourced, Discontinued, Modified or Never Undertaken

Interpersonal Exchange

Hochschild (1979) explained that during interpersonal exchanges with others we keep a mental ledger of what our feeling rules tell us is owed: what the other person expects to receive, and what is owed in return. If this exchange remains in balance, the status quo should be maintained.

In the caregiving arrangement, both the caregiver and care recipient are giving and receiving emotional 'gifts' with the other, or engaging in 'emotional reciprocity' (Mac Rae 1998). In the parent-daughter relationship, feeling rules may tell a daughter she 'owes' her parents a kind and loving heart, or at least acceptance and tolerance. The parent expects to receive this. In return the daughter is 'owed,' for example, a positive self-image and possibly some warm feelings or appreciation from the parent. However, as the parents' needs increase and more care is required, emotions can become strained, parents may be unable or unwilling to reciprocate, and the exchange can be thrown out of balance.

The literature has suggested that this 'unbalanced emotional exchange' is particularly pronounced when the care recipient is cognitively impaired (Chien et al. 2006; Mac Rae 1998; Simpson and Acton 2013; Yan and Kwok 2011). Mac Rae (1998), for example, found that individuals with dementia require more understanding and emotional investment the worse they become. However, due to the nature of their illness they may be less capable of expressing appreciation, or may even display aggressive behaviour toward their caregiver. The caregiver must then simultaneously deal with the negative emotions of the care recipient while controlling her or his own emotions.

Exchange theory posits that once a relationship becomes unbalanced a change of behaviour in those who feel they are giving more than they are receiving is likely to result (Allen 2010). Among the daughters in this book, caregiver stress was frequently the cause of care imbalance. The first change to occur from this was most often the employment of a domestic helper to assume the daughter's caregiving responsibilities, if financially feasible. If this remedy became too burdensome, one of two outcomes was probable: a wish for the parent to die or institutionalisation of the parent. Ying, a Hong Kong Baby Boomer, expressed her desire to be freed from caregiving:

> Well, I accept the fact that I have to live in that situation until mom pass away or unless she gets better which...would be a miracle. So, until she passed away...sometimes I would pray that God would release me by taking Mom to you. (Ying)

Chenguang, a mainland Baby Boomer whose mother had Alzheimer's disease, and who had already hired a domestic helper, reflected on the alternative:

> So, after my father is gone away, if my mother's mind is completely gone, maybe we have to choose to get her to the nursing home at that time. Because, what can I do? I can't follow her around, look after her all the time. (Chenguang)

Disability of the Parent Care Recipient

For many of these women, particularly in Hong Kong and Singapore, when it became impossible or impractical for the family to care for a parent alone, a domestic helper might first be sought. Yuet's criteria were similar to many of the daughters when it came to hiring an FDH or CDH to care for a disabled parent:

> ...because it takes a longer time to take care of [the parent] ... so, if more than one month, two months, is [disabled] it takes more effort to take care of them. So, they may think it is better to have a helper. (Yuet)

Eventually, placing the parent into a nursing home could be the only remaining option. The litmus test appeared to be the point at which the parent required professional care beyond the family's or the helper's abilities, or specialised equipment was needed that could not fit into the family home. The extreme physical disability of the care recipient was universally cited as the reason for institutionalisation, even for parents with dementia. Ning, for example, institutionalised her uncle after he had a stroke and lost his sight:

> The maid couldn't take care of him and the two others [aunts] at home. He hasn't had any sight anymore. Then whenever he went to [the] toilet [or to] bathe, [he] needed the nurse to do it. That would be too much for her. And…there is no place for a second maid. It's [her flat] too small. (Ning)

In Huan's case, her mother-in-law needed to be hoisted onto a stretcher for bathing:

> Yeah, they got a stretcher. They got a big room. And then they got a skilled person to take her [to] the bath. They got an electric bed. They can raise her up and down, alright? Got the facility. (Huan)

Even with a domestic helper, caregiving could become impossible if the helper did not get enough rest:

> The servant sleeps with her in the same room. And then she's incontinent… I can't ask the servant in the middle of the night…[to] change the diapers. She must get some sleep, enough sleep. That's a problem. (Huan)

Interestingly, physical disability could also be cited when the real reason was something else. For example, one daughter whose father was unpleasant and difficult to manage said she had moved him into a flat by himself with an FDH. Then she added that 'the final plan will be sending [dad] to a nursing home… in *view of the recent decline* in the past few months… actually the temper thing I can tolerate'. (Meiying, Hong Kong Baby Boomer)

Conflict Avoidance

One of the major themes heard from these daughters, regardless of where they lived, was the need to avoid conflict and maintain harmony within the family. Both the daughters and their parents, as related by their daughters, appeared to share the same view. Anticipating the time when caring for a parent might become necessary, Wenling explained why hiring a domestic helper had become more accepted in Kunming:

> But it gets more and more common because our parents they also have their life and sometimes we think if we live with our parents now it will cause more conflict. So, you can pay your money and find some not your relatives, family members. Then you can reduce this problem. (Wenling)

Helpers Viewed as More Professional and Emotionally Predisposed to Caregiving

Some of the daughters compared their own skills and emotional capacity for caregiving with experienced domestic helpers. Yuet, for example, reflected on the reasons professionals might be hired, but warned about the problem inherent in it:

> It's common only when they think the family member is really busy and cannot make any contribution. And also, some of the rich people will think it is better to have the helper because they are much more professional. But, it's always a question, professional. (Yuet)

Yan spoke to the emotional component of caregiving, explaining why hiring a helper is better for the care recipient:

> I don't like this work, take care of [the] old one. I think it's good to take care of old people. It's good work. It's great work. [However,] my patience is not well…. For example, I take care of my parents I am not patient. So, I think maybe I do this work, it's not good. A good housekeeper…I think it's very great if enough patience. Chinese woman, if they haven't a good education not another choice. Now take care of old, salary is good…. A lot of women do it. Second… a lot are warm hearted…a lot of women [are] patient, careful. So, the first, warm hearted, is important [to] take care of [the] old. If you [are] warm hearted but you haven't patience, you don't like this job. Warm hearted is very good. (Yan)

Daughters' Needed or Wanted to Work

As discussed previously, some of the daughters were unwilling to quit their jobs. Women, like Lihwa, Wenling, Luli and Lian, preferred working to staying at home. Lian, for example, returned to work from maternity leave a month early and said she could not wait to go to work on Monday mornings. She stated that she was not interested in housework and did not feel 'fulfilled' staying at home. Further, being self-sufficient was important to her:

> If I become a stay-at-home mom, then financially I will be totally dependent on my husband, [and] feel very insecure…I don't want to add stress on him and also knowing my husband, he will have a lot of expectations if I'm a stay-at-home-mom. (Lian)

However, for others, the income they earned supported not only themselves, but their families. They could not quit, even if their parents expected them to. Yan described this situation:

> My parents don't like it, you know [an outside person in their house]…. they think we have children. You must take care of us. If we have children, don't need it [housekeeper]. So, the Chinese children is very tired, especially we have work, we have a job. The job is especially, I'm busy. So, I couldn't take care of them, [I don't] have a lot of time. (Yan)

Chunhua related the challenge that was common among most of the women interviewed for this book, trying to find a balance:

> We have to find a solution for it…. This very much depends on our time. For example, I need to still work for eight hours a day, then I can't contribute eight hours a day [to my parents], but I can do that after the work. Probably I would need a helper for this eight hours or whatever support for this eight hours. So, … on one hand is their need and on the other hand is also the ability to coordinate the resources to support them. (Chunhua)

Regardless of how filial she was, when a daughter was the sole support of her family, particularly if she was a single woman, she could not permanently stop working. If she could not afford a domestic helper and her parent was disabled, her only alternative could be institutionalisation. After three years caring for her mother at home, Li, for example, had to return to work to pay for her parents' care and living expenses in addition to her own. Li's mother was in a wheelchair and needed help with bathing. Her father was too ill to care for his wife. Li recalled:

> I couldn't afford to hire a person to take care of her, and also I have to go out to work, and I have little time to take care of her. I think this is safer for her to stay at the nursing home. (Li, Hong Kong Baby Boomer)

Previously, negative relational motivation was discussed as a reason for declining to undertake the support or care of a parent. However, as seen above, there were other circumstances preventing daughter caregiving. Beyond that, the fact that daughters could unilaterally exercise choice in care decisions evidences the substantial normative change occurring within these Asian cultural settings.

Normative Influences Underpinning the Decision to Institutionalise a Parent

> Actually, most of the old people, the last step is in the nursing house. Become more and more. Of course, everybody's young people is busy now, have no time to take care of them. (Chenguang)

The Influence of Traditional Norms

In traditional families like Huan's, daughters or daughters-in-law carefully negotiated the decision to institutionalise parents, ensuring that it was made and approved by the family. Although family members might have been unwilling to care for the parents themselves, they could nonetheless oppose institutionalisation, expecting others to assume the responsibility.

This was the case with many of these daughters, but it can be seen specifically in the example of Huan. Four years before her mother-in-law required institutionalisation, Huan had her placed on a waiting list for a good nursing home. When it became clear that nursing home care was imminent, opposition arose from Huan's sister-in-law. Huan immediately involved her husband who in turn spent six months consulting with his siblings. When an opening finally did occur and action was required, Huan deferred to her husband again. She refused to make the decision alone, explaining that, 'If she [mother-in-law] goes to the nursing home… and [she] dies suddenly, then I will be… responsible for all the fault… A lot of blame will be putting on me'. A 'trial period' was arranged and Huan was charged with implementing it:

> If she can stay in a nursing home for one month and is still ok, not pass away, then we will continue. [I] observe. And every day I go to the nursing home and sit there from nine to nine and see all the workers, how they treat my mother-in-law. (Huan)

Huan sat in the nursing home for two months making sure her mother-in-law was properly cared for. Gradually, her domestic helper replaced her. The helper spent 10–12 hours a day, every day, caring for the old woman in the facility for the next three years until Huan's mother-in-law died.

The Influence of Government Support on the Decision to Outsource Care

Government pensions are a relatively recent phenomenon in Singapore, Hong Kong and especially in mainland China. However, they have already been fostering normative change. Particularly in the mainland, elderly parents have become more self-sufficient than they were previously. Some have been able to take care of themselves with little or no help from their children until they have reached the last stages of their lives. Pensions have allowed them to live independently, in their own homes in their home towns and near their friends, even if their children have moved away. Many of the daughters, particularly in Kunming, said their parents preferred this. Luli, whose parents lived in their home town, some distance from her, articulated this very clearly:

And now I think in big cities, actually we do not need to support our parents financially as most of them, most of the elderly they have the pension and they also have their own house. We do not need to support them [with] money, we do not give them a house. They have their own. So, I think now what we need to do is spend time and take care of them, communicate with them. Mostly, I think they may need emotional, spiritual care. Just as my parents, they do not want to live with me and my husband and my child as they think we are different generations, we have different interests and what we love are different. If they live with us it's not the life they want. They just live at my home town. They have their friends. They have the things they love to do. So, I think from this point I do not force them to live with me. I do not say come here and I will take care of you. I will give you something. No, I don't think this is a kind of filial piety. I think, just obey them and let them to be happy. This is also some kind of filial piety. (Luli)

As seen from Luli's comments, emotional support has become more important than instrumental support. Yun described what that meant to her:

I think it's not because when they need you and you will like to go visit them. It's because you think about them and then you go to visit them. And, if they need your help and I think [it] pretty much depends on what they wanted, if they wanted me to [provide] financial support, I will do as well. If they don't want financial support, they just want me to be with them, and I will go stay with them. Yeah, and also I talk about my life with them. It's kind of also, I think emotional support to let them know I'm ok, I'm doing well and how's the grandchildren doing, those kinds of things. And also, sometimes [I] ask [for] some suggestions from them, if I am confused and if I have any problem.... They are very happy to help. (Yun)

According to the daughters, pensions were influential making in long term care decisions, both for their parents and for themselves. Repeatedly they commented on the positive aspects of care homes and how important it was for the government to build and support them. They also cited abuses by family members, especially extended family, stealing from the elderly under the auspices of providing care. This is elder abuse. Controlling their own funds and health care decisions, with support from their children, was one way of preventing this.

The One Child Policy, Single Daughters and Daughters with Only Children

As discussed in the Introduction to this book, Chinese families in Hong Kong, Singapore and mainland China have all become smaller since the end of the Second World War. Among the 64 Baby Boomer and Gen X daughters, four were only children (all in mainland China), 25 had no children (20 of these women had never married) and 18 had only one child. In Hong Kong and Singapore, singlehood and one-child families were a choice, heavily influenced by socio-economic conditions. Conversely, between 1978 and 2013 mainland China legislated and enforced its One Child Policy under which most urban families were forbidden to have a second child. Whether by choice or by law, smaller families have resulted in substantial normative change.

First, as seen in the literature and among virtually all the interviewed daughters, these generations of women were willing to institutionalise themselves rather than burden their children. The following are some of their statements:

> I want to go to the old, the old palace.... I said to my husband, we are old more and more. We go to [the] old palace. Yes. We needn't my daughter take care of me all day, all [the] time. She is tired; very, very tired. If I love her I will not do that to her....So now I'm worried about my retired life. I think maybe if I sick I have a daughter, only one child. She wants to work a job. She have her family. She have her children. She must take care of them. It's cruel. Too much cruel. (Yan, Gen X, Kunming)

> I will expect myself to take care of myself when I'm getting old...I will send in myself to the nursing home. (An, Gen X, Hong Kong)

I have to say that if I am having a poor health condition, I will sign myself Into an institution rather than stay with my kids.... If I had to be taken care of by my kids, their life will be disturbed and both of us won't be happy. (Bo, Gen X, Hong Kong)

These women were also mindful of the importance of taking care of themselves to postpone nursing home admission or the need for care from their child. Yan articulated this when she said, 'I think I must exercise, [be] strong. I [take] care of myself. She [her daughter] needs to have her own life'. Chunhua expressed a similar sentiment:

First, I don't want to burden [my son] and second I want to have my own life as much as possible. So, this way, for example, my husband and I, we try to do exercise and to ensure that we keep our health condition. (Chunhua)

Second, in some families the only child was a girl. Girls who had become 'like sons' and cared for their parents 'like a son' might also inherit when their parents died, just as if they had been the eldest son.

Finally, their own family home was often considered by these daughters to be an asset to support their old age, rather than to be bequeathed to their child, as tradition previously dictated. As Yan said, 'I think I need to go, I want to go, I like to go to the old place, the home, use my house for support when I am old'.

Outsourced Care Destigmatised

If a stigma existed in the past about outsourcing parent care, among these daughters it no longer appeared to. The use of domestic helpers by the Hong Kong and Singapore women was widespread at all stages of support and care, and it was growing in mainland China. Further, all of the daughters, regardless of where they were from, and even if they had mixed emotions about it, viewed institutionalisation as a viable, practical, and often necessary, option. As Huan said:

Of course, she [her mother-in-law] don't like [it] because it's a different environment… It's very heart breaking for me actually. And I still [have] some bad feeling. Am I doing the right thing for her at that moment…you got tears and you got cries…but you can't help [it]. (Huan)

Although it was not something most of them welcomed, in most cases making the decision to institutionalise a parent did not appear to be averse to culturally acceptable norms in these generations of women. As Jai pointed out, 'I didn't have to take care of my mom. I could have put her in a nursing home. That is still fulfilling my duty because she is still having care'.

One reason nursing home placement has become more acceptable is that the quality has been improving. According to Chenguang, in Kunming for example, 'now the nursing home condition has become better and better. Some of them, if you pay more money is high enough, you can get a good grade, a high grade'.

Some of the daughters even started thinking about nursing home placement well in advance because good nursing homes had waiting lists lasting several years:

I would think about…one day [when] she is less mobile…So what sort of hospital she should enter and does she need any nursing home, etc. You know that sort of thing I always have in my mind as well…If…all the ordinary helpers cannot take good care [of her] …then she may need to go to the nursing home. And, even on that, I pick the nursing home already. (Lihwa)

Most important, once a parent was institutionalised, continued support from the family was crucial. Although normative change had modified traditional filial obligation, providing a helper alone was still not an acceptable substitute for the patient's children:

[The] helper in the hospital [is common] and [not opposed to] the Chinese tradition. [However,] even for my grandma when she was really ill…she was lucky to have nine daughters and sons, so they were able to take shifts. They took shifts to take care of her during her last time and it's from shame if they have a lot of children and they use a helper to take care of her in the last time. (Yuet)

Caring for Institutionalised Parents Without a Domestic Helper

Among these women, continued support for long-term institutionalised family members was common. Four of the seven daughters continued to be active in their family member's life by supplementing professional care following permanent hospital or nursing home admission. As previously seen with Huiqing in Chap. 4 and Rou in Chap. 6, the time management and physical challenges associated with this type of care are severe. Imagine then how much worse it is when supplemental care continues for an indeterminate period of time. This is what happened to Li.

Li had always lived with her parents and had been supporting both them and her brother since she was 19. Eleven years before I interviewed Li, her mother had been confined to a wheelchair. At the time, Li worked during the day and cared for her mother at night in their home. However, she often had to leave work to take her mother to the hospital. At the same time, Li's father was also in poor health, which meant she was frequently caring for both parents at the same time. She described it:

> My mother and my father always go to the hospital. Sometime two of them went to the hospital. I have to take care of one and then later on I go to another room to take care of [the other]. (Li)

In this way, for three years Li cared for her parents by herself, with intermittent but frequent hospitalisations of both. During this time, the contract she was working under expired, and while looking for a new job, she took time off to take care of her mother full time:

> This year she is very weak. Always [I] have to go to the hospital. If I have to work then I cannot always apply [for] the leave to take care of my mother. [If] I have no work then I can take my full time to take care of her. (Li)

Li recalled how, when her mother was hospitalised she fed her lunch and dinner every day and also looked after her father who was in and out of the nursing home. Shuttling between the hospital and the nursing home, perhaps several times a day, Li said she was very tired and stressed. She explained what it was like:

Maybe my mother live in the hospital I have to look after my mother and then later on I went to the [nursing home] to see my father. If my father lives in the hospital I have to [go] to the [nursing] home to see my mother. Every day [it was] like this. (Li)

When her mother could no longer eat or bathe without the use of medical apparatus, the decision was made to permanently place her in a nursing home. Li explained why she did this:

Because she don't want to eat and… because… I do not have the apparatus to help the elderly people…[and] I am thinner than my mother. I have not the strength to…bathe, to wash the hair, and to do all these. (Li)

Li noted that she never considered hiring a domestic helper because her home was too small and she believed that helpers did not have the same knowledge as hospital staff. She thought it was safer to institutionalise her mother. Besides, she indicated she could not afford a helper and she had to go back to work.

After she returned to work, Li visited her mother on weekends and cared for her father at home. Within four years, her father lost the ability to walk and he was also permanently placed in a nursing home. For several months, Li went to see him every day during her lunch hour and on her way home from work until he adjusted to living in the facility.

Li's mother died after spending eight years in the nursing home. Her father was still institutionalised at the time Li and I spoke. She said she was visiting him every night, feeding him his dinner and remaining with him until he fell asleep, around 10:00 p.m.

Li said she had no choice but to institutionalise her parents. She noted that she had 'to accept this' no matter how long it lasted, and added: 'I will not give up myself, because nobody will help you. [It] is only you [who can] help yourself'.

Stories told by the other caregiving daughters were similar to Li's. Chunhua related that she cooked and visited her mother in the hospital every day for five years. Ning recalled years of visiting her aunts and uncle when they were intermittently hospitalised. Sometimes all three kin were in different hospitals and she described having to shuttle between them.

For two years, Yow alternated with her sister-in-law, accompanying her mother-in-law to dialysis treatments from 7 a.m. to 11 p.m. as many as three times a week, and more often when her condition worsened and she was hospitalised. All of these women described how stressed they were during these times.

Conditions were different when a domestic helper was hired to become the primary caregiver. This is discussed below.

Employing a Domestic Helper

Domestic helpers (FDHs/CDHs) were employed at all stages of the typology. Over 30 daughters hired them to care for their nuclear families and their parents at one time or another. In Hong Kong and Singapore, the ability to hire a helper was facilitated by the government, who ensured the cost remained low. The daughters reported paying the FDHs they employed the equivalent range of 150–300 pounds British Sterling per month. In mainland China, where wages were not subsidised and CDHs did not always live with their employers, wages could be proportionally higher.

In some instances, married daughters related that their domestic helpers had initially been hired to care for their children or household. However, if their parents were living with them, the helper's duties might be expanded to include elder support and eventually caregiving as the parents aged. In the case of the unmarried daughters in Singapore and Hong Kong, most continued to live with their parents into adulthood, and an FDH might be hired to help with domestic chores while the daughter was working. Alternatively, if parents were living separately, as their needs and dependency increased, the daughters and their siblings (when they had them) might contribute financially to a helper hired to assist, and later provide full time care for their parents in their parents' own homes.

In the case of temporary care, the daughters might send their own helpers to their parents' home or instruct them to care for a parent while he or she was recuperating in the daughter's home. FDHs were generally unavailable for part time employment in Singapore or Hong Kong because they were retained on the basis of a two-year contract.

Among the daughters interviewed for this book, the decision to employ a helper was generally made by her, sometimes in consultation with her husband or siblings, depending on where care was to be provided. Seven of the daughters reported employing a helper to be the full-time caregiver of a family member in their own home or an institution. In two cases the helper did both sequentially. Another nine daughters spoke about hiring a domestic helper to live with their parents in the parents' home. Five of the six FDHs interviewed for this research also said they cared for the elderly parents of their employer.

In the remainder of this chapter, the discussion of full-time care by domestic helpers is advanced from the perspective of both the daughter-employer and the helper.

Issues Between Employers and Domestic Helpers

The difficult lives of foreign domestic helpers have been well documented in the literature. However, not all have lived under egregious circumstances. Among the small group of FDHs (N = 6) interviewed for this book, some had good relationships with their employers and others experienced troubling conditions. Some had affection for individual members of the families they cared for. Conversely, three of the FDHs interviewed had sexual advances made toward them by the husband of the household, and one received money for sexual favours. More of the FDHs however, reported issues arising from their perceived low status in the household or their caregiving activities.

From the onset of caregiving, many of the daughters explained that they expected their helper to learn and understand the condition of the care recipient. These daughters also spoke of providing skills training for their helper relevant to the care she was to undertake. Further, the daughters expressed a desire for their helpers to adopt their caregiving philosophies, like Huan, who listed her requirements:

> You must prepare their mind, alright, to accept this patient…If you can… do this work, stay on. If you don't, just leave it, just go away. I have to… train you up. Otherwise, you can't help me. (Huan)

Even with training, however, problems could arise in the course of everyday caregiving, especially if the parent was cognitively impaired. Ya and her FDH, Bonnie elaborate the point. Like Huan, Ya said she explained her requirements for caregiving to Bonnie, before the latter ever commenced her caregiving duties of Ya's mother:

> We already told her before she joined us that she [mom] has dementia. You must learn to accept…and don't take it with heart or whatever [if] she scolds you…She [may] just call you [something bad and the] next moment she could be good to you. She can't even remember what she says. So, I explain to her and make her know this is a sickness, that none of us can help her… So, we expect the maid to solve [the problems and] to get along well with her. (Ya)

Living together in the same household, Ya described how her mother picked on Bonnie for small things, making sure 'that she's not lazy' and scolding her because 'she wants her way'. Ya said her mother was also 'paranoid and fearful' about what Bonnie might do to her. She had read in the newspaper about how 'some maids poison you or they urinate on the food and let you eat', so her mother 'would not eat until I eat with her'. Meanwhile, the helper, Bonnie, was forced to contend not only with the mother's dementia but also with her incontinence and prolapse. Ya said her mother refused to wear a diaper, so Ya installed a rubber sheet on her bed. When the weather was hot, her mother complained and Ya removed it. That meant Bonnie had to change and wash the bed linens one or more times a day. According to Ya, her mother had accused Bonnie of stealing the rubber sheet because she had forgotten why it was missing. Ya explained how every day there was an incident between her mother and Bonnie. She had become the mediator, making her 'stressed on both sides', even though, she noted, her mother accused her of siding with Bonnie against her.

Ya's situation is just one example. However, it shows the kind of mistrust and tension that could, and often did result when the helper was expected to assume the role of the caregiving daughter. It should also be noted that living apart from the parent and helper did not completely relieve the daughter of the caregiving burden. Although Ya and Bonnie lived with Ya's mother, daughters like Chenguang, whose parents lived in their own home, were still required to constantly mediate between the impaired parent and the helper. Chenguang, whose mother also had dementia, sounded very much like Ya when speaking about her mother and the helper. She recalled how her mother was obsessed with the helper, and related incidents in which the helper was accused of stealing from her mother, having an affair with her father, and even trying to kill Chenguang's mother. Like Ya, Chenguang was accused of siding with the helper against her mother. She said she could not count the number of housekeepers she had hired who had quit because they could not bear the mother's treatment. Chenguang reported feeling angry, but said she 'should do my filial respect', so she gave up trying to change her mother, kept quiet and tried to 'do as my mother likes' to 'keep her happy'.

Domestic helpers caring for family members play a unique role. By assuming the caregiving burden they help to maintain family harmony and balance. However, they also affect the daughter-parent relationship in profound ways, as seen below.

Daughters, Parents and Foreign Domestic Helpers

In this section, two narratives are presented to illustrate the daughter-parent relationship when a domestic helper has become the primary caregiver. The first is told from the perspective of the Chinese daughter. The second is told from the perspective of a Filipina FDH.

Transition from Home to Nursing Home Care

Yuan had always been close to her mother, and as a single working woman she had continued to live with her into adulthood. Shortly after the turn of the millennium she noticed a change in her mother's behaviour, prompting her 'to find a maid'. Susan, a Filipina, was hired and remained with Yuan for the next 11 years.

In the beginning, Yuan's mother was ambulatory, but as she became weaker, Susan gradually assumed more responsibility until she assisted with bathing, grooming, walking, and transfers. Providing hands-on care was a full time job. However, the mother's mental condition also continued to worsen, especially at night. Yuan noted how she regularly pulled the drawers out of her dresser, took them to the living room and threw the clothes on the floor, claiming they were not hers. Then she would turn on the television and yell at it. When her mother began to hallucinate and wander, Yuan had her tested. The diagnosis was mild to moderate dementia.

Explaining her mother's deterioration, Yuan recalled how one night she returned home to find her missing. She was finally located in the car park of their building at 1:00 a.m. in her nightgown. After that, Susan was moved into the mother's room to prevent her from wandering and to help with toileting in the night. Yuan's mother had begun to wear a diaper, and she had also become more aggressive and bad tempered, yelling at Susan and Yuan. She had begun to throw things, including food, and was becoming difficult to control. She walked around shouting all night and tried to get out of the house, so that Susan had to get up to calm her. Yuan observed that her mother's erratic nocturnal behaviour was lasting longer and becoming more frequent, spilling over into the daytime. Her mother had been attending day-care three days a week, but Yuan said every few weeks she was told to bring her home because she was disrupting the other patients. According to Yuan, Susan began to complain about the workload and stress.

Eleven years after Yuan hired Susan, she quit. In the final year of her employment, Yuan's mother had been institutionalised. Susan spent eight, hours a day caring for her in the nursing home, with Yuan visiting her mother two to three times a week.

Yuan's Coping Strategy Earlier in her life, Yuan had worked as a special needs teacher. Like Huan, she returned to the skill sets she had learned at that time and implemented them with her mother:

> Say sometimes [they are] like banging on the floor, or banging on the wall, when I was a special school teacher, I had to handle these sorts of behaviours. So, I'm not really that upset…because *I think I can remove my role as a daughter to be a teacher or care worker or a therapist*. (Yuan; *Emphasis added*)

Focusing on her role as a professional, Yuan said, 'that's why I can play with her, especially nowadays...I *can change my mode*'. She had also begun a course in music therapy to work with her mom. Otherwise, Yuan added, her social life had not been substantially affected by caregiving, and her work hours were flexible so she could schedule around her mother's care. She acknowledged, however that because she had to work fewer hours she had accepted a lower position, indicating that was a big adjustment. Beyond that, she said she could 'cope quite well'.

How Yuan's FDH Affected Her Ability to Cope Throughout the 11 year caregiving experience with Yuan's mother, it appeared to be Susan who endured most of the direct stress and burden. In Yuan's words, whereas she [Yuan] could sleep through the night with minor interruptions, Susan had to maintain constant vigilance, often losing sleep. Susan also spent more time with Yuan's mother than Yuan did, being subjected to more emotional outbursts and abusive behaviour. Additionally, Susan was carrying out what might be considered unpleasant tasks such as diaper changing. After ten years, she began to complain of the stress and had to be induced to renew her contract. In her final year, when Susan took a month's holiday, Yuan assessed that she could not manage alone and that was the impetus to institutionalise her mother.

If Yuan's situation is compared to Li's or Ai's, the difference an FDH makes becomes evident. The FDH becomes a buffer between the daughter and her parent, absorbing the worst aspects of caregiving. The following is an FDH's account of caregiving from her perspective.

An FDH's Perspective on Caregiving and Daughter-Parent Relationships

Nancy was a 33-year-old never married Filipina who had worked for three families. The following discussion relates to Nancy's first and second employers, both of whom were Chinese.

Family 1 Nancy first came to Singapore to live with a three-generation family, caring for their young children and assisting the wife's parents, who were both healthy. She was placed under the supervision of the grandmother.

Nancy related how her day began at 5:00 a.m. She tried to arise before the grandmother because if the grandmother awoke first Nancy would only be given two pieces of bread and a cup of coffee for breakfast. For lunch Nancy said she was given one package of noodles to eat. At din-nertime, she was not allowed to dine at the table, and was only given scraps of food. She described how a neighbour maid snuck leftovers to her through the gate at night. In the six months she worked for this fam-ily, Nancy said she lost 20 kg.

Throughout the day, the grandmother followed Nancy around the house, forcing her to clean and re-clean the same things until the grand-mother was satisfied. If any dust was found when the grandmother ran her finger over the furniture, she wiped it on Nancy's face. The grand-mother told Nancy she must do every task exactly as she would. Even washing the dishes, Nancy was instructed on how to dispense the soap onto the plate. She was required to scrub the floors of the three-storey home on her hands and knees, and was not allowed to use a mop. Laundry, Nancy remembered, was done by hand rather than in the wash-ing machine, with the grandmother standing over her supervising.

At the end of her 18-hour day, Nancy slept on the floor under the din-ing room table. In the middle of the night the grandmother often awak-ened her, yelling at Nancy to find her medicine. Nancy claimed she did not know where the medicine was kept, and when she could not locate it, the grandmother became angry, one time throwing a chair at her.

Nancy's employer informed her that she did not get along with her mother either. Nonetheless, Nancy was told to be patient because the grandmother was old. In Nancy's words, neither her employer nor the grandmother showed any concern for her. At one point Nancy said she broke both her feet and was not given medical care. She remarked that she felt like she was in prison and said she was treated 'like an animal'.

At the end of six months Nancy gave up, stating that she was afraid of her emotions and worried that if she stayed she might hurt the grandmother. She asked to go home, but the employer-daughter refused to sign her release papers, telling Nancy she had invested too much time training her. Nancy had to pay the Philippine agency six-months wages for sending her to Singapore, so in the end, she went through this experience earning nothing.

Family 2 Nancy went back to the Philippines but returned to Singapore four years later to care for another family with two elderly grandparents and two young children. The grandfather had colon cancer and was unable to eat, so Nancy fed him through a tube. She bathed him, lifted him and changed his diaper. Nancy described him as being 'like a baby'.

When the grandfather was still alive, Nancy fed the grandmother and administered her medicine. Following the grandfather's death, the grandmother developed dementia. Nancy said the grandmother tried to leave the house, became bad tempered and threw tantrums, adding, 'she [was] always angry with me'. Her anger could escalate to the point of shouting, banging her head against the wall, and throwing things. If Nancy responded, she said it became worse.

The grandmother also had chronic urine infections, requiring her to wear a catheter. However, she kept pulling it out so Nancy had to take her to the hospital twice a day to replace it. Upon the grandfather's death, Nancy was also moved into the grandmother's room where she slept on a foam mattress on the floor next to the grandmother's bed. Nancy described what it was like:

> [After the grandfather] died she become very worse already. She doesn't know where is the toilet. She passes urine in the room. Of course, ... I need to clean that one because we cannot sleep together because the smell is there and then I clean [in] the middle of the night...[I] change the bed. Sometimes [it is] not in the bed, [but] in the floor also. She [is] confused... We try to put [a] diaper [on her] but she takes [it] out... She says, 'why [do] I [need to] put this one [on]?' Because she doesn't know...Then [it is] no use, even [if] you put the diaper on, because she takes [it] out and then she sleeps. (Nancy)

At night, the grandmother talked in her sleep, calling out the name of her late husband and waking Nancy up. Nancy worked 17 hours a day and under the best of circumstances said she only slept five hours a night. She claimed she was constantly exhausted because in addition to caring for the elderly woman and the two children, she did the housework and cooking. Nancy said she never got out of the house except for one day off a month, and remarked that her employers never spoke to her except to tell her what to do. According to Nancy, the only person who showed her any kindness or appreciation was the grandfather, and Nancy was happy to do anything for him. When he died, Nancy said the job became more difficult and she became homesick, recalling how she cried and prayed.

After two and a half years, Nancy broke her contract. The grandmother was passing urine in the bed every night, interrupting Nancy's sleep to change the sheets. Nancy said the daughter-wife was jealous of her because the children thought Nancy was their mother. However, according to Nancy, what finally put her over the edge was fear. One day the grandmother gave a pair of scissors to the toddler. Nancy said she reported the incident to the daughter, however the daughter refused to put latches on the cupboards or take any safety precautions. Alarmed, Nancy said she assessed that if something happened she would be blamed, especially because the daughter had asked Nancy not to tell the husband about the scissors. Nancy explained that the husband did not like his mother-in-law and the daughter had told her he would become angry.

The Daughter-Parent Relationship Nancy related that the husband in the family would not eat with his mother-in-law, so the grandmother ate alone. She said, 'That's why she feels she's nothing... that's why the [grandmother], she [is] always in the room...that is why the dementia becomes very worse, because...they don't talk to her'.

Nancy observed that the employer-daughter only spent 20 minutes a day with her mother, even though she worked from home. When the daughter went out the grandmother would shout at Nancy, asking where her daughter was, when she was coming back and why she [the grandmother] could not go with her. Nancy said in a one hour period she might ask these questions twenty times. Sometimes, Nancy recalled, she would give the grandmother the phone to call her daughter: 'and then she called, [and in] just one minute put down the phone, [and then] she [would] ask again, where [did the] daughter go, because she forget already...she scream, she shout...she scold me upside down. I don't bother her because I know she's sick already'. Nancy added:

> That's why the [grandmother], she always says to me, she doesn't like them. Better she die. That's why [it is] very hard. I feel [the grandmother] she feels the loneliness. Also, sometimes...I explain to her [but] she doesn't understand because I'm the helper only, but...she needs attention [the daughter] cannot give to her. That's why the [grandmother]...she tells [me] ...I want to die already. No use the life is like this. (Nancy)

This theme was repeated over and over. The grandmother told Nancy that she wanted to jump out of the window and die.[1] Nancy tried to tell the daughter-employer how lonely and unhappy her mother was, but the daughter countered: 'What to do? I have work. I cannot monitor them every minute every day. I need to earn money also. She has a lot of medicine. I need to pay, I need to work'.

Other FDHs Mary, another Filipina FDH, had similar experiences to Nancy's. However, Mary continued in employment with the same family for 22 years. During this time, she cared for three young boys and elderly grandparents living in the daughter's three-generation household. The grandfather had cancer and emphysema. For six years, the last three of which he was disabled, she administered his medicines, bathed and dressed him, assisted with transfers and walking, and fed him with a spoon. For 16 years, she also took care of the grandmother. Mary explained that during the first 14 years, the grandmother followed her around the house all day, nagging, irritable, abusive and disrespectful. Like Nancy and Susan, the grandmother threw things at Mary. During the last two years of the grandmother's life, Mary administered her medications, bathed and dressed her, assisted with toileting and toileting clean up, and fed the grandmother through a tube. Describing the daughter-parent relationship, Mary said that both the husband and the wife worked until 19:00 each day and there was little contact between the grandparents and the other family members. At night, the grandparents ate alone then went to bed. Mary did say that the daughter appeared to be concerned for her parents' well-being and interfaced with Mary on a regular basis to ensure the household ran smoothly. Both grandparents remained at home until their deaths.

Neither Mary nor Nancy cared for their employers' parents in the nursing home. However, like Lola in Chap. 4, Rachael, another Hong Kong Filipina, did. As with Lola, Rachael's employer lived apart from her parents and Rachael was sent to clean for them. Later, her duties expanded to caring for the elderly couple every day. The grandmother had Alzheimer's disease and Rachel bathed and fed her, changed her diaper and accompanied her to day-care. Eventually the grandmother was institutionalised. Rachael continued to care for the grandfather, including accompanying him every day to visit and care for his wife in the nursing home. When he was also institutionalised, Rachael cared for both grandparents from nine to four every day. Their daughter, who lived part time in Canada, visited them for an hour on Saturdays, when she was in town. At the time of her interview, Rachel said the grandmother no longer recognised her daughter, but she still knew Rachael. She added that she loved the grandparents and felt like they were family members.

Foreign Domestic Helpers and Emotion Work

Six FDHs were interviewed for this book. Four articulated that they had good relationships with their employers. However, the relationships appeared to be asymmetrical and fraught with conditions. Principal among these was that the FDHs were required to be obedient, respectful, and in control of their emotions at all times, often under stressful circumstances. Mary, talking about the grandmother she cared for, expressed a common sentiment:

> Especially the old woman…she doesn't care at all whether you will be hurt…because maybe she feels like you are nobody in the house…So, I will just say if that is the case, so be it. I cannot control anything. I can also not command her to do this or to do that or…follow what I want because I am only the maid here. (Mary)

A major theme emerging from the FDH interviews was how fearful they *all* were of losing control. Indeed, during the months I resided in Asia doing research for this book, stories regularly appeared in the newspapers about helper injustice and suicide, in addition to misconduct and abuses. By way of example, here is what one domestic helper said in her interview:

> Every night…when the lady is out because she likes to play mahjong. Then my boss [is] always at home naked, walking [around] naked…Sometimes he [employer husband] doesn't like to work. He wants to have sex with me, And, I said no. I said no. I said no sir, don't do this to me or else I'm going to kill myself or else I'm going to kill you too. (Sophie)

Regardless of how fond the domestic helpers were of their employers or care recipients, or how close to them they were, all of them did extensive emotion work. Their objectives varied from maintaining an appropriate and acceptable display, generating feelings of warmth they believed they *should* have, or most often suppressing anger. Repeatedly, statements were made like: 'If I am angry, I just keep quiet. I didn't talk'. (Heather)

All the domestic helpers had similar coping strategies. Perhaps because of their religious upbringing, the most common emotion work was prayer. Mary, for example, said it was the 'number one' thing she did to cope because she did not want 'to do wrong'. Later, she added:

> I have to believe in what you call prayers you see, because in prayers, within these long years that I've been here, only my prayers [are] helping me… I can feel it, you know. So, even though sometimes I have experience, other people will just criticise you…or say something at your back, I can still move on like this, you know. (Mary)

Mary's coping strategy had two additional components: splashing water on her face, and thinking happy thoughts. She conjured up images of her children back home, whereas other helpers spoke of the homes they were building in the Philippines with the money they earned and how they could educate their children. This was all deep acting, psychologically transferring loving thoughts of their own families onto those they had to love or at least care about. It suggested that under such circumstances caregiving might be difficult or impossible without it.

Conclusion

Outsourced care is the fourth and last stage of the typology of support and care. This chapter initially explored the dilemma over outsourcing care before examining why care might be discontinued or modified, or the daughters might decline to provide it.

Interpersonal exchange was the first area to be examined. Hochschild (1979) explained that in our interpersonal exchanges we keep mental ledgers of debits and credits with the objective of maintaining a balance between them. Framing rules and feeling rules tell us what is owed and what is expected in return. Applied to this group of women, as care became more burdensome and the rewards diminished, the exchange between the caregiver and care recipient could become unbalanced. An unbalanced exchange was likely to result from caregiver stress, particularly if the care recipient was cognitively impaired. Once the exchange became imbalanced, the first modification of the caring arrangement was most often the employment of a domestic helper. Alternatively, the caregiver might attempt to continue the arrangement but wish the parent would die to relieve the caregiver's stress. If care with the assistance of a domestic helper became impossible, institutionalisation of the parent might become necessary. Although this was accepted as 'giving care', and thus complying with norms of filial obligation, it was generally treated as a last resort. Usually, only when the care recipient needed special equipment or professional supervision was it considered.

Exchange was discussed in the context of existing care arrangements. If care was being contemplated but had not been implemented, other considerations could intervene. To preserve family harmony, some daughters said they preferred to hire a paid helper rather than move in with their parents to provide care. Others pointed to the better skills and compassion of professional caregivers. Finally, if the daughter was the sole support of her parents or preferred to work and provide financial support rather than hands-on care (with or without a helper), she might be unwilling or unable to provide instrumental care.

The normative influences related to institutionalisation were also discussed. The influence of traditional norms could still be seen through the collective nature of decision making, particularly when nursing home placement was being considered. Daughters and daughters-in-law were reluctant to expose themselves to the possibility of blame from other family members in the event something went wrong. The influence of contemporary norms was observed in the growing importance of government pensions, allowing the elderly to remain independent. It was also seen in the daughters' willingness to institutionalise themselves when they reached old age. Most of the daughters expected this, rather than being cared for at home. They suggested that perhaps they would use their homes to pay for their care rather than leave their property to their children. Finally, nursing home placement was losing its stigma. Homes could even be looked at long before they were necessary, and parents could be placed on waiting lists for the better institutions. However, it was still important for adult children to provide care for institutionalised parents.

Attention was then redirected to what happened when domestic helpers became the primary caregivers of elderly parents. As with institutional placement, the employment of helpers was indicative of the influence of contemporary norms on filial responsibility.

Care by outsourcing daughters, even after a family member had been institutionalised, was prevalent among these women. How they coped without help from a domestic helper was illustrated through the story of Li, an unmarried, Baby Boomer who cared for both her father and her mother at home and then later in the nursing home and hospital. Li had no help and most of the time she worked, because she was the sole support of her family. Her story showed how difficult and stressful trying to work and provide care without help could be. Even after her parents were institutionalised she shuttled back and forth to the hospital and nursing home during and after work, feeding and comforting them. Other respondents told similar stories about caring for institutionalised parents, reporting heavy stress. Their reward came from fulfilling their duty, and knowing they had tried to improve on their family member's difficult circumstances.

The employment of foreign domestic helpers was then considered, and some of the issues between the daughter-employers and their domestic helpers were presented. Specific examples of the conflict and tension that could arise were seen through the challenges faced by Ya, Chenguang and their helpers.

To illustrate the relationship between a daughter, her parent and domestic helper, Yuan's narrative was presented. Yuan was an unmarried, working professional whose mother slid into dementia over a period of eleven years. During this time, Yuan became increasingly dependent on her helper, Susan, to care for her mother. In Susan's final year working for Yuan, the mother was institutionalised, and she remained in the nursing home even after Susan retired, with Yuan visiting her two to three times a week.

Yuan's narrative allowed us to see her coping strategy and Susan's effect on Yuan's ability to cope. Yuan professed to have nominal stress with her mother due to her experience working with emotionally disabled children. However, Susan was the one enduring the direct brunt of caregiving, including sleep deprivation and emotional abuse from someone she was not related to. This led to Nancy's narrative, offering an FDH's perspective.

Nancy was a Gen X Filipina who worked for three different families. In the first two situations, she cared for her employers' home, children and elderly grandparents under what she perceived as stressful and difficult conditions. From Nancy's story one could see the physical and emotional strain that helpers could be placed under, and how they might become fearful of the circumstances of their employment.

Nancy's story also provided another glimpse into how the presence of a domestic helper could affect the daughter-parent relationship. In the second family she worked for, there was barely any contact between the employer-daughter and her mother. The grandmother was distraught and angry over her neglect and often spoke of killing herself. When Nancy tried to relay this to her employer, she was rebuffed by the daughter's explanation that she had no time to monitor her elderly parents.

Other domestic helpers told stories similar to Nancy's, of both mistreatment by employers and the employers' distant relationships with their parents, even when living in the same home. These other helpers also spoke of caring for the elderly parents in their own homes and in nursing homes. The theme emerging from their observations was one of working women with young families, busy lives, and very little time or interest in caring for their elderly parents. In at least one instance, Rachael the helper became closer to the grandparents she cared for than their own daughter and family.

The other thing seen through the domestic helpers was how they did emotion work to suppress anger and generate positive displays, in addition to bolstering their ability to cope. One important commonality among all of them was the fear of losing control.

The employment of and dependency on foreign domestic helpers is part of a greater normative change occurring in Asian Chinese families. This is discussed in the next and final chapter.

Notes

1. The mother in law of one of the women interviewed for this book actually did jump out of the window of a twelfth story high rise to her death.

References

Allen, K. (2010). *Classical sociological theory* (2nd ed.). Los Angeles: Pine Forge Press.

Chien, W.-T., Norman, I., & Thompson, D. R. (2006). Perceived benefits and difficulties experienced in a mutual support group for family carers of people with schizophrenia. *Qualitative Health Research, 16*(7), 962–981.

Hochschild, A. R. (1979). Emotion work, feeling rules and social structure. *American Journal of Sociology, 85*(3), 551–575.

Mac Rae, H. (1998). Managing feelings: Caregiving as emotion work. *Research on Aging, 20*(1), 137–160.

Simpson, C., & Acton, G. (2013). Emotion work in family caregiving for persons with dementia. *Issues in Mental Health Nursing, 34*(1), 52–58.

Yan, E., & Kwok, T. (2011). Abuse of older Chinese with dementia by family caregivers: An inquiry into the role of caregiver burden. *International Journal of Geriatric Psychiatry, 26*(5), 527–535.

9

Discussion and Conclusion

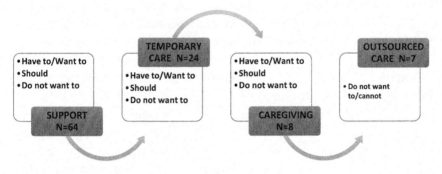

Image of the typology of support and care

This book began with the overarching question: Why are contemporary Chinese daughters still willing to undertake traditional parent caregiving activities considering their self-sufficient, modern lifestyles and attitudes, and what are their coping strategies for accommodating the tension and conflict involved with discharging filial obligation?

To gain insight into this question, between 2011 and 2017, 67¹ Chinese women and six Filipina domestic helpers were interviewed in Hong Kong, Singapore and Kunming, Yunnan province, mainland

© The Author(s) 2018
P. O'Neill, *Urban Chinese Daughters*, St Antony's Series,
https://doi.org/10.1007/978-981-10-8699-1_9

China. Analysis was then conducted within the theoretical framework of symbolic interactionism, Arlie Hochschild's theory of emotion work, and conceptual models underpinning motivation for caregiving.

Almost immediately, it became clear that what the daughters referred to as 'caregiving' made no distinction between support behaviour such as visiting with young and active parents, and hands-on instrumental care of elderly, disabled or cognitively impaired parents. To remedy any potential confusion arising from this ambiguity, a stage model of parental need and care intensity was developed, arrayed by increasing levels of parent disability and need, and corresponding levels of daughter commitment and involvement. This was denominated the *typology of support and care*, and it distinguished between four stages, or 'types' of support and care. As depicted above, these stages or types included support provided to healthy independent parents; temporary care offered in times of parents' acute heath emergencies; hands-on, long-term caregiving performed for unhealthy, dependent parents; and finally, parent care outsourced to domestic helpers (FDHs/CDHs), other family members or care institutions.

Having established a means of differentiating between adult children interacting with able-bodied parents and those actually providing or having provided hands-on care for disabled parents, caregiving motivations and coping strategies were addressed. Drawing from the conceptual and theoretical framework supported by the literature, the typological model was further elaborated. A central aim of the research was to more fully understand why Chinese daughters were willing to support and care for their elderly parents, how they managed potential tensions in discharging filial obligation, and why they might discontinue or decline to undertake support and care. That is, it set out to learn what norms and values were motivating-indeed compelling Chinese daughters to provide support and care for their elderly parents, despite the pressures of outside employment, the difficulty of the tasks, the demands on their time and resources, and the toll on their physical and psychological health, and further, what could undermine these motivating norms and values, leading to a discontinuation of or refusal to provide support or care. It also sought to understand the process of discharging care and how conflicts experienced in caregiving could be resolved.

To this end, three key analytical categories related to motivations and their underlying norms and values, plus the processes of emotional coping, were incorporated into the typology. These categories were defined and labelled: conceptual norms of motivation, including structural norms of filial obligation ['*I have to*'] and relational norms of affection, gratitude and reciprocity ['*I want to*']; a theoretical approach to managing tension and conflict in the discharge of filial obligation ['*I should want to*']; and conceptual and theoretical underpinnings explaining unwillingness or inability to provide support and care ['*I do not want to/I cannot*'].

Through this process, it became possible to explore what was driving support and care and to better understand how the daughters interviewed for this book managed support and caregiving as parental need changed. Four strands of research questions were generated:

1. Why would filial obligation remain a strong normative value among modern Chinese women and why would they be willing to provide support and care for ageing parents?
2. Is there a relationship between how daughters feel toward their parents and in-laws and the amount and quality of support and care they are willing to provide to them? If so, does this represent a shift from traditional Chinese values of filial obligation?
3. How do modern Chinese women negotiate the actual discharge of support and caregiving?
4. If filial obligation remains a strong normative value among Chinese daughters, why would they delegate caregiving responsibilities to foreign domestic helpers or other helpers and be willing to place elderly parents in nursing homes?

In this chapter, the key empirical findings are revisited to shed light on the research questions and to demonstrate how these findings add to the existing discourse on Asian caregivers. This is followed by a discussion of the policy implications associated with the changing roles and status of Chinese daughters. The book concludes with some remarks from the author.

Understanding the Current Caregiving Paradigm of Chinese Families in Hong Kong, Singapore and Mainland China

All four of the research questions grew out of the central paradox between traditional Chinese values and the modern lifestyles of Chinese women. This chapter begins by reviewing the findings from the empirical analysis addressing this paradox in the context of the book's conceptual and theoretical framework and previous research on family caregiving in Asia.

Filial obligation remains a strong normative value among the modern Chinese women in this book because, in the first instance, for the two core generations (1946–1980) of daughters represented here, it was taught to them by their parents. Traditional Chinese values, espousing duty to one's family, were conveyed explicitly or implicitly to the daughters, then reinforced directly or indirectly through a variety of mechanisms that could include school, cinema, friends and family, community, government policy, social engineering, and even the Christian religion. Most of the daughters also learned family responsibility associated with female gender roles at a very early age. The accumulated information was then amalgamated and internalised, no doubt facilitated by the long history of Confucianism and filial piety associated with Chinese families and culture. Hochschild (1983) called these internalised norms *framing rules*, or the meanings and interpretations individuals give to the situations they are in. They become the attitudinal and behavioural standards one strives to meet.

As a result of their upbringing, most of the daughters said they were very 'Chinese' or 'traditional' in their thinking. However, traditional Chinese values did not mean the same thing to everyone. For some daughters, they were synonymous with filial piety, whereas others had never heard the term 'filial piety' *'xiao'* or *'xiaoshun'*.

Filial piety has continued to be central to the Chinese caregiving discourse, and it has been broadly construed as a structural norm. However, some recent studies have asserted that it has always had moral and relational overtones and that this, or its financial aspects, might be all that remain (Lee and Kwok 2005; Lieber et al. 2004; Ng et al. 2002; Wong and Chau 2006). These kinds of findings have given way to considerable debate among Asia scholars over the forces 'eroding' or transforming filial piety and what this has meant for intergenerational relationships within Chinese families. However, no accord has been achieved, and thus, within the academic community, the nature and importance of filial piety to Chinese family caregiving is presently unclear.

Ambiguity over the definition and relevance of filial piety was similarly reflected in the lack of consensus among the women in this book. When they were asked what it meant to them, the responses of those who understood the term ranged from 'you just say yes to everything', to having a bond, respect, meals together, hospital visits, honouring one's parents, obedience, love, caring for parents, even thinking for one's parents. The only reasonable explanation for this is that, in the symbolic interactionist tradition, filial piety, or more accurately, filial obligation, among these women was individually interpreted and ascribed personal meaning and definition. This was based on what they were taught and observed in their childhood families, then modified by exposure to contemporary norms and modern lifestyles experienced outside the family.

Despite the myriad discrepant views of what filial *piety* was, among these women commitment to filial *obligation* was robust. Likely due to the strength of early family ties and a supporting cultural environment in which structural norms could be effectively disseminated, filial obligation remained an integral part of the daughters' internalised system of values. Having established this, it is now possible to ask how this commitment translated into a **willingness to provide support and care for ageing parents.**

In addressing this question, it might be prudent to return momentarily to the filial piety discussion, because one has to wonder where traditional filial piety and familism intersect. If the structural elements of filial piety, such as ancestor worship, arranged marriages, and female dependency have dissipated, as the daughters claimed, then an argument could reasonably be made that it might have been responsibility for the well-being of the family unit alone, rather than a superimposed ideology, that was underpinning the adult daughters' willingness to discharge filial obligation. This was reflected in the interviews, and it is an important distinction because, if true, the quality and nature of parent-child relationships, together with learned family values, could be driving filial obligation more than outside pressure to conform to historical Chinese structural norms. This is not to infer that the latter have vanished. However, even if they are merely debilitated, it would essentially represent a transposition of the Confucian structure and a concession to contemporary norms advocating independent thought.

In line with this way of thinking, some of the literature has suggested that relational norms are stronger motivators than duty for initiating and continuing family support and care (Croll 1995; Horowitz and Shindelman 1983: 18; Lyonette and Yardley 2003; Wong and Chau 2006). What emerged from the interviews, however, was not quite as straight forward as that.

First, as explained in Chap. 5, most of the daughters interviewed were incapable of disentangling their sense of duty, gratitude, and love for their parents. This was understandable from the perspective of traditional Chinese values, where overt expressions of affection have been uncommon. The implicit nature of relational norms among the daughters thus served to overlay their sense of duty in many instances, with the end result being an indivisible composite of feeling and obligation. That is no doubt why duty, affection and gratitude rarely appeared alone as drivers of support and caregiving for *one's own parents*. This, of course, was not true of in-laws, but that is discussed below.

Second, as seen throughout the empirical chapters, but particularly in Chap. 7, because these daughters lived in transitioning societies, there was potential for tension and conflict between the traditional norms they were raised with and the influence of contemporary norms. As Ai explained, she grew up with a strong commitment to her family, but education gave her a desire for independence. When her mother developed dementia and Ai forfeited her freedom to care for her, elements of her personal value system clashed and she had to choose between duty generated by love and gratitude, and her desire to live life on her own terms.

This raises a third point. Motivation for providing care to elderly parents or in-laws could change in the process of discharging it, related to the amount of stress and what the caregiving daughter did to try to overcome her desire to be relieved of caregiver burden. The latter is discussed below. What is important here is that whatever else motivated the Chinese daughters in this study to provide support or care for their families, either initially or in the process of carrying it out, one thing above all else appeared to have underpinned it: self-image.

The concept of Face, tied to self-image, has profound historical roots in the Chinese context, and it was a deeply imbedded value among the families of the women interviewed for this book in addition to the women themselves. Face extended into all aspects of expected behaviour within the Chinese community, including support and caregiving.

Holroyd (2001), Mac Rae (1998), and Aronson (1990), all wrote about how self-image is fundamental to female caregiving. One can see how this could be particularly compelling in Chinese families where, for centuries, the only value a daughter had was derived from caring for others. Going beyond the concept of Face, Holroyd (2001: 1127) pointed out that for the traditional Chinese daughter, her ability to implement 'what is considered right and ought to be done', was a condition precedent to earning her rightful place within her family and the wider world; her 'personhood'. Sustaining this meant subordinating self-interest to personhood at all times. Holroyd described this as a cultural model.

Due to the changing nature of filial piety, the cultural model, in the strict Confucian sense Holroyd portrayed it, might not be a perfect fit with what is happening today. Although it is a Western perspective, Aronson's (1990: 70, 72) approach could be slightly more relevant. She proposed that women have a tendency to align their own values with prevailing ideologies and then judge themselves by them. One could argue that Chinese women, whose cultural norms have historically forged and imposed strong gender roles on them, have not substantially altered the image of themselves as being subservient and responsible for the family. Having already internalised these self-expectations when young, the daughters in this book could have been placed in the position of accepting filial obligation or, as Aronson suggested, potentially feeling shame and guilt for failing to live up to these internalised assumptions originating in traditional Chinese ideology.

The daughters in this book were highly invested in living up to what they believed a good daughter or a good caregiver should be; and guilt was a prominent theme. Thus, whereas structural and relational filial norms might have been underpinning motivations for caregiving, self-image is more likely to have acted as the enforcer of filial obligation, ensuring that its discharge conformed to one's individual framing rules, or the interpretation of cultural expectations each daughter had determined she must live by to be free from guilt and shame.

With this in mind, it is possible to examine the *relationship between how the daughters felt toward their parents and in-laws and the amount and quality of support and care they were willing to provide to them.* At the centre of this was the changing roles and status of the Chinese daughters. Simply put, once they began to earn enough money to become self-sufficient, the traditional caregiving paradigm as it related to their natal families and their husbands' families shifted. The affection and gratitude daughters reported feeling for their families of origin, and the commitment and responsibility they said they had toward them, was not duplicated in their relationships with parents-in-law. This manifested at all stages of the typology for these women.

At the support stage the daughters spent more time with their own families and less time with their in-laws. Few were living with their in-laws and more were remaining single, continuing to reside with their families of origin. Daughters who lived with their natal families either permanently or prior to marriage, provided financial support to their parents, alone or in conjunction with their siblings, thereby shifting daughter-parent dependency from a downward to an upward construct. Many married daughters who worked also continued to contribute money to their parents' support, even though culturally, they were not morally obligated to do so. Conversely, they did not provide financial support to their in-laws.

At the temporary care stage, daughters exhibited more concern and patience with their own parents and more willingness to sacrifice for them, even at their own expense. For example, they were more likely to bring home cooked meals to their hospitalised parents, but not to their in-laws, or to take leave from work for their parents.

The importance of relationships could also be seen during periods of illness or recuperation of elderly family members in the daughter's own home. Daughters indicated that parents-in-law were invited out of a desire to help their husbands, or duty, not out of affection for their in-laws. This position has been supported in the literature (Wong 2000) and illustrated by the fact that domestic helpers, rather than daughters-in-law, were the primary caregivers of *all* parents-in-law in this book. In contrast, some daughters providing in home care for their own parents did so themselves, without help from an FDH or CDH. Further, although there were time limitations imposed on both parents and in-laws, and all were eventually returned to their own homes, stress was more associated with the termination of in-law care than it was for parents. In that regard, greater emotion work was reported in the context of caring for in-laws versus one's own family.

The daughters' statements, that mothers and daughters preferred to care for each other rather than in-laws, further highlighted the growing emphasis on relationships and the paradigm shift away from structural norms. Similarly, sentiments concerning mother-daughter affection have been expressed in the Asian caregiving literature where stories of unhappy relationships between daughters-in-law and mothers-in-law have also appeared (Lee 2014; Long et al. 2014). Affection for one's own family, thus, might be considered a more natural state than the previous construct of 'marrying out', in which daughters were denied membership in their natal families, and where bonding and affection between daughters and their parents were not allowed to develop organically.

At both the temporary care and caregiving stages of the typology, *all* care for in-laws was motivated by duty, whereas care for most parents continued to be motivated by combinations of duty, affection and gratitude. Once caregiving became more demanding and longer in duration, the difference between how daughters felt about their own parents and their in-laws, and its effect on the quality and quantity of care became even more pronounced. As a practical matter, this meant daughters were more willing to provide long-term, hands-on care for their own parents, but not their in-laws, and to endure greater caregiver burden, as demonstrated by Ai and Li. Only one daughter, Huan, provided long-term care for her in-laws, and that was with the help of three FDHs. Further, Huan acknowledged that in addition to duty, caregiving was tied to her husband's approval, which was essential to her self-image and well-being.

In the literature, duty has been more closely aligned with financial, rather than emotional or instrumental support (Lee and Kwok 2005; Ng et al. 2002), and this was often the case between the daughters in this book and their in-laws. However, financial arrangements, with nothing more, were also observed among the daughters and their own parents where the childhood relationship had been strained, distant or characterised by violence. Further, estranged fathers and mothers were offered no support whatsoever by the daughters in this book, not even financial.

Beyond structural and relational norms, structural impediments such as employment status and geographic distance could also be implicated in the quality and quantity of support and care. However, the degree to which structural impediments disrupted family relationships appeared to be guided by intention. Daughters could and did use distance and work as excuses to minimise contacts with their in-laws, when they wanted to. In contrast, they rarely allowed these obstacles to deter them from outings and meals with their families of origin, and never allowed them to interfere in times of emergencies. Moreover, regular telephone contact with parents took place regardless of the daughters' personal circumstances. The same effort was not made for in-laws.

All of this represented *a shift from traditional Chinese values*, not only because relational, rather than structural norms, appeared to be stronger drivers of the quality and quantity of care, but also because there was choice where none existed before. This was evident in the case of Sheu-Fuh and Bik, who not only declined to provide care but even refused to maintain contact with their mothers. It was also reflected in the number of daughters electing singlehood, the dearth of intergenerational households and the increased bargaining power exercised by daughters with husbands over limiting or discontinuing parent-in-law support and care.

Given that this was how these Chinese daughters felt about their parents and in-laws and the support and care owed to them, *how did these modern Chinese women negotiate the actual discharge of support and caregiving?* Here the difference between support and caregiving within the greater family structure must be clearly distinguished.

Support required very little commitment of time and emotional investment. It could be argued that its primary purpose was to preserve family unity, and in particular, the parent-child relationship. Whereas filial obligation motivated by structural and relational norms was a factor in providing support, it was not severely tested. Further, although emotion work was performed to maintain balance in the relationship and a willingness to continue it, avoidance was also a viable strategy, especially with regard to in-laws, but also for daughters co-residing with parents.

In contrast, considerable hardship could be associated with caregiving, particularly if it was prolonged. The strength of filial obligation norms could be critically challenged, given that avoidance was unlikely to be a preferred option. Regardless of how strongly affection and gratitude were implicated with caregiving, at its core it was duty, inextricably entwined with one's self-image that appeared to hold the caregiving arrangement together. In this regard, emotion work took on new meaning. It might be performed to preserve the relationship and caring arrangement; to control one's emotions to endure the burden; to resolve conflict between one's duty and desires; and to serve as a restraint on a potential impulse to harm the care recipient out of frustration or anger.

One could also argue, that the more emotionally invested these adult daughters were in their parents, the more difficult caregiving could become, particularly if the parent was cognitively impaired (Horowitz and Shindelman 1983: 18; Lyonette and Yardley 2003). Where affection and gratitude were inducing care by these daughters, there was more emotional strain, less inclination to quit, and greater effort exerted to find new ways to continue, even if the daughter's own health and well-being were sacrificed for the sake of the parent. Daughters might also have had to emotionally adjust to the parents' decline, perhaps view them in a revised context, and for daughters with demented parents, possibly grieve for the loss of a beloved person whose personality had changed.

In addition to the emotion work performed by the daughters to manage support and caregiver burden, other strategies made use of included joining support groups, meeting with friends, seeking professional advice, reading self-help books, walking, and relying on religion. The resolution of conflict related to the nature and extent of support and care to be provided could also be postponed by, for example, accepting overseas employment. Many, but not all, of the daughters also employed domestic helpers (FDHs/CDHs) to assist with full time caregiving, especially in Singapore and Hong Kong. This leads to the final research question: *If filial obligation has remained a strong normative value among Chinese daughters, why would they delegate caregiving responsibilities to foreign domestic (or other) workers and be willing to place elderly parents into nursing homes?*

In the words of the daughters, the employment of domestic helpers and the institutionalisation of parents in nursing homes, fulfilled their filial obligation because both were 'providing care'. Domestic helpers in fact, had not only become culturally acceptable within the Hong Kong and Singapore Chinese communities, they were indispensable to the contemporary caregiving paradigm. Due to the paucity of social welfare services, without helpers, single caregiving daughters with severely impaired parents might have been unable to work, as would married daughters sandwiched between children, parents and jobs who might find it too difficult to juggle these multiple roles and obligations.

There was a lot at stake for a woman who left employment. Particularly in mainland China, there was a strong likelihood she would barred from re-entering the workforce if she was out of work for too long. In such cases, the gains she had achieved through education and hard work, including independence and financial self-sufficiency, would be forfeited. The monetary contributions made to both her parents and, if married, to her nuclear family, would also cease. Without their daughters' monetary contributions, some parents would be deprived of an important source of financial support in their old age. Further, becoming dependent herself, an unemployed daughter would be likely to lose her status and bargaining power within the family. The daughters did not show any indication that these were conditions they would favour or wish to return to.

Institutionalising parents and parents-in-law was another solution, and although these daughters agreed it was normatively acceptable, it was still considered to be a last resort. Most of the daughters were reluctant to place their own parents into nursing homes unless they were unable to physically accommodate the demands of care or their parents were so cognitively impaired they were uncontrollable. The exception to this was where the parent-child relationship was unsatisfactory. Additionally, nursing home placement for in-laws did not appear to face the same resistance. However, daughters were not generally included in decisions over in-law institutionalisation; nor did they want to be.

Contributing to the Chinese Caregiving Discourse

Up until now, most of the contemporary Chinese caregiver literature can best be described as falling into two basic categories: studies exploring the degree to which adult Asian children have relied on filial piety as a motivation for caregiving, and those examining the ways in which caregivers have coped with the discharge of filial obligation. In the first case, the discussion of filial piety has nearly always begun with an effort to redefine it in the context it has been understood by the authors. This book has taken a different approach, suggesting that the filial piety debate might be outdated, and that it could be familism rather than filial piety that is presently driving parental support and care in Asian Chinese families.

Past research investigating the discharge of care has primarily focused on carers of dementia patients, how they have managed stress, and in the family context, how the relationship between a parent and child might have affected the caregiving arrangement. However, unlike this book, prior caregiver studies have not differentiated between the demands of short-term and long-term care, nor the disparities in the levels of stress between the caregivers of cognitively impaired versus disabled parents. As observed, there were important distinctions between all these factors that affected the care decisions of these daughters, such as who care would be provided to, where care would be administered, by whom care would be delivered, and how long caregiving would last.

Caregiving duration and stress could additionally influence whether a caregiver's motivation for providing care was modified in the process of discharging it. A change in motivation could shift the way caregiving was managed, affect the long-term health consequences for the caregiver, or determine whether care would be outsourced. This has not previously been considered.

If the literature has been unsuccessful at differentiating between how the caregiving experience might change once it is underway, or between temporary and long-term care, even more often it has failed to discriminate between those who have actually been providing hands-on care and those who have only considered it prospectively. To better understand these differences a new instrument was created for this book. The typology of support and care has facilitated a more accurate analysis of caregiving attitudes and behaviour as parents' need and dependency have grown. By clearly demarcating between support for healthy parents, and temporary and long-term care of infirm parents, the typology has shown that what has been perceived as 'caregiving' might actually have been two different constructs: support and care. There are implications from this, because what adult children are willing to do for their parents when the demands are few (support) may change as the requirements of caregiving increase, particularly if long-term care has commenced.

In this book, caregiving has been approached from a new perspective: the changing roles and status of Chinese daughters. Initiating the study from this point of view has allowed it to explore how the transitioning nature of Chinese society in Hong Kong, Singapore and mainland China has influenced the daughters' attitudes and behaviour in relation to their families and their lives in general, in addition to the caregiving paradigm.

Examining filial obligation in the context of personally interpreted norms, or as Hochschild (1983) called them, 'framing rules' and 'feeling rules', has also made it possible to probe more deeply into how internalised filial obligation norms intersected with the daughters' self-image. By using this approach, this book has not only been able to confirm the importance of relationships to caregiving, but also to show that motivation related to support and caregiving is more complex and individual than previously believed. The interaction between self-image and normative motivations of support and care have transcended and expanded the previous conceptual framework.

The exploration of filial obligation from the perspective of personally interpreted norms has additionally uncovered a possible nexus between contemporary Asian norms and caregiver burden. Some daughters explained that living in a time of transition created conflict between their own needs and lifestyles and the needs and traditional expectations of their parents. How tension and conflict were resolved depended almost entirely on the daughters' expectations of themselves and what they had to do to avoid guilt and shame, even if that meant self-sacrifice or enduring the love-hate construct called 'caring dilemma'.

Dealing with feelings and emotions in the context of support and caregiving was a salient theme among these women, and one of the principal areas of exploration was whether Hochschild's (1983) theory of emotion work could be expanded to the Chinese caregiving community. The findings from this book suggest that emotion work is appropriate and useful in the Asian Chinese setting both for situations involving support and hands-on care. Control over emotions has historically been a taught behaviour in Chinese families, learned when children were young. According to most of the daughters, challenging parental authority through outward demonstrations of emotion was culturally unacceptable and considerable effort was exerted to avoid it. The narratives demonstrated how emotion work was used to conform to appropriate behaviour, in addition to justifying, initiating or sustaining support or care.

In the process of exploring emotion work, another normative shift became apparent: the daughters' reliance on the Christian religion and prayer as a means of bridging the gap between what they actually felt and what they believed they should feel. The emergence of Christianity within the Chinese community might also have further implications for caregiving, because those with low structural or relational norms of filial obligation could nonetheless be motivated to provide support and care out of a belief that they were supported by God, or that biblical commandments compelled them to honour their parents.

One of the most crucial, yet unexpected, findings to emerge from this research was the daughters' reliance on domestic helpers and the importance of helpers to the current caregiving paradigm. As discussed, the employment of FDHs was likely to be what enabled the adult daughters to provide support and caregiving for elderly parents in Singapore and Hong Kong while remaining in employment. The hiring of domestic helpers was not as pronounced in mainland China. However, it was on the rise. The other difference was that, due to language and cultural differences, the Kunming daughters employed family members or local women, sometimes from the rural area, rather than foreigners.

Finally, a new cultural paradigm could be emerging from this research with implications for caregiving in the Chinese context, and that is that these daughters did not want to impose the burden of filial obligation on their own children; nor did they expect their children to take care of them in their own old age. Nearly all the daughters indicated they would institutionalise themselves before they would appeal to their children for help. The daughters were, therefore, declining to transmit to their children the very values with which they were raised.

Policy Implications

The changing roles and status of Chinese daughters; the preference for their natal families rather than their in-laws, or their choice not to marry; their tendency for fewer children; their predilection for work and the importance of the income they earn to themselves and their families; their disinclination to transmit norms of filial obligation to their children; their reliance on domestic helpers; plus the greater longevity and needs of their parents; the current dearth of elderly services; and the inadequacy of pensions and health insurance in Singapore, Hong Kong and mainland China all beg the issue of how elderly Chinese parents will be cared for in the future.

In this regard, there were some differences between Hong Kong and Singapore, on the one hand and mainland China on the other. In the former, all the daughters had at least one sibling to share the support and care of their parents. In the mainland, 44% were only children. In Hong Kong and Singapore, 45% of the daughters had no children, 18% had only one child and 36% were single. In mainland China, all the daughters were married and all of them had at least one child.[2]

For the married and childless, only their spouse may be available to care for them in old age. For those electing singlehood, there may be no one at all to take care of them. In any event, the daughters said they did not expect to be cared for by their children. However, what happens if they are taking care of their own parents when they reach retirement age?[3] The resources they have set aside for their own care might need to be diverted to their parents, or even to their grandparents. Remember the expression: '4-2-1', meaning one child taking care of two parents and four grandparents (Zhan 2004).

Prior to their own retirement, single women who are the only child of elderly parents may have to choose whether to remain in employment as their parents' health care needs increase. If they drop out of the workforce, their ability to support their parents indefinitely and achieve financial security for their own old age may be jeopardised or even extinguished. The only viable alternative may be to leave elderly parents at home alone or to outsource their care.

Married daughters without siblings may be forced to choose between caring for their own parents or their in-laws or try to care for both. Families with sons and not daughters may receive financial, but not instrumental or emotional support if there is no daughter-in-law willing to provide the latter. Within the Chinese culture, there is no actual precedent of males providing hands-on care. The moral obligation historically imposed on sons to care for their parents has more accurately been the duty of their wives to perform the manual labour while sons assumed financial responsibility for the extended family and other duties unrelated to care.

Ultimately, the continuation of family elder care presumes that daughters will still be willing to undertake it. Most of the interviewed daughters, who were among the current generations of caregivers, were disinclined to leave employment for caregiving, even though they insisted their families were important. The negative consequences for daughters leaving employment, as discussed earlier, may additionally extend to the government. For example, lower fertility portends declining numbers of individuals available to join the workforce in the future. Women may be needed to fill jobs. Jobs also generate taxable income to support social welfare programmes, and create purchasing power that benefits what in Hong Kong, Singapore, and increasingly in mainland China, have become consumer economies. Further, women in unemployment are not earning pension and health care benefits, however modest, which may result in future dependency on the government if there is no one to care for them.

The reliance of daughters on domestic helpers who act as surrogates for them is without a doubt what enables the vast majority of the women in

Hong Kong and Singapore to work. However, the importation and employment of FDHs depends on several factors, including government policies promoting their use, tacit approval of conditions favourable to employers, keeping costs low, and forcing FDHs to leave when their employment is terminated.

What is often overlooked is that access to FDHs also relies on conditions in the home countries of these women, such as high unemployment, inadequate wages, and poor economies. As long as FDHs can make more money abroad than in their countries of origin they will most likely continue to endure the difficult conditions under which they live and work outside. However, should circumstances improve at home, the number of those seeking overseas employment could diminish. If that were to happen, under the existing 'family first' policies of Hong Kong and Singapore, one could argue that a serious crisis could result. If FDHs were to be removed from the caregiving paradigm, who or what would take their place? It is entirely possible that large numbers of elderly parents would be institutionalised and more women would leave the workforce. Hong Kong and Singapore should not wait to see if this transpires.

A further shift in policy enabling elderly people to become even more self-sustaining and one that supports families through shared care responsibilities is urgently needed. The family can remain the primary caregiver of their elderly parents. However, given the structural and normative changes occurring in Singapore, Hong Kong and mainland China it is highly unlikely that families, principally daughters, can continue to bear the caregiving burden alone. Pensions, social security and insurance targeted at adequate income and health care for seniors should be expanded and enhanced so that they are not dependent on their families for financial support. Seniors who achieve greater independence are more likely to have a better quality of life, and their children may experience less stress, which, the literature has suggested, creates happier and more harmonious families (Cheng et al. 2008; Ng et al. 2002).

More social welfare programmes and care services, distributed by the government at the local level, with greater support from the business community and NGOs, also need to be expanded to enable elderly people to remain in their own homes. Finding new ways to honour, assist and respect older people and the families who care for them, is a challenge. However, it should be regarded as no less than a moral obligation by the societies in which they live.

The Final Word

Urban Chinese daughters in Singapore, Hong Kong and mainland China have come a long way since Lee Choo Neo wrote about them 100 years ago (Cheng 1977). Unlike then, they now have the right to be educated, employed as professionals, and lead self-sufficient, independent lives, if that is their choice. Their monetary contributions to their parents, and even their siblings, make them valuable assets, and have helped them achieve greater status within their families. Nonetheless, traditional expectations concerning filial obligation continue to be imposed on Chinese daughters by their families, their governments, and themselves.

The world and Chinese families, however, are different than they were a century ago. It is more difficult today to manage the demands on one's life and resources, including time. Given this, it may be problematic, if not impossible, for Chinese daughters to sustain indefinitely the many roles they must often assume, particularly if any disruption occurs to the supply of domestic helpers. Looking to the future then, one must ask: How much of the caregiver burden in an ageing society will Chinese daughters be asked to assume, and what will be the personal cost to them to remain filial daughters?

Notes

1. There were 64 women born between 1946 and 1980; three women born before 1946 and six Filipina domestic helpers. The three oldest women were not included in the analysis but were interviewed for comparison.
2. Interestingly, 22% had two children and both were Gen X. Fifty-five percent of the mainland women had sons.
3. Even though some parents of the women interviewed for this book, and the women themselves, had pensions, these have largely been viewed as inadequate.

References

Aronson, J. (1990). Women's perspectives on informal care of the elderly: Public ideology and personal experience of giving and receiving care. *Ageing and Society, 10*(1), 61–84.

Cheng, S.-H. (1977). Singapore women: Legal status, educational attainment, and employment patterns. *Asian Survey, 17*(4), 358–374.

Cheng, S.-T., Chan, W., & Chan, A. M. (2008). Older people's realisation of generativity in a changing society: The case of Hong Kong. *Ageing and Society, 28*(5), 609–627.

Croll, E. J. (1995). *Changing identities of Chinese women; rhetoric, experience and self-perception in twentieth-century China.* Hong Kong: Hong Kong University Press.

Hochschild, A. (1983, 2012). *The managed heart: Commercialization of human feeling.* Berkeley: University of California Press.

Holroyd, E. (2001). Hong Kong Chinese daughters' intergenerational caregiving obligations: A cultural model approach. *Social Science & Medicine, 53*(9), 1125–1134.

Horowitz, A., & Shindelman, L. W. (1983). Reciprocity and affection. *Journal of Gerontological Social Work, 5*(3), 5–20.

Lee, K. S. (2014). Gender, care work, and the complexity of family membership in Japan. In S. Harper (Ed.), *Critical readings on ageing in Asia* (pp. 853–876). Leiden: Brill. Reprinted from *Gender & Society* (2010) 24(5), 647–671.

Lee, W. K.-M., & Kwok, H.-K. (2005). Differences in expectations and patterns of informal support for older persons in Hong Kong: Modification to filial piety. *Ageing International, 30,* 188–206.

Lieber, E., Nihura, K., & Mink, I. T. (2004). Filial piety, modernization, and the challenges of raising children for Chinese immigrants: Quantitative and qualitative evidence. *Ethos, 32*(3), 324–347.

Long, S. O., Campbell, R., & Nishimura, C. (2014). Does it matter who cares? A comparison of daughters versus daughters-in-law in Japanese elder care. In S. Harper (Ed.), *Critical readings on ageing in Asia* (pp. 1373–1390). Leiden: Brill. Reprinted from *Social Science Japan Journal* (2009) 12(1), 1–21.

Lyonette, C., & Yardley, L. (2003). The influence on carer wellbeing of motivations to care for older people and the relationship with the care recipient. *Ageing and Society, 23*(4), 487–506.

Mac Rae, H. (1998). Managing feelings: Caregiving as emotion work. *Research on Aging, 20*(1), 137–160.

Ng, A. C. Y., Phillips, D. R., & Lee, W. K.-m. (2002). Persistence and challenges to filial piety and informal support of older persons in a modern Chinese society: A case study in Tuen Mun, Hong Kong. *Journal of Aging Studies, 16*(2), 135–153.

Wong, O. M. H. (2000). Children and children-in-law as primary caregivers: Issues and perspectives. In W. T. Liu & H. Kendig (Eds.), *Who should care for the elderly* (pp. 297–321). Singapore: Singapore University Press.

Wong, O. M. H., & Chau, B. H. P. (2006). The evolving role of filial piety in eldercare in Hong Kong. *Asian Journal of Social Science, 34*(4), 600–617.

Zhan, J. H. (2004). Socialization or social structure: Investigating predictors of attitudes toward filial responsibility among Chinese urban youth from one- and multiple-child families. *International Journal of Aging and Human Development, 59*(1), 105–124.

References

Aboderin, I. (2006). *Intergenerational support and old age in Africa.* New Brunswick: Transaction Publishers.

Allen, K. (2010). *Classical sociological theory* (2nd ed.). Los Angeles: Pine Forge Press.

Appelrouth, S., & Edles, L. D. (2007). *Sociological theory in the contemporary era.* Los Angeles: Pine Forge Press.

Aronson, J. (1990). Women's perspectives on informal care of the elderly: Public ideology and personal experience of giving and receiving care. *Ageing and Society, 10*(1), 61–84.

Au, A., Li, S., Leung, P., Pan, P.-C., Thompson, L., & Gallagher-Thompson, D. (2010). The coping with caregiving group program for Chinese caregivers of patients with Alzheimer's disease in Hong Kong. *Patient Education and Counselling, 78,* 256–260.

BBC World Asia. (2013, March 25). Hong Kong court denies domestic workers residency. *BBC News China.* Retrieved online August 10, 2013, from www.bbc.co.uk/news/world-asia-china-21920811

Berman, H. J. (1987). Adult children and their parents: Irredeemable obligation and irreparable loss. *Journal of Gerontological Social Work, 10*(1-2), 21–34.

Blake, C. F. (1994). Foot-binding in neo-Confucian China and the appropriation of female labor. *Signs: Journal of Women in Culture and Society, 19,* 676–712.

© The Author(s) 2018
P. O'Neill, *Urban Chinese Daughters,* St Antony's Series,
https://doi.org/10.1007/978-981-10-8699-1

Blumer, H. (1969). *Symbolic interactionism: Perspective & method.* Berkeley: University of California Press.

Bolton, S. C. (2000). Who cares? Offering emotion work as a 'gift' in the nursing labour process. *Journal of Advanced Nursing, 32*(8), 580–586.

Bolton, S. C., & Boyd, C. (2003). Trolley dolly or skilled emotion manager? Moving on from Hochschild's managed heart. *Work, Employment & Society, 17,* 289–308.

Brant, M., Haberkern, K., & Szydlik, M. (2009). Intergenerational help and care in Europe. *European Sociological Review, 25*(5), 585–601.

Brody, E. M. (1985). Parent care as a normative family stress. *The Gerontologist, 25*(1), 19–29.

Cahill, S., & Eggleston, R. (1994). Managing emotions in public: The case of wheelchair users. *Social Psychology Quarterly, 57,* 300–312.

Cai, F., Giles, J., O'Keefe, P., & Wang, D. (2012). *The elderly and old age support in rural China.* Washington, DC: The World Bank.

Chan, A. (1999). The role of formal versus informal support of the elderly in Singapore: Is there substitution? *Southeast Asian Journal of Social Science, 27*(2), 87–110.

Chan, S. W.-C. (2010). Family caregiving in dementia: The Asian perspective of a global problem. *Dementia and Geriatric Cognitive Disorders, 30,* 469–478.

Chan, R. K. H. (2011). Patterns and paths of child care and elder care in Hong Kong. *Journal of Comparative Social Welfare, 27*(2), 155–164.

Chan, H., & Lee, R. P. L. (1995). Hong Kong families: At the crossroads of modernism and traditionalism. *Journal of Comparative Family Studies, 26*(1), 83–99.

Chan, A. C. M., & Lim, M. Y. (2004). Changes of filial piety in Chinese societies. *International Scope Review, 6*(11), 1–16.

Chan, S. S. C., Viswanath, K., Au, D. W. H., Ma, C. M. S., Lam, W. W. T., Fielding, R., Leung, G. M., & Lam, T.-H. (2011). Hong Kong Chinese community leaders' perspectives on family health, happiness and harmony: A qualitative study. *Health Education Research, 26*(4), 664–674.

Chappell, N. L., & Funk, L. (2012). Filial responsibility: Does it matter for care-giving behaviours? *Ageing and Society, 32*(7), 1128–1146.

Chen, L. (2011). Elderly residents' perspectives on filial piety and institutionalization in Shanghai. *Journal of Intergenerational Relationships, 9*(1), 53–68.

Chen, L., & Han, W.-J. (2016). Shanghai: Front-runner of community-based elder in China. *Journal of Aging & Social Policy, 28*(4), 292–307. https://doi.org/10.1080/08959420.2016.1151310.

Chen, S. X., Bond, M. H., & Tang, D. (2007). Decomposing filial piety into filial attitudes and filial enactments. *Asian Journal of Social Psychology, 10*(4), 213–223.

Cheng, S.-H. (1977). Singapore women: Legal status, educational attainment, and employment patterns. *Asian Survey, 17*(4), 358–374.

Cheng, S.-T. (1993). The social context of Hong Kong's booming elderly home industry. *American Journal of Community Psychology, 21*(4), 449–467.

Cheng, S.-T., Chan, W., & Chan, A. M. (2008). Older people's realisation of generativity in a changing society: The case of Hong Kong. *Ageing and Society, 28*(5), 609–627.

Cheng, Y., Rosenberg, M. W., Wang, W., Yang, L., & Li, H. (2012). Access to residential care in Beijing, China: Making the decision to relocate to a residential care facility. *Ageing and Society, 32*, 1277–1299. https://doi.org/10.1017/So144686X11000870.

Cheng, T. C., Ip, I. N., & Kwok, T. (2013a). Caregiver forgiveness is associated with less burden and potentially harmful behaviours. *Aging & Mental Health, 17*(8), 930–934.

Cheng, T. C., Lam, L. C. W., Kwok, T., Ng, N. S. S., & Fung, A. W. T. (2013b). Self-efficacy is associated with less burden and more gains from behavioural problems of Alzheimer's disease in Hong Kong Chinese caregivers. *The Gerontologist, 53*, 71–80.

Cheung, C.-K., & Chow, E. O.-W. (2006). Spilling over strain between elders and their caregivers in Hong Kong. *International Journal of Aging and Human Development, 63*(1), 73–93.

Cheung, C.-K., & Kwan, A. Y.-H. (2009). The erosion of filial piety by modernisation in Chinese cities. *Aging and Society, 29*, 179–198.

Cheung, F., & Wu, A. M. S. (2013). Emotional labour and successful ageing in the workplace among older Chinese employees. *Ageing and Society, 33*(6), 1036–1051.

Chien, W.-T., Norman, I., & Thompson, D. R. (2006). Perceived benefits and difficulties experienced in a mutual support group for family carers of people with schizophrenia. *Qualitative Health Research, 16*(7), 962–981.

Chilcott, J. H. (1998). Structural functionalism as a heuristic device. *Anthropology & Education Quarterly, 29*(1), 103–111.

Chiu, S. W. K., Choi, S. Y. P., & Kwok-fai, T. (2005). Getting ahead in the capitalist paradise: Migration from China and socioeconomic attainment in colonial Hong Kong. *International Migration Review, 39*(1), 203–227.

Choi, J. (2008). Work and family demands and life stress among Chinese employees: The mediating effect of work-family conflict. *The International Journal of Resource Management, 19*(5), 878–895.

Chong, E. (2013, July 19). Myanmar maid jailed for abusing employer's mum who suffers from dementia. *Singapore Straits Times*. Retrieved online August 12, 2013, from www.straitstimes.com/.../myanmar-maid-jailed-abusing-employers-mum-who -suffers-dementia-2013071

Chou, K.-L. (2009). Number of children and upstream intergenerational financial transfers: Evidence from Hong Kong. *Journal of Gerontology: Social Sciences, 65B*, 227–235.

Chou, R. J.-A. (2011). Filial piety by contract? The emergence, implementation, and implications of the "family support agreement" in China. *The Gerontologist, 51*, 3–16.

Chou, K.-L., & Cheung, C. K. (2013). Family-friendly policies in the workplace and their effect on work-life conflicts in Hong Kong. *The International Journal of Human Resource Management, 24*, 3872–3885.

Chou, K.-L., Chow, N. W. S., & Chi, I. (2004). Preventing economic hardship among Chinese elderly in Hong Kong. *Journal of Aging & Social Policy, 16*(4), 79–97.

Chow, N. (1991). Does filial piety exist under Chinese communism? *Journal of Aging and Social Policy, 3*(1/2), 209–225.

Chow, N. (2006). The practice of filial piety and its impact on long term care policies for elderly people in Asian Chinese communities. *Asian Journal of Gerontology & Geriatrics, 1*(1), 31–35.

Chung, T. Y. R., Pang, K. L. K., & Tong, Y. W. J. (2010). *Work-life balance survey of the Hong Kong working population 2010*. (Tech. Rep.). Hong Kong: The University of Hong Kong Public Opinion Programme.

Churton, M., & Brown, A. (2010). *Theory and method* (2nd ed.). Basingstoke: Palgrave Macmillan.

Cicirelli, V. G. (1983). Adult children's attachment and helping behavior to elderly parents: A path model. *Journal of Marriage and the Family, 45*(4), 815–825.

Cicirelli, V. G. (1993). Attachment and obligation as daughters' motives for caregiving behavior and subsequent effect on subjective burden. *Psychology and Aging, 8*(2), 144–155.

Clark, T. N. (1972). Structural-functionalism, exchange theory, and the new political economy: Institutionalization as a theoretical linkage. *Social Inquiry, 42*(3–4), 275–298.

Constable, N. (1996). Jealousy, chastity, and abuse: Chinese maids and foreign helpers in Hong Kong. *Modern China, 22*(4), 448–479.

Constable, N. (1997). *Maid to order in Hong Kong: stories of migrant workers*. New York: Cornell University Press.

Cook, S., & Dong, X.-y. (2011). Harsh choices: Chinese women paid work and unpaid care responsibilities under economic reform. *Development and Change, 42*(4), 947–965.

Coombes, L., Allen, D., Humphrey, D., & Neale, J. (2009). In-depth interviews. In J. Neal (Ed.), *Research methods for health and social care* (pp. 197–210). Basingstoke: Palgrave Macmillan.

Croll, E. J. (1995). *Changing identities of Chinese women; rhetoric, experience and self-perception in twentieth-century China.* Hong Kong: Hong Kong University Press.

Croll, E. J. (2006). The intergenerational contract in the changing Asian family. *Oxford Development Studies, 34*(4), 473–491.

Del Corso, A., & Lanz, M. (2013). Felt obligation and the family life cycle: A study on intergenerational relationships. *International Journal of Psychology, 48*, 1196–1200.

Deutsch, F. M. (2006). Filial piety, patrilineality, and China's one-child policy. *Journal of Family Issues, 27*(3), 366–389.

DeVault, M. L. (1999). Comfort and struggle: Emotion work in family life. *Annals of the American Academy of Political and Social Science, 56*, 52–63.

Dikötter, F. (2013). *The tragedy of liberation: A history of the Chinese revolution 1945–1957.* London: Bloomsbury Press.

Dikötter, F. (2016). *The cultural revolution: A people's history 1962–1976.* London: Bloomsbury Press.

Dixon, N. (1995). The friendship model of filial obligation. *Journal of Applied Philosophy, 12*(1), 77–87.

Du, P. (2013). Intergenerational solidarity and old-age support for the social inclusion of elders in mainland China: The changing roles of family and government. *Ageing and Society, 33*(01), 44–63.

Elman, B. A. (2013). The civil examination system in late imperial China, 1400–1900. *Frontiers of History in China, 8*(1), 32–50.

Erickson, R. J. (1993). Reconceptualizing family work: The effect of emotion work on perceptions of marital quality. *Journal of Marriage and Family, 55*(4), 888–900.

Erickson, R. J. (2005). Why emotion work mattes: Sex, gender, and the division of household labour. *Journal of Marriage and the Family, 67*(2), 337–351.

Evans, S. (2008). The introduction of English-language education in early colonial Hong Kong. *History of Education, 37*(3), 383–408.

Fenby, J. (2008). *History of modern China: The fall and rise of a great power 1850 to the present.* London: Penguin Books.

Finch, J., & Mason, J. (1993). *Negotiating family responsibilities*. Abingdon: Routledge.

Fincher, L. H. (2014). *Leftover women*. London/New York: Zed Books.

Finley, N. J., Roberts, M. D., & Banahan, B. F. (1988). Motivators and inhibitors of attitudes of filial obligation toward aging parents. *The Gerontologist, 28*(1), 73–78.

Fong, P. E., & Lim, L. (1982). Foreign labour and economic development in Singapore. *International Migration Review, 16*(3), 548–576.

Foster, D., & Ren, X. (2015). Work-family conflict and the commodification of women's employment in three Chinese airlines. *The International Journal of Resource Management, 26*(12), 1568–1585. https://doi.org/10.1080/095851 92.2014.949621.

Fu, T.-h. (2014). Do state benefits impact on intergenerational family support? The case of Taiwan. In S. Harper (Ed.), *Critical Readings on Ageing in Asia* (pp. 1419–1432). Reprinted from Intergenerational Relationships (2008) *6*(3), 339–354.

Ghy, T., & Woo, J. (2009). Elder care: Is legislation of family responsibility the solution? *Asian Journal of Gerontology and Geriatrics, 4*(2), 72–75.

Goh, D. P. S. (2009). Chinese religion and the challenge of modernity in Malaysia and Singapore: Syncretism, hybridisation and transfiguration. *Asian Journal of Social Science, 37*(1), 107–137.

Gomes, C. (2011). Maid-in-Singapore: Representing and consuming foreign domestic workers in Singapore cinema. *Asian Ethnicity, 12*(2), 141–154.

Graham, E., Teo, P., Yeoh, B. S. A., & Levy, S. (2002). Reproducing the Asian family across generations: 'Tradition,' gender and expectations in Singapore. *Asia Pacific Population Journal, 17*(2), 60–86.

Hashimoto, A., & Ikels, C. (2005). Filial piety in changing Asian societies. In M. L. Johnson (Ed.), *The Cambridge handbook of age and ageing* (pp. 437–442). Cambridge: Cambridge University Press.

Hatton, C. (2013). New China law says children 'must visit parents'. *BBC News*.www.bbc.co.uk/news/world-asia-china

HelpAge International. (2013). *Ageing population in Myanmar*. http://ageingasia.org/category/ageing-population/

HelpAge International. (2014). *Ageing population in Myanmar*. http://ageingasia.org/category/ageingpopulation-myanmar/

Hess, B. B., & Waring, J. M. (1978). Changing patterns of aging and family bonds in later life. *The Family Coordinator, 27*(4), 301–314.

Ho, S. C., Chan, A., Woo, J., Chong, P., & Sham, A. (2009). Impact of caregiving on health and quality of life: A comparative population-based study of caregivers for elderly persons and non-caregivers. *Journals of Gerontology (Biological Sciences and Medical Sciences), 64A*(8), 873–879.

Hochschild, A. R. (1979). Emotion work, feeling rules and social structure. *American Journal of Sociology, 85*(3), 551–575.

Hochschild, A. (1983, 2012). The managed heart: Commercialization of human feeling. Berkeley: University of California Press.

Hochschild, A. R. (with Machung, A.). (1989, 2012). *The second shift: Working families and the revolution at home.* New York: Viking Penguin, Inc.

Holroyd, E. (2001). Hong Kong Chinese daughters' intergenerational caregiving obligations: A cultural model approach. *Social Science & Medicine, 53*(9), 1125–1134.

Holroyd, E. (2003a). Hong Kong Chinese family caregiving: Cultural categories of bodily order and the location of self. *Qualitative Health Research, 13*(2), 158–170.

Holroyd, E. (2003b). Chinese family obligations toward chronically ill elderly members: Comparing caregivers in Beijing and Hong Kong. *Qualitative Health Research, 13*(3), 302–318.

Holroyd, E. A., & Mackenzie, A. E. (1995). A review of the historical and social processes contributing to care and caregiving in Chinese families. *Journal of Advanced Nursing, 22*, 473–479.

Hong, Y.-H., & Liu, W. T. (2000). The social psychological perspective of elderly care. In W. T. Liu & H. Kendig (Eds.), *Who should care for the elderly* (pp. 165–179). Singapore: Singapore University Press.

Hong Kong Community Business Online. *Work-Life Balance.*http://www.communitybusiness.org/focus_areas/WLB.htm

Horowitz, A., & Shindelman, L. W. (1983). Reciprocity and affection. *Journal of Gerontological Social Work, 5*(3), 5–20.

Housing Development Board. (2017). Living with/near parent or married child. http://www.hdb.gov.sg/cs/infoweb/residential/buying-a-flat/resale/living-with-near-parents-or-married-child

Hsu, H.-C., Lew-Ting, C.-Y., & Wu, S.-C. (2014). Age, period, and cohort effects on the attitude toward supporting parents in Taiwan. In S. Harper (Ed.), *Critical readings on ageing in Asia* (pp. 1373–1390). Leiden: Brill. Reprinted from *The Gerontologist* (2001) *41(6)*, 742–750.

Hu, Y. (2016). Impact of rural-to-urban migration on family and gender values in China. *Asian Population Studies, 12*(3), 251–272. https://doi.org/10.1080/17441730.2016.1169753.

Huang, S., & Yeoh, B. S. A. (2007). Emotional labour and transnational domestic work: The moving geographies of maid abuse in Singapore. *Mobilities, 2*(2), 195–217.

Huat, C. B. (2009). Being Chinese under official multiculturalism in Singapore. *Asian Ethnicity, 10*(3), 239–250.

Ikels, C. (1993). Settling accounts: The intergenerational contract in an age of reform. In D. Davis & S. Harrell (Eds.), *Chinese families in the post-Mao era* (pp. 307–333). Berkeley: University of California Press.

Inland Revenue Authority of Singapore. (2017). Parent relief. https://www.iras.gov.sg/IRASHome/Individuals/Locals/Working-Out-Your-Taxes/Deductions-for-Individuals/Parent-Relief-/-Handicapped-Parent-Relief/

Ip, G. S. H., & Mackenzie, A. E. (1998). Caring for relatives with serious mental illness at home: The experiences of family carers in Hong Kong. *Archives of Psychiatric Nursing, 12*(5), 288–294.

Izuhara, M. (2010). Housing, wealth and family reciprocity in East Asia. In M. Izuhara (Ed.), *Ageing and intergenerational relations* (pp. 77–94). Bristol: Policy Press.

Jang, S.-N., Avendano, M., & Kawachi, I. (2012). Informal caregiving patterns in Korea and European countries: A cross-national comparison. *Asian Nursing Research, 6*(1), 19–26.

Keay, J. (2009). *China, a history*. New York: Basic Books.

Keller, S. (2006). Four theories of filial duty. *The Philosophical Quarterly, 56*(223), 254–274.

Khalik, S. (2009, August 17). Government may act against children who dump their elderly parents. *Singapore Straits Times*. http://news.asiaone.com/News/the+Straits+Times/Story/A1Story20090817-161452.html

Kim, T.-H., & Han, S.-Y. (2013). Family life of older Koreans. In J.-N. Bae, J.-M. Kyung, Y.-K. Roh, J.-C. Sung, & Y.-H. Won (Eds.), *Ageing in Korea, today and tomorrow* (pp. 68–93). Seoul: Federation of Korean Gerontological Societies.

Koh, E. M. L., & Tan, J. (2000). Favouritism and the changing value of children: A note on the Chinese middle class in Singapore. *Journal of Comparative Family Studies, 31*, 519–528.

Kornreich, Y., Veretinsky, I., & Potter, P. B. (2012). Consultation and deliberation in China: The making of China's health-care reform. *The China Journal, 68*, 176–203.

Kruml, S. M., & Geddes, D. (2000). Exploring the dimensions of emotional labour: The heart of Hochschild's work. *Management and Communication Quarterly, 14*, 8–49.

Kua, E. H. (1989). Psychological distress of families caring for the frail elderly. *Singapore Medical Journal, 30*(1), 42–44.

Kuah, K.-E. (1990). Confucian ideology and social engineering in Singapore. *Journal of Contemporary Asia, 20*(3), 371–383.

Lam, R. C. (2006). Contradictions between traditional Chinese values and the actual performance: A study of the caregiving roles of the modern sandwich generation in Hong Kong. *Journal of Comparative Family Studies, 37*(2), 299–318.

Lan, P.-C. (2006). *Global Cinderellas: Migrant domestics and newly rich employers in Taiwan.* Durham: Duke University Press.

Lau, P. W. L., Cheng, J. G. Y., Chow, D. L. Y., Ungvari, G. S., & Leung, C. M. (2009). Acute psychiatric disorders in foreign domestic workers in Hong Kong: A pilot study. *International Journal of Social Psychiatry, 55*(6), 569–576.

Law, W.-W. (2007). Schooling in Hong Kong. In G. Postiglione & J. Tan (Eds.), *Going to school in East Asia* (pp. 86–121). Westport: Greenwood Publishing.

Law of the People's Republic of China on Protection of The Rights and Interests of the Elderly, Chapter II: Maintenance and support by families. (1996). Retrieved online September 14, 2014, from http://www.china.org.cn/ english/government/207403.htm

Lee, W. K.-M. (2000). Women employment in colonial Hong Kong. *Journal of Contemporary Asia, 36,* 246–264.

Lee, K. S. (2014). Gender, care work, and the complexity of family membership in Japan. In S. Harper (Ed.), *Critical readings on ageing in Asia* (pp. 853–876). Leiden: Brill. Reprinted from *Gender & Society* (2010) 24(5), 647–671.

Lee, W. K.-M., & Kwok, H.-K. (2005a). Differences in expectations and patterns of informal support for older persons in Hong Kong: Modification to filial piety. *Ageing International, 30,* 188–206.

Lee, W. K.-M., & Kwok, H.-k. (2005b). Older women and family care in Hong Kong: Differences in filial expectation and practices. *Journal of Women and Aging, 17*(1-2), 129–150.

Lee, J., & Yip, N.-M. (2006). Public housing and family life in East Asia: Housing and social change in Hong Kong 1953–1990. *Journal of Family History, 31,* 66–82.

Lei, L. (2013). Sons, daughters and intergenerational support in China. *Chinese Sociological Review, 45*(3), 26–52.

Li, D. (2004). Gender inequality in education in rural China. In T. Jie, Z. Bijun, & S. L. Mow (Eds.), *Holding up half the sky: Chinese women, past, present and future* (pp. 159–171). New York: Feminist Press of the City University of New York.

Li, M., & Bray, M. (2006). Social class and cross-border higher education: Mainland Chinese students in Hong Kong and Macau. *Journal of International Migration and Integration, 7*(4), 407–424.

Li, L. W., Long, Y., Essex, E. L., Sui, Y., & Gao, L. (2012). Elderly Chinese and their family caregivers' perceptions of good care: A qualitative study in Shandong, China. *Journal of Gerontological Social Work, 55*(7), 609–625.

Lieber, E., Nihura, K., & Mink, I. T. (2004). Filial piety, modernization, and the challenges of raising children for Chinese immigrants: Quantitative and qualitative evidence. *Ethos, 32*(3), 324–347.

Lin, J.-P., & Yi, C.-C. (2011). Filial norms and intergenerational support to aging parents in China and Taiwan [special issue]. *International Journal of Social Welfare, 20*(Supp.s1), S109–S120.

Liu, t.-s. (2003). A nameless but active religion: An anthropologist's view of local religion in Hong Kong and Macau. *The China Quarterly, 174*, 373–394.

Liu, T., & Sun, L. (2016). Pension reform in China. *Journal of Aging & Social Policy, 28*(1), 15–28.

Lo, S. (2003). Perceptions of work-family conflict among married female professionals in Hong Kong. *Personnel Review, 32*(3), 376–390.

Long, S. O., Campbell, R., & Nishimura, C. (2014). Does it matter who cares? A comparison of daughters versus daughters-in-law in Japanese elder care. In S. Harper (Ed.), *Critical readings on ageing in Asia* (pp. 1373–1390). Leiden: Brill. Reprinted from *Social Science Japan Journal* (2009) *12(1)*, 1–21.

Luk, W. S.-C. (2002). The home care experience as perceived by the caregivers of Chinese dialysis patients. *International Journal of Nursing Studies, 39*(3), 269–277.

Lyonette, C., & Yardley, L. (2003). The influence on carer wellbeing of motivations to care for older people and the relationship with the care recipient. *Ageing and Society, 23*(4), 487–506.

Mac Rae, H. (1998). Managing feelings: Caregiving as emotion work. *Research on Aging, 20*(1), 137–160.

MacKenzie, A. E., & Holroyd, E. E. (1996). An exploration of the carers' perceptions of caregiving and caring responsibilities in Chinese families. *Journal of Nursing Studies, 33*(1), 1–12.

Malhotra, C., Malhotra, R., Ostbye, T., Matchar, D., & Chan, A. (2012). Depressive symptoms among informal caregivers of older adults: Insights from the Singapore survey on informal caregiving. *International Psychogeriatrics, 24*(8), 1335–1346.

McMillan, A. F., & Danubrata, E. (2012, October 1). Old age in China is a fledgling business opportunity. *The New York Times.* http://www.nytimes.com/2012/10/02/business/global/old-age-in-ch...

Mehta, K. (1999). Intergenerational exchanges: Qualitative evidence from Singapore. *Southeast Asian Journal of Social Science, 27*(2), 111–122.

Mehta, K. K., & Ko, H. (2004). Filial piety revisited in the context of modernizing Asian societies. *Geriatrics and Gerontology International, 4*(Supp. 4), S77–S78.

Mehta, K., Osman, M. M., & Lee, A. E.-Y. (1995). Living arrangements of the elderly in Singapore: Cultural norms in transition. *Journal of Cross-Cultural Gerontology, 10*(1-2), 113–143.

MetLife Mature Market Institute, National Alliance for Caregiving and University of Pittsburgh Institute of Aging. (2010). *The MetLife study of working caregivers and employer health care costs; new insights and innovations for reducing health care costs for employers.* https://www.metlife.com/assets/cao/mmi/publications/studies/2010/mmi-working-caregivers-employers-health-care-costs.pdf

Mingxia, C. (2004). The marriage law and the rights of Chinese women in marriage and the family. In T. Jie, Z. Bijun, & S. L. Mow (Eds.), *Holding up half the sky: Chinese women, past, present and future* (pp. 159–171). New York: Feminist Press of the City University of New York.

Ministry of Community Development, Youth and Sports, Singapore. (2007). Inaugural study confirms positive benefits of work-life harmony to individuals and business: MCYS Media Release No. 43/2007: app.msf.gov.sg/portals/0/summary/publication/43-20071.pdf

Moir, J. (2012, June 29). Families dump elderly in hospitals. *South China Morning Post.* www.scmp.com/article/119179/families-dump-elderly-hospitals

Mok, K. H. (2016). Massification of higher education, graduate employment and social mobility in the greater China region. *British Journal of Sociology of Education, 37*(1), 51–71. https://doi.org/10.1080/01425692.2015.1111751.

Montgomery, R. J. V., & Kosloski, K. (2009). Caregiving as a process of changing identity: Implications for caregiver support. *Generations: Journal of the American Society on Aging, 33*(1), 47–52.

Moskowitz, S. (2002). Adult children and indigent parents: Intergenerational responsibilities in international perspective. *86 Marquette Law Review 401.*

Mrsnik, M. (2010, October 10). *Standard & poor's: Global aging 2010: An irreversible truth.* Council on foreign Relations. http://www.cfr.org/aging/standard-poors-global-aging-2010-irrever...

Ng, A. C. Y., Phillips, D. R., & Lee, W. K.-m. (2002). Persistence and challenges to filial piety and informal support of older persons in a modern Chinese society: A case study in Tuen Mun, Hong Kong. *Journal of Aging Studies, 16*(2), 135–153.

Ngan, R., & Cheng, I. C. K. (1992). The caring dilemma, stress and needs of carers for the Chinese frail elderly. *Hong Kong Journal of Gerontology, 6*(2), 34–41.

Ngan, R., & Wong, W. (1996). Injustice in family care of the Chinese elderly in Hong Kong. *Journal of Aging & Social Policy, 7*(2), 77–94.

Nip, P. T. K. (2010). Social welfare development in Hong Kong. Changes and challenges in building a caring and harmonious society. *Asia Pacific Journal of Social Work and Development, 20*(1), 65–81.

Office of the High Commissioner on Human Rights. (2009). *Responses to the office of the United Nations High Commissioner for Human Rights.*www.ohchr. org/Documents/Issues/EPoverty/casher/Korea.pdf

Olsen, R. E. (2011). Managing hope, denial or temporal anomie? Informal cancer carers' accounts of spouses' cancer diagnoses. *Social Science & Medicine, 73*(6), 904–911.

Parliament of Singapore. (1994, July 25–27) Maintenance of Parents Bill – Second Reading. Parliamentary Debates Singapore: Official Report. Singapore: Singapore National Printers. In P. A. Rozario & S.-I. Hong (2011) Doing it 'right' by your parents in Singapore: A political economy examination of the maintenance of parents act of 1995. *Critical Social Policy, 31*(4), 607–627.

Parrott, T. M., & Bengtson, V. L. (1999). The effects of earlier intergenerational affection, normative expectations, and family conflict on contemporary exchanges of help and support. *Research on Aging, 21*(1), 73–105.

Pei, X., & Tang, Y. (2012). Rural old age support in transitional China: Efforts between family and state. In S. Chen & J. L. Powell (Eds.), *Aging in China: Implications to social policy of a changing economic state* (International perspectives on aging 2, pp. 61–81). doi: https://doi.org/10.1007/978-1-4419-8351-0_5. Springer Science=Business Media LLC 2012.

Pereira, A. A. (2005). Religiosity and economic development in Singapore. *Journal of Contemporary Religion, 20*(2), 161–177.

Peterson, G. (2008). To be or not to be a refugee: The international politics of the Hong Kong refugee crisis, 1949–1955. *The Journal of Imperial and Commonwealth History, 36*(2), 171–195.

Pierce, J. L. (1995). *Gender trials: Emotional lives in contemporary law firms.* Berkeley: University of California Press.

Pinay, B. (2012, Mid-March). *Two Filipinas thought to have jumped off employers' flat; Investigation on.* Sun Internet Edition. http://www.sunweb.com.hk/Story.asp?hdnStoryCode=7230&

Pong, S.-l. (1991). The effect of women's labor on family income inequality: The case of Hong Kong. *Economic Development and Cultural Change, 40*(1), 131–152.

Post, D. (2004). Family resources, gender, and immigration: Changing sources of Hong Kong educational inequality, 1971–2001. *Social Science Quarterly, 85*(5), 1238–1258.

Qian, Y., & Qian, Z. (2015). Work, family and gendered happiness among married people in urban China. *Social Indicators Research, 121*, 61–74. https://doi.org/10.1007/s11205-014-0623-9.

Rajakru, D. (1996). The state, family and industrial development: The Singapore case. *Journal of Contemporary Asia, 26*(1), 3–27.

Republic of China (Taiwan) Ministry of the Interior. (2012). *Senior citizens welfare act*. http://www.moi.gov.tw/english/english_law/law_detail. aspx?sn=180

Rickles-Jordan, A. (2007). Filial responsibility: A survey across time and oceans. *Marquette Elder's Advisor, 9*(1), 183–204.

Rozario, P. A., & Hong, S.-l. (2011). Doing it "right" by your parents in Singapore: A political economy examination of the Maintenance of parents act of 1995. *Critical Social Policy, 31*(4), 607–627.

Rozario, P. A., & Rosetti, A. L. (2012). "Many helping hands": A review and analysis of long-term care policies, programs, and practices in Singapore. *Journal of Gerontological Social Work, 55*(7), 641–658.

Rubin, H. J., & Rubin, I. S. (1995). *Qualitative interviewing: The art of hearing data*. Thousand Oaks: Sage Publishing.

Rudolph, J. (1998). Reconstructing collective identities: The Babas of Singapore. *Journal of Contemporary Asia, 28*(2), 203–232.

Salaff, J. W. (1976). Working daughters in the Hong Kong Chinese family: Female filial piety or a transformation in the family power structure? *Journal of Social History, 9*(4), 439–466.

Salaff, J. W. (1995). *Working daughters of Hong Kong: Filial piety or power in the family* (Rev ed.). New York: Columbia University Press.

Seng, L. K. (2009). Kampong, fire, nation: Towards a social history of postwar Singapore. *Journal of Southeast Asian Studies, 40*(3), 613–643.

Shang, X., & Wu, X. (2011). The care regime in China: Elder and child care. *Journal of Comparative Social Welfare, 27*(2), 123–131. https://doi.org/10.10 80/17486831.2011.567017.

Silverstein, M., & Bengtson, V. L. (1997). Intergenerational solidarity and the structure of adult child-parent relationships in American families. *American Journal of Sociology, 103*(2), 429–460.

Silverstein, M., Parrott, T. M., & Bengtson, V. L. (1995). Factors that predispose middle-aged sons and daughters to provide social support to older parents. *Journal of Marriage and the Family, 57*(2), 465–476.

Silverstein, M., Conroy, S. J., Wang, H., Giarrusso, R., & Bengtson, V. L. (2002). Reciprocity in parent-child relations over the adult life course. *Journals of Gerontology: Social Sciences, 57B*(1), S3–S13.

Silverstein, M., Conroy, S. J., & Gans, D. (2012). Beyond solidarity, reciprocity and altruism: Moral capital as a unifying concept of intergenerational support for older people. *Ageing and Society, 32*(7), 1246–1262.

Simpson, C., & Acton, G. (2013). Emotion work in family caregiving for persons with dementia. *Issues in Mental Health Nursing, 34*(1), 52–58.

Singapore Attorney General's Chambers. Maintenance of Parents Act, Chapter 167B, original enactment: Act 35 of 1995; revised edition 1996: Singapore statutes online: statutes.agc.gov.sg/.../cgi_getdata.pl?actno...MAINTENANCE%20 OF% 20PARENTS%20ACT%0A

Singapore Business Review. (2013, June 22). *Singapore offers third best work-life balance in Asia.*http://sbr.com.sg/economy/news/singapore-offers-third-best-work-life-balance-in-asia

Singapore Management University Social Sciences & Humanities. (2008). *The confucian filial duty to care for elderly parents* (Working Paper Series, Paper no. 02-2008, 1-26). Singapore: Williams, J., & Mooney, B.

Song, E. K. W. (2007). Ignoring "history from below": People's history in the historiography of Singapore. *History Compass, 5*(1), 11–25.

Stein, C. H., Wemmerus, V. A., Ward, M., Gaines, M. E., Freeberg, A. L., & Jewell, T. C. (1998). Because they're my parents: An intergenerational study of felt obligation and parental caregiving. *Journal of Marriage and the Family, 60*(3), 611–622.

Steinberg, R. J., & Figart, D. M. (1999). Emotional labour since the managed heart. *Annals of the American Academy of Political and Social Science, 561*, 8–26.

Stuifbergen, M. C., & Van Delden, J. J. M. (2011). Filial obligations to elderly parents: A duty to care? *Medicine Health Care and Philosophy, 14*(1), 63–71.

Suanet, B., Van Groenou, M. B., & Van Tilburg, T. (2012). Informal and formal home-care use among older adults in Europe: Can cross-national differences be explained by societal context and composition? *Ageing and Society, 32*(3), 491–515.

Sullivan, P. L. (2005). Culture, divorce, and family mediation in Hong Kong. *Family Court Review, 43*(1), 109–123.

Sung, K.-t. (2000). An Asian perspective on aging east and west: Filial piety and changing families. In V. L. Bengtson, K.-D. Kim, G. C. Myers, & K.-S. Eun (Eds.), *Aging in east and west: Families, states and the elderly* (pp. 41–58). New York: Springer Publishing Co.

Sung, K.-t. (2001). Elder respect: Exploration of ideals and forms in East Asia. *Journal of Aging Studies, 15*(1), 13–26.

Tan, E. K. B. (2003). Re-engaging Chineseness: Political, economic and cultural imperatives of nation-building in Singapore. *The China Quarterly, 175*, 751–774.

Tang, C. S.-K. (2009). The influence of family-work role experience and mastery of psychological health of Chinese employed mothers. *Journal of Health Psychology, 14*(8), 1207–1217.

Tang, C. S.-K., Wu, A. M. S., Yeung, D., & Yan, E. (2009). Attitudes and intention toward old age home placement: A study of young adult, middle-aged, and older Chinese. *Ageing International, 34*(4), 237–251.

Teo, Y. (2010). Shaping the Singapore family, producing the state and society [special issue]. *Economy and Society, 39*(3), 337–359.

Teo, P., Graham, E., Yeoh, B. S. A., & Levy, S. (2003). Values, change and intergenerational ties between two generations of women in Singapore. *Ageing and Society, 23*(3), 327–247.

Teo, P., Mehta, K., Thang, L. L., & Chan, A. (2006). *Ageing in Singapore, service needs and the state.* Oxford: Routledge.

Thomas, E. (1990). Filial piety, social change and Singapore youth. *Journal of Moral Education, 19*(3), 192–205.

Thomas, C., Morris, S. M., & Harman, J. C. (2002). Companions through cancer: The care given by informal carers in cancer contexts. *Social Science & Medicine, 54*(4), 529–544.

Tonkens, E. (2012). Working with Arlie Hochschild: Connecting feelings to social change. *Social Politics, 19*(2), 194–218.

Tse, M. M. Y., Lai, C., Lui, J. Y. W., Wong, E. K., & Yeung, S. Y. (2016). Frailty, pain and psychological variables among older adults living in Hong Kong nursing homes: Can we do better to address multimorbidities? *Journal of Psychiatric and Mental Health Nursing, 23,* 303–311.

Turner, J. H., & Stets, J. E. (2005). *The sociology of emotions.* New York: Cambridge University Press.

Verbrugge, L. M., & Chan, A. (2008). Giving help in return: Family reciprocity by older Singaporeans. *Ageing & Society, 28*(1), 5–34.

Walker, A. J., Pratt, C. C., Shin, H.-Y., & Jones, L. L. (1990). Motives for parental caregiving and relationship quality. *Family Relations, 39*(1), 51–56.

Wallace, R. A., & Wolf, A. (2006). *Contemporary sociological theory: expanding the classical tradition* (6th ed.). Princeton: Pearson/Prentice Hall.

Wallhagen, M. I., & Strawbridge, W. J. (1995). My parent-not myself: Contrasting themes in family care. *Journal of Aging and Health, 7*(4), 552–572.

Wang, J., & Wu, B. (2017). Domestic helpers as frontline workers in China's home-based elder care: A systematic review. *Journal of Women & Aging, 29*(4), 294–305. https://doi.org/10.1080/08952841.2016.1187536.

Wang, L.-Q., Chien, W.-T., & Lee, I. Y. M. (2012). An experimental study on the effectiveness of a mutual support group for family caregivers of a relative with dementia in mainland China. *Contemporary Nurse, 30*(2), 210–224. https://doi.org/10.5172/conu.2012.40.2.210.

Wang, P., Yap, P., Koh, G., Davies, J., Dalakoti, M., Fong, N.-P., Tiong, W. W., & Luo, N. (2016). Quality of life and related factors of nursing home residents in Singapore. *Health and Quality of Life Outcomes, 14*, 112–121. https://doi.org/10.1186/s12955-016-0503-x.

Wanhua, M. (2004). The readjustment of China's higher education structure and women's higher education. In T. Jie, Z. Bijun, & S. L. Mow (Eds.), *Holding up half the sky: Chinese women, past, present and future* (pp. 159–171). New York: Feminist Press of the City University of New York.

Wen, Y., & Hanley, J. (2015). Rural-to-urban migration, family resilience, and policy framework for social support in China. *Asian Social Work and Policy Review, 9*, 18–28.

Wharton, A., & Erickson, R. J. (1993). Managing emotions on the job and at home: Understanding the consequences of multiple emotional roles. *The Academy of Management Review, 19*(3), 457–486.

Whitbeck, L. B., Simons, R. L., & Conger, R. D. (1991). The effects of early family relationships on contemporary relationships and assistance patterns between adult children and their parents. *Journals of Gerontology, Social Sciences, 46*(6(Supp. 6)), S330–S337.

Whitbeck, L., Hoyt, D. R., & Huck, S. M. (1994). Early family relationships, intergenerational solidarity, and support provided to parents by their adult children. *Journal of Gerontology, Social Sciences, 49*(4(Supp. 2)), S85–S94.

Whyte, M. K. (2004). Filial obligations in Chinese families: Paradoxes of modernization. In C. Ikels (Ed.), *Filial piety: Practice and discourse in contemporary East Asia* (pp. 106–127). Stanford: Stanford University Press.

Wicclair, M. R. (1990). Caring for frail elderly parents: Past parental sacrifices and the obligations of adult children. *Social Theory and Practice, 16*(2), 163–189.

Wong, A. K. (1981). Planned development, social stratification, and the sexual division of labor in Singapore. *Signs: Journal of Women in Culture and Society, 7*(2), 434–452.

Wong, S.-I. (1986). Modernization and Chinese culture in Hong Kong. *The China Quarterly, 106*, 306–325.

Wong, O. M. H. (2000). Children and children-in-law as primary caregivers: Issues and perspectives. In W. T. Liu & H. Kendig (Eds.), *Who should care for the elderly* (pp. 297–321). Singapore: Singapore University Press.

Wong, T.-H. (2003). Education and state formation reconsidered: Chinese school identity in postwar Singapore. *Journal of Historical Sociology, 16*(2), 237–265.

Wong, O. M. H. (2005). Gender and intimate caregiving for the elderly in Hong Kong. *Journal of Aging Studies, 19*(3), 375–391.

Wong, O. M. H., & Chau, B. H. P. (2006). The evolving role of filial piety in eldercare in Hong Kong. *Asian Journal of Social Science, 34*(4), 600–617.

Woo, J., Ho, S. C., Lau, J., & Yuen, Y. K. (1994). Age and marital status are major factors associated with institutionalization in elderly Hong Kong Chinese. *Journal of Epidemiology and Community Health, 48*(3), 306–309.

Xiao, Y. & Cooke, F.L. (2012) Work-life balance in China? Social policy, employer strategy nd individual coping mechanisms. Asia Pacific Journal of Human Resources, 50, 6-22, DOI: 19.1111/j.1744-7941.2011.00005.x.

Xie, Y., & Zhu, H. (2009). Do sons or daughters give more money to parents in urban China? *Journal of Marriage and the Family, 71*(1), 174–186.

Xu, B. (2016). A silver lining to China's ageing population. *Australian Business Review; Business Spectator.* Retrieved from http://www.businessspectator.com. au/article/2016/1/27/china/silver-lining-chinas-ageing-population

Xu, G., & Wang, J. (2015). Primary health care, a concept to be fully understood and implemented in current China's health care reform. *Family Medicine and Community Health, 3*(3), 41–51.

Yan, E., & Kwok, T. (2011). Abuse of older Chinese with dementia by family caregivers: An inquiry into the role of caregiver burden. *International Journal of Geriatric Psychiatry, 26*(5), 527–535.

Yan, E., Tang, C. S.-K., & Yeung, T. D. (2002). No safe haven: A review on elder abuse in Chinese families. *Trauma, Violence & Abuse, 3*(3), 167–180.

Yeh, S.-H., Johnson, M. A., & Wang, S.-T. (2002). The changes in caregiver burden following nursing home placement. *International Journal of Nursing Studies, 39*(6), 591–600.

Yeh, K.-H., Yi, C.-C., Tsao, W.-C., & Wan, P.-S. (2013). Filial piety in contemporary Chinese societies: A comparative study of Taiwan, Hong Kong and China. *International Sociology, 28*(3), 277–296. https://doi.org/10. 1177/0268580913484345.

Yen, C.-H. (1981). Early Chinese clan organizations in Singapore and Malaya, 1819-1911. *Journal of Southeast Asian Studies, 12*(1), 62–92.

Yeoh, B. S. A., & Huang, S. (2010). Foreign domestic workers and home-based care for elders in Singapore. *Journal of Aging & Social Policy, 22*(1), 69–88.

Yeoh, B. S. A., Huang, S., & Devasahayam, T. W. (2004). Diasporic subjects in the nation: Foreign domestic workers, the reach of law and civil society in Singapore. *Asian Studies Review, 28*(1), 7–23.

Yin, L. C. (2003). Do traditional values still exist in modern Chinese societies? The case of Singapore and China. *Asia Europe Journal, 1*(1), 43–59.

Yip, K.-S. (2004). A critical review of family caregiving of mental health consumers in Hong Kong. *Journal of Family Social Work, 7*(3), 71–89.

Yip, P. S. F., & Lee, J. (2002). The impact of the changing marital structure on fertility of Hong Kong SAR. *Social Science & Medicine, 55*(12), 2159–2169.

Yongping, J. (2004). Employment and Chinese women under two systems. In T. Jie, Z. Bijun, & S. L. Mow (Eds.), *Holding up half the sky: Chinese women, past, present and future* (pp. 159–171). New York: Feminist Press of the City University of New York.

Yoon, G., Eun, K.-S., & Park, K.-S. (2000). Korea: Demographic trends, sociocultural contexts, and public policy. In V. L. Bengtson, K.-S. Eun, K.-D. Kim, & G. C. Myers (Eds.), *Aging in east and west; families, states and the elderly* (pp. 121–137). New York: Springer Publishing.

Young, A. (1992). A tale of two cities: Factor accumulation and technical change in Hong Kong and Singapore. *NBER Macroeconomics Annual, 7*, 13–54.

Yu, X. (2004). The status of Chinese women in marriage and family. In T. Jie, Z. Bijun, & S. L. Mow (Eds.), *Holding up half the sky: Chinese women, past, present and future* (pp. 159–171). New York: Feminist Press of the City University of New York.

Yu, A. (2015, June 16). Hongkongers have worst work-life balance in Asia-Pacific as 77pc take calls on holiday. *South China Morning Post.* http://www.scmp.com/news/hong-kong/economy/article/1822705/hongkongers-have-worst-work-life-balance-asia-pacific-77pc

Zhan, J. H. (2004). Socialization or social structure: Investigating predictors of attitudes toward filial responsibility among Chinese urban youth from one- and multiple-child families. *International Journal of Aging and Human Development, 59*(1), 105–124.

Zhan, J. H., & Montgomery, R. J. V. (2003). Gender and elder care in China: The influence of filial piety and structural constraints. *Gender and Society, 17*(2), 209–229.

Zhan, H. J., Ba, G. L., Guan, X., & Bai, H.-g. (2006a). Recent developments in institutional elder care in China. *Journal of Aging & Social Policy, 18*(2), 85–108.

Zhan, H. J., Liu, G., & Guam, X. (2006b). Willingness and availability: Explaining new attitudes toward institutional elder care among Chinese elderly parents and their adult children. *Journal of Aging Studies, 20*, 279–290.

Zhan, H. J., Feng, X., & Luo, B. (2008). Placing elderly parents in institutions in urban China: A reinterpretation of filial piety. *Research on Aging, 30*(5), 543–571.

Zhan, H. J., Feng, Z., Chen, Z., & Feng, X. (2011). The role of the family in institutional long-term care: Cultural management of filial piety in China.

International Journal of Social Welfare, 20, s121–s134. https://doi. org/10.1111/j.1468-2397.2011.00808.x.

Zhang, H. (2017). Recalibrating filial piety: Realigning the state, family and market interests in China. In G. Santos & S. Harrell (Eds.), *Transforming patriarchy: Chinese families in the twenty-first century* (pp. 234–250). Seattle/ London: University of Washington Press.

Zhang, L. J., Gu, P. Y., & Hu, G. (2008). A cognitive perspective of Singaporean primary school pupils use of reading strategies in learning to read English. *British Journal of Educational Psychology, 78*(2), 245–271.

Zhang, N. J., Guo, M., & Zheng, X. (2012). China: Awakening giant developing solutions to population aging. *The Gerontologist, 52*(5), 589–596.

Zhang, M., Foley, S., & Yang, B. (2013). Work-family conflict among Chinese married couples: Testing spillover and crossover effects. *The International Journal of Resource Management, 24*(17), 3213–3231. https://doi.org/10.108 0/09585192.2013.763849.

Zhou, Y. (1997). Labor migration and returns to rural education in China. *American Journal of Agricultural Economies, 79*(4), 1278–1287.

Online Statistics

Hong Kong

Hong Kong Census and Statistics Department, special administrative region. (2015, September 25). *Population projections 2015–2064.* http://www.censtatd.gov.hk/hkstat/sub/sp190.jsp?productCode=B1120015

Hong Kong Census and Statistics Department, special administrative region. (2017, May 19). *Statistics on domestic households.* https://www.censtatd.gov. hk/hkstat/sub/sp150.jsp?tableID=005&ID=0&productType=8

Hong Kong Housing Authority. Housing in Figures. (2016). https://www.housingauthority.gov.hk/en/common/pdf/about-us/publications-and-statistics/ HIF.pdf

Hong Kong immigration department. (2016a). *Foreign domestic helpers.* http:// www.immd.gov.hk/eng/faq/foreign-domestic-helpers.html#eligibility

Hong Kong immigration department. (2016b). *Practical guide for employment of foreign domestic helpers.* http://www.labour.gov.hk/eng/public/wcp/ FDHguide.pdf

Hong Kong Monthly Digest of Statistics. (2015). *Marriage and divorce trends in Hong Kong.* https://www.censtatd.gov.hk/hkstat/sub/sp160. jsp?productCode=FA100055

Hong Kong: The facts. (2014, June). http://www.gov.hk/en/about/abouthk/factsheets/docs/population.pdf

Social indicators of Hong Kong. (2017a). http://www.socialindicators.org.hk/en/indicators/education/7.7

Social indicators of Hong Kong. (2017b). http://www.socialindicators.org.hk/en/indicators/elderly/31.12

Women and men in Hong Kong, key statistics. (2014). *Table 4.49, foreign domestic helpers by nationality and sex.* http://www.statistics.gov.hk/pub/B11303032014AN14B0100.pdf

Women and men in Hong Kong key statistics. (2016). *Labour force participation rate.* http://www.statistics.gov.hk/pub/B11303032016AN16B0100.pdf

Women and men in Hong Kong key statistics, Education. (2016). http://www.statistics.gov.hk/pub/B11303032016AN16B0100.pdf

Women and men in Hong Kong key statistics Marriage, fertility and family conditions. (2016). http://www.censtatd.gov.hk/hkstat/sub/sp180.jsp?productCode=B1130303

Mainland China

China Statistical Yearbook. (2016). *Household population, sex ratio, and household size by region, 2015 (Sect. 2–10).* http://www.stats.gov.cn/tjsj/ndsj/2016/indexeh.htm

China Statistical Yearbook, Sect. 2-4. (2016). *National Bureau of statistics of China.* http://www.stats.gov.cn/tjsj/ndsj/2016/indexeh.htm

China Statistical Yearbook, Sect. 2-5. (2016). *National Bureau of statistics of China.* http://www.stats.gov.cn/tjsj/ndsj/2016/indexeh.htm

People's Daily Online. (2010, September 26). *Chinese delay average age of marriage, first child.* http://en.people.cn/90001/90782/7151025.html

People's Republic of China. (2010). *Population census (Table 5-4, Chapter 5, Part 1).* http://www.stats.gov.cn/tjsj/pcsj/rkpc/6rp/indexch.htm

People's Republic of China, Ministry of Education. (2017). http://www.moe.edu.cn/publicfiles/business/htmlfiles/moe/moe_2803/200907/49979.html

Statista. (2017). *Number of elderly people living in nursing homes in China from 2009 to 2014.* https://www.statista.com/statistics/251943/number-of-elderly-persons-in-nursing-homes-in-china/

Women and Men in China, Facts and Figures. (2012). *National Bureau of statistics, tabulation on the 2010 population census of the People's Republic of China, 2012.* http://www.unicef.cn/en/uploadfile/2014/0109/20140109030938887.pdf

Singapore

Housing Development Board. (2016). *Living with/near parent or married child.* http://www.hdb.gov.sg/cs/infoweb/residential/buying-a-flat/resale/living-with-near-parents-or-married-child

Inland Revenue Authority of Singapore. (2017). *Patent relief.* https://www.iras.gov.sg/IRASHome/Individuals/Locals/Working-Out-Your-Taxes/Deductions-for-Individuals/Parent-Relief-/-Handicapped-Parent-Relief/

Ministry of Community Youth and Development. (2007). Committee on Ageing Issues. *Study of national work-life harmony.* https://www.msf.gov.sg/.../Media%20Release_Research%20on%20Work-   Life%20Harmony%20%28final%20version%29.pdf

Ministry of Education Singapore. (2017). *Compulsory education.* https://www.moe.gov.sg/education/education-system/compulsory-education

Ministry of Manpower. (2016a). *Labour force in Singapore.* http://stats.mom.gov.sg/iMAS_PdfLibrary/mrsd_2016LabourForce_survey_highlights.pdf

Ministry of Manpower. (2016b). *Strategies for work-life harmony.* http://www.mom.gov.sg/employment-practices/good-work-practices/work-life-strategies

Ministry of Manpower. (2017a). *Work permit for FDW, eligibility and requirements.* http://www.mom.gov.sg/passes-and-permits/work-permit-for-foreign-domestic-worker/eligibility-and-requirements

Ministry of Manpower. (2017b). *Employment act, who it covers.* http://www.mom.gov.sg/employment-practices/employment-act/who-is-covered

Ministry of Manpower. (2017c). *Checklist for employers of FDWs.* http://www.mom.gov.sg/~/media/mom/documents/work-passes-and-permits/checklist-hiring-fdw-english.pdf?la=en

Ministry of Manpower. (2017d). *Levy concession for a foreign domestic worker.* http://www.mom.gov.sg/passes-and-permits/work-permit-for-foreign-domestic-worker/foreign-domestic-worker-levy/levy-concession#for-aged-persons

Ministry of Manpower, Singapore. (2014, June). http://www.mom.gov.sg/statistics-publications/others/statistics/Pages/ForeignWorkforceNumbers.aspx

Statistics Singapore. (2011/09). *The elderly in Singapore.* https://www.singstat.gov.sg/docs/default-source/default-document-library/publications/publications_and_papers/population_and_population_structure/ssnsep11-pg1-9.pdf

Statistics Singapore. (2014). *Population Trends 2014. Life Expectancy.* http://www.singstat.gov.sg/publications/publications_and_papers/population_and_population_structure/population2014.pdf

Statistics Singapore. (2016a). *Population trends*. http://www.singstat.gov.sg/publications/publications-and-papers/population-and-population-structure/population-trends

Statistics Singapore. (2016b). *Births and deaths, life tables 2015–2016*. http://www.singstat.gov.sg/publications/publications-and-papers/population#births_and_deaths

Statistics Singapore. (2016c). *Marriages and divorce*. http://www.singstat.gov.sg/publications/publications-and-papers/marriages-and-divorces/marriages-and-divorces

Statistics Singapore. (2017a). *Education and literacy*. http://www.singstat.gov.sg/statistics/latest-data#20

Statistics Singapore. (2017b). *Households*. http://www.singstat.gov.sg/statistics/latest-data#22

Statistics Singapore. (2017c). *Households*. http://www.singstat.gov.sg/statistics/latest-data#22

Other

Central Intelligence Agency The World Factbook. (2016). https://www.cia.gov/library/publications/the-world-factbook/fields/2256.html

United Nations Department of Economic and Social Affairs Population Division. (2015). *World population ageing 2015*. Retrieved from http://www.un.org/en/development/desa/population/publications/pdf/ageing/WPA2015_Report.pdf

United Nations Population Fund. (2011). *UNFPA annual report 2011*. Retrieved from http://www.unfpa.org/publications/unfpa-annual-report-2011

United Nations World Population Ageing 1950-2050. (2016). www.un.org/esa/population/publications/worldageing19502050/pdf/180singa.pdf

United Nations World Population Division Department of Economic and Social Affairs, Population Division. (2008). *World population prospects. The 2008 revision*. Retrieved from www.un.org/esa/population/publications/wpp2...

World Bank. (2014). *Fertility rate, total (births per woman) data/table*. Retrieved from http://data.worldbank.org/indicator/SP.DYN.TFRT.IN?order...

World Bank. (2016). *Population ages 65 and above (% of total)*. Retrieved from http://data.worldbank.org/indicator/SP.POP.65UP.TO.ZS

Index[1]

---

[1] Note: Page numbers followed by 'n' refer to notes.

© The Author(s) 2018
P. O'Neill, *Urban Chinese Daughters*, St Antony's Series,
https://doi.org/10.1007/978-981-10-8699-1